Newborn and Infant Nutrition: A Clinical Perspective

Newborn and Infant Nutrition: A Clinical Perspective

Editor: Karol Prosser

AMERICAN
MEDICAL PUBLISHERS
www.americanmedicalpublishers.com

AMERICAN
MEDICAL PUBLISHERS
www.americanmedicalpublishers.com

Cataloging-in-Publication Data

Newborn and infant nutrition : a clinical perspective / edited by Karol Prosser.
p. cm.
Includes bibliographical references and index.
ISBN 978-1-63927-753-7
1. Newborn infants--Nutrition. 2. Infants--Nutrition. 3. Newborn infants—Diseases--Nutritional aspects.
4. Newborn infants—Diseases--Diagnosis. 5. Newborn infants—Diseases--Treatment. I. Prosser, Karol.
RJ216 .N49 2023
649.33--dc23

American Medical Publishers,
41 Flatbush Avenue,
1st Floor, New York,
NY 11217, USA

ISBN 978-1-63927-753-7 (Hardback)

Contents

Preface

It is often said that books are a boon to mankind. They document every progress and pass on the knowledge from one generation to the other. They play a crucial role in our lives. Thus I was both excited and nervous while editing this book. I was pleased by the thought of being able to make a mark but I was also nervous to do it right because the future of students depends upon it. Hence, I took a few months to research further into the discipline, revise my knowledge and also explore some more aspects. Post this process, I begun with the editing of this book.

Infancy is the time of rapid growth after the fetal period. This stage of life requires optimized nutrition in order to achieve proper growth and organ development. The amount of nutrition needed to support and maintain adequate growth and optimal health, while maintaining homeostasis with other nutrients is determined by the individual requirements of infants. Nutritional needs differ during infancy and growth patterns are directly related to optimal nutrition. In the first six months, breast milk is the best source of nutrition for infants. Human milk may have particular advantages for premature infants due to the interrelationships between host defense, nutritional support and gastrointestinal development. Carbohydrates and protein, folate, calcium, zinc, fat and iron are a few of the nutrients that infants require to grow and stay healthy. This book unravels the recent studies on the role of nutrition in newborn and infant health. It consists of contributions made by international experts. The extensive content of this book provides the readers with a thorough understanding of the subject.

I thank my publisher with all my heart for considering me worthy of this unparalleled opportunity and for showing unwavering faith in my skills. I would also like to thank the editorial team who worked closely with me at every step and contributed immensely towards the successful completion of this book. Last but not the least, I wish to thank my friends and colleagues for their support.

Editor

The Pattern of Complementary Foods in American Infants and Children Aged 0–5 Years Old—A Cross-Sectional Analysis of Data from the NHANES 2011–2014

Elieke Demmer [1], Christopher J. Cifelli [1,*], Jenny A. Houchins [1] and Victor L. Fulgoni III [2]

[1] National Dairy Council, 10255 West Higgins Road, Suite 900, Rosemont, IL 60018-5616, USA; eliekedemmer@gmail.com (E.D.); jenny.houchins@dairy.org (J.A.H.)
[2] Nutrition Impact, LLC, Battle Creek, MI 49014, USA; VIC3RD@aol.com
* Correspondence: chris.cifelli@dairy.org

Abstract: Proper nutrition early in life can influence children's present and future health. While several authoritative sources provide eating/food recommendations, only a few studies have assessed whether these recommendations are followed. The goal of this paper was to examine food and nutrient intakes on any given day during infancy and early childhood among various ethnicities. Twenty-four-hour dietary recall data of 0–5 years-old children (n = 2431) from the National Health and Nutrition Examination Survey (NHANES) 2011–2014 was used to estimate intakes of nutrients and food groups and prevalence of inadequate intake. Data was analyzed separately for various age groups and ethnicities, and differences in means by age and or race/ethnicity were determined by t-tests with $p < 0.05$ as significant. The results indicate that intakes of all food groups were expectedly low at 0–11 months, increased with age, and were influenced by race/ethnicity. Mixed dish consumption, which also increased with age, made substantial contributions to children's food group intakes. However, there was a substantial percentage of the population among all age and race/ethnic groups who did not consume the recommended amounts for each food group and had inadequate intakes of key nutrients, such as calcium, vitamin D, and vitamin E. Non-Hispanic black children consumed less dairy and more protein foods, and a significantly greater proportion of these children had inadequate intakes of calcium and vitamin D compared to their peers. In conclusion, the results from this study suggest that a substantial population of American infants and children from 0 to five years of age did not meet food group recommendations and had inadequate intakes of key nutrients such as calcium, vitamin D, and vitamin E from foods.

Keywords: dairy; protein; vegetable; added sugar; calcium; vitamin D; vitamin E

1. Introduction

Proper nutrition early in life can affect development and help set the stage for future eating habits that can influence nutrition status for a lifetime [1]. As such, the American Academy of Pediatrics (AAP) states that "an important goal of early childhood nutrition is to ensure children's present and future health by fostering the development of healthy eating behaviors" and that "appropriate feeding behavior is vital in promoting healthy growth and development but also in engendering healthy behavior and habits that can prevent the advent of chronic disease" [2]. While several authoritative sources provide recommendations on what, when, and how much children should be eating [2,3], few studies have assessed whether these recommendations are followed, how these food choices impact nutrient intake, and what, if any, differences exist among race/ethnic groups. Ethnic disparities in dietary patterns are reflective of biological, cultural, and food practice differences that are further modified by social, economic, and environmental factors [4,5]. Given that the 2020 Dietary Guidelines for Americans (DGA) will include the first two years of life for the first time [6,7], it is critical to understand the eating behaviors and patterns of this young population. One specific question posed by the joint United States Department of Agriculture (USDA) and Health and Human Services "Pregnancy and Birth to 24 Months project" is "What is the relationship between complementary feeding and micronutrient status" [8].

The AAP recommends human milk as the sole source of nutrients for healthy term infants with iron-fortified formula as the appropriate substitute for human milk [2]. While the AAP supports exclusive breastfeeding for approximately six months, it recognizes that infants may be developmentally ready to accept complementary foods at four to six months of age [2]. Complementary foods are defined as nutrient- and energy-containing solid or semi-solid foods fed to infants in addition to human milk and formula [2]. The introduction of complementary foods prior to four months of age is thought to contribute to later overweight status [9–12]. While single-grain fortified infant cereal is often the first complementary food introduced, there is no medical evidence that introducing solid foods in any order has any advantage. As such, the AAP recommends that single-ingredient foods from any food group can be introduced at this time [2]. In fact, previous research has shown that after six months of age, infants accept cereals and meats equally well [13].

Energy requirements of toddlers are difficult to estimate, and the appropriateness of energy intake is best judged by growth [2]. It has been estimated that between 12–24 months of age, 49–63% of energy comes from table foods [14]. While most American toddlers' diets contain adequate amounts of protein and carbohydrate, findings from the 2008 Feeding Infants and Toddlers Study (FITS) suggest that nearly 25% of toddlers had intakes of fat below recommended levels [15]. The AAP recommends against fat or cholesterol restrictions for infants younger than two years, when rapid growth and neurologic development requires high energy intakes, unless a concern for obesity or family history of cardiovascular disease exists [16].

The goal of this paper was to examine what American infants and children from 0–5 years are eating, what they consume on any given day during infancy and childhood, how these food choices influence nutrient intake, and to determine if differences exist among ethnic groups at this young and important age.

2. Methods

2.1. Subjects

Data from National Health and Nutrition Examination Survey (NHANES), a large dietary survey of a nationally representative sample of the U.S. population, was used to assess dietary intakes and introduction of complementary foods to children of ethnic subgroups in the U.S. population [17]. The present analysis combined two NHANES datasets (NHANES 2011–2012 and 2013–2014). Dietary data (24-h recalls provided by parents/caretakers) from children aged five years and younger (n = 2431; 1290 from NHANES 2011–2012 and 1141 from 2013–2014) were included (Table 1), which represents over 22 million U.S. children aged 0–5 years [18]. Children with incomplete or unreliable data (as determined by the USDA) were excluded from the analysis (n = 507) as were those consuming breast milk (n = 260); the latter were excluded so as not to overestimate those with nutrient inadequacy given we do not have data on the amount of breastmilk consumed. All parents/caretakers or proxies provided written informed consent, and the Research Ethics Review Board at the NCHS approved the survey protocol. Analysis of de-identified data from the survey is exempt from the federal regulations for the protection of human research participants. Analysis of restricted data through the NCHS Research Data Center is also approved by the NCHS ERB. This study did not require further institutional review as this was the analysis of secondary data without any personal identifiers.

Table 1. Sample sizes by age and race/ethnicity, NHANES 2011–2014.

	0–11 Months	12–23 Months	2–3 Years	4–5 Years
All	526	394	836	675
Non-Hispanic White	145	91	197	133
Non-Hispanic Black	122	85	210	156
Hispanic	158	131	244	223
Asian	25	33	78	72

2.2. Estimation of Intake

Dietary intake data were obtained via 24-h dietary recall interviews with caretakers of children using an Automated Multiple-Pass Method [19]. Complementary food intake was assessed using USDA food codes corresponding to What We Eat In America (WWEIA), the dietary intake component of NHANES [20]. Food subgroups and all baby foods (USDA food category starting with 90) were reassigned to broader food group categories (e.g., 'banana baby food: fruit' was added to the 'fruit' group) [20]. Energy and nutrient intake from foods were determined using respective Food & Nutrient Database for Dietary Studies (FNDDS) for each NHANES cycle [21,22] available from total nutrients intake files. Use of supplements was not included in these analyses. Intake of MyPlate servings [23] was calculated using the Food Patterns Equivalents Databases (FPED) 2011–2012 and 2013–2014 for NHANES 2011–2012 and 2013–2014 dietary data, respectively. The number of MyPlate servings was aggregated over all foods consumed during the 24-h recall to calculate the daily intakes of MyPlate food groups.

2.3. Statistical Analyses

SAS 9.2 (SAS Institute, Cary, NC, USA) and SUDAN 11 were used with NHANES design aspects and sampling weights to ensure nationally representative estimates. Usual nutrient intakes of energy and nutrients were determined using the National Cancer Institute method using both days of dietary intake [24]. The percentage of the population below the Estimated Average Requirement (EAR) was assessed. Amounts of MyPlate food groups consumed and the percent of the population not meeting the age specific recommendations for various food groups [3,25] were also computed. Covariates used for the usual intake models were dietary recall number (1 or 2) and day of recall coded as weekday or weekend (Fri, Sat, and Sun). Separate analyses were conducted for the following age groups in the U.S. population (males and females combined): 0–11 months, 12–23 months, 2–3 years, and 4–5 years; and self-identified ethnic groups (males and females combined): non-Hispanic whites (NH-whites), non-Hispanic blacks (NH-blacks), Hispanics, and Asians (all of which are sampled to be nationally representative). Mean amounts and standard errors (SE) were determined with "Proc Surveymeans" procedure, while for analyses of ethnicity by age, "Proc Surveyreg" procedure was used with age (in months), gender, race/ethnicity and family poverty income ratio included as covariates; differences in means and least square means by age and ethnicity were determined by t-tests while differences in percentages below recommendations were assessed with the Z-statistic. $p < 0.05$ as deemed significant.

3. Results

Reported intakes of various food groups among children analyzed by age are presented in Table 2. Regardless of ethnicity, intake of all food groups among 0–11 months-old children was low. Intake of total dairy increased as children got older, with a maximum average intake of 2.44 cup equivalents among those aged 12–23 months; after 23 months of age, dairy consumption began to decrease. Protein and grain intake increased as children got older. The amount of fruit consumed increased to a little above 1 cup per day when children were 12–23 months-old and then decreased after three years of age. Vegetable consumption increased with age, although the amounts consumed were consistently very low, never getting above 0.7 cups per day. The consumed amounts of solid fats, oils, and added sugars quickly increased as children got older. The largest increase in intake of various food groups (~800% increase in dairy, ~447% increase in protein, ~250% increase in grains and fruits intake) was noted between the ages 0–11 months and 12–23 months. Similarly, intake of solid fat and added sugar increased by more than 500% between age groups 0–11 months and 12–23 years. Mixed dish consumption, which also increased with age, made substantial contributions to children's food intake. Among 4–5 year-old children, mixed dishes contributed 16% of dairy intake (52% of cheese intake, data not shown), 27% of protein intake, 31% of grains and vegetables intake, and 45% of solid fat intake (Table 2).

Table 2. Amount of food consumed per food group, NHANES 2011–2014.

	0–11 Months (Mean ± SE)	12–23 Months (Mean ± SE)	2–3 Years (Mean ± SE)	4–5 Years (Mean ± SE)
Total Dairy [1] (cups eq.)	0.27 ± 0.03	2.4 ± 0.10	2.2 ± 0.08	2.0 ± 0.09
Mixed dishes	0.02 ± 0.005	0.18 ± 0.03	0.23 ± 0.02	0.32 ± 0.02
Total Protein [2] (oz. eq.)	0.36 ± 0.04	2.0 ± 0.11	2.7 ± 0.11	3.0 ± 0.18
Mixed dishes	0.09 ± 0.01	0.49 ± 0.04	0.59 ± 0.04	0.81 ± 0.08
Total Grains [3] (oz. eq.)	0.85 ± 0.07	3.1 ± 0.13	4.5 ± 0.14	5.5 ± 0.15
Mixed dishes	0.19 ± 0.03	0.98 ± 0.10	1.3 ± 0.09	1.7 ± 0.09
Total Fruit [4] (cups eq.)	0.34 ± 0.03	1.2 ± 0.06	1.4 ± 0.07	1.2 ± 0.07
Mixed dishes	0.01 ± 0.003	0.001 ± 0.001	0.001 ± 0.0004	0.001 ± 0.001
Total Vegetables [5] (cups eq.)	0.26 ± 0.02	0.47 ± 0.04	0.56 ± 0.03	0.66 ± 0.05
Mixed dishes	0.04 ± 0.01	0.18 ± 0.02	0.17 ± 0.01	0.21 ± 0.02
Solid Fats [6] (g)	1.1 ± 0.15	8.3 ± 0.89	13.0 ± 0.77	17.0 ± 0.68
Mixed dishes	0.67 ± 0.12	4.4 ± 0.52	6.5 ± 0.49	7.8 ± 0.47
Oils [7] (g)	0.74 ± 0.15	4.5 ± 0.28	7.0 ± 0.33	8.9 ± 0.50
Mixed dishes	0.43 ± 0.08	1.8 ± 0.17	2.1 ± 0.13	2.8 ± 0.20
Added Sugars [8] (tsp eq.)	0.33 ± 0.06	2.6 ± 0.35	4.3 ± 0.24	6.2 ± 0.30
Mixed dishes	0.02 ± 0.01	0.12 ± 0.02	0.26 ± 0.02	0.40 ± 0.05

SE, Standard Error; eq, equivalents. [1] Total Dairy include: Milk, flavored milk, dairy drinks and substitutes, total cheese, total yogurt, dairy from mixed dishes, dairy from snacks and sweets; [2] Protein include: meats, poultry, seafood, eggs, cured meats/poultry, plant-based protein foods, baby food meat, protein from mixed dishes, protein from snacks and sweets; [3] Grains include (whole and refined): cooked grains, breads, rolls, tortillas, quick breads and bread products, ready-to-eat cereals, cooked cereals, baby food cereals, baby food grains, grains from mixed dishes, grains from snacks and sweets; [4] Total Fruits include: whole fruit, 100% fruit juice, baby food fruit, fruit from mixed dishes, fruit from snacks and sweets; [5] Vegetables include: vegetables excluding potatoes and legumes, white potatoes, 100% vegetables juice, baby food vegetables, vegetables from mixed dishes, vegetables from snacks and sweets; [6] Solid fats include: butter and animal fats, margarine, cream cheese, sour cream, whipped cream, cream and cream substitutes, mayonnaise, salad dressings and vegetable oils, solid fat from mixed dishes, solid fat from snacks and sweets; [7] Oils include: whipped cream, cream and cream substitutes, mayonnaise, salad dressings and vegetable oils, oils from mixed dishes, oils from snacks and sweets; [8] Added Sugars include: sugars and honey, sugar substitutes, jams, syrups, toppings, added sugars from mixed dishes, added sugar from snacks and sweets.

Intakes of food groups among children differed by ethnicity (Table 3). NH-black children ages 12–23 months, 2–3 years, and 4–5 years consumed significantly less dairy than NH-white and Hispanic children. After 1 year of age, dairy consumption was consistently the lowest among NH-black children. However, the prevalence of cheese consumption among NH-black children was similar to NH-white and Hispanic children (data not shown). Asian children consumed more yogurt than the other ethnic groups (data not shown). Older NH-white and Hispanic children (2–3 years and 4–5 years of age) consumed significantly less protein foods than NH-black children. At 4–5 years of age, Asian children consumed significantly less fruit than NH-white children. Intake of added sugars among 4–5-year-old children was more than the American Heart Association's (AHA's) recommended daily limit of 6 teaspoons [26] for all ethnicities except for Hispanic children, who consumed significantly less added sugar at this age than their NH-white and NH-black peers (Table 3). Intake of grains, vegetables and solid fat were not significantly different among ethnic groups.

Table 3. Amount of food consumed per food group by age and ethnicity, NHANES 2011–2014.

	0–11 Months LSM ± SE	**12–23 Months LSM ± SE**	**2–3 Years LSM ± SE**	**4–5 Years LSM ± SE**
Total dairy [1] (cup eq.)				
Non-Hispanic white	0.38 ± 0.05 [a]	2.6 ± 0.21 [b]	2.2 ± 0.14 [b]	2.1 ± 0.19 [b]
Non-Hispanic black	0.22 ± 0.06 [ab]	1.8 ± 0.16 [a]	1.6 ± 0.14 [a]	1.5 ± 0.11 [a]
Hispanic	0.16 ± 0.05 [b]	2.5 ± 0.11 [b]	2.4 ± 0.13 [b]	2.2 ± 0.12 [b]
Asian	0.15 ± 0.10 [b]	2.3 ± 0.32 [ab]	2.4 ± 0.32 [b]	2.1 ± 0.21 [b]
Total Protein [2] (oz. eq.)				
Non-Hispanic white	0.45 ± 0.06 [a]	2.0 ± 0.20	2.5 ± 0.16 [a]	2.8 ± 0.29 [a]
Non-Hispanic black	0.44 ± 0.14 [ab]	2.0 ± 0.28	3.3 ± 0.27 [bc]	3.9 ± 0.32 [b]
Hispanic	0.21 ± 0.04 [b]	2.0 ± 0.13	2.6 ± 0.14 [a]	2.8 ± 0.19 [a]
Asian	0.38 ± 0.17 [ab]	1.5 ± 0.27	2.7 ± 0.49 [ac]	2.5 ± 0.29 [a]
Total grain [3] (oz. eq.)				
Non-Hispanic white	0.85 ± 0.10	3.2 ± 0.19	4.2 ± 0.14	5.3 ± 0.26
Non-Hispanic black	0.89 ± 0.15	3.3 ± 0.17	4.6 ± 0.22	5.5 ± 0.30
Hispanic	0.95 ± 0.11	2.9 ± 0.26	4.7 ± 0.28	5.6 ± 0.23
Asian	0.68 ± 0.20	3.3 ± 0.41	5.1 ± 0.54	4.8 ± 0.49
Total fruits [4] (cup eq.)				
Non-Hispanic white	0.38 ± 0.04 [a]	1.2 ± 0.13	1.4 ± 0.12	1.7 ± 0.10 [a]
Non-Hispanic black	0.25 ± 0.04 [bc]	1.4 ± 0.15	1.4 ± 0.14	1.7 ± 0.13 [ac]
Hispanic	0.34 ± 0.05 [ab]	1.2 ± 0.09	1.3 ± 0.11	1.3 ± 0.10 [a]
Asian	0.17 ± 0.06 [c]	1.0 ± 0.17	1.4 ± 0.19	0.85 ± 0.14 [bc]
Total vegetables [5] (cup eq.)				
Non-Hispanic white	0.27 ± 0.02	0.45 ± 0.06	0.51 ± 0.04	0.67 ± 0.08
Non-Hispanic black	0.23 ± 0.04	0.48 ± 0.06	0.56 ± 0.04	0.76 ± 0.07
Hispanic	0.28 ± 0.03	0.48 ± 0.04	0.64 ± 0.06	0.64 ± 0.05
Asian	0.26 ± 0.11	0.56 ± 0.12	0.52 ± 0.08	0.68 ± 0.08
Solid fats [6] (g)				
Non-Hispanic white	1.2 ± 0.26	8.7 ± 1.51	12.4 ± 1.3	17.8 ± 0.9
Non-Hispanic black	0.96 ± 0.19	8.8 ± 1.31	14.5 ± 0.9	17.4 ± 1.5
Hispanic	0.88 ± 0.17	7.7 ± 1.10	14.4 ± 0.8	17.4 ± 1.1
Asian	1.2 ± 0.82	5.1 ± 1.33	12.6 ± 1.5	15.4 ± 2.6
Oils [7] (g)				
Non-Hispanic white	0.82 ± 0.26	4.2 ± 0.43	6.1 ± 0.37 [a]	8.3 ± 0.79 [ab]
Non-Hispanic black	0.60 ± 0.21	6.0 ± 0.93	8.3 ± 0.67 [bc]	11 ± 1.1 [b]
Hispanic	0.85 ± 0.16	4.6 ± 0.50	7.9 ± 0.75 [bc]	8.1 ± 0.68 [a]
Asian	0.91 ± 0.47	4.0 ± 0.90	7.7 ± 1.51 [ac]	8.6 ± 1.09 [ab]
Added sugars [8] (tsp eq.)				
Non-Hispanic white	0.31 ± 0.08 [ab]	2.8 ± 0.77	4.5 ± 0.36	7.4 ± 0.51 [bc]
Non-Hispanic black	0.27 ± 0.09 [ab]	2.1 ± 0.52	4.8 ± 0.44	6.1 ± 0.43 [bc]
Hispanic	0.50 ± 0.16 [a]	2.4 ± 0.34	4.1 ± 0.33	4.5 ± 0.26 [a]
Asian	0.07 ± 0.11 [b]	1.5 ± 0.60	4.1 ± 0.56	7.0 ± 2.27 [ac]

[a,b,c] Least square means with different superscripts are significantly different by race/ethnicity within age groups, $p < 0.05$. LSM, Least Squares Mean; SE, Standard Error; eq, equivalents; [1] Total Dairy include: Milk, flavored milk, dairy drinks and substitutes, total cheese, total yogurt, dairy from mixed dishes, dairy from snacks and sweets; [2] Protein include: meats, poultry, seafood, eggs, cured meats/poultry, plant-based protein foods, baby food meat, protein from mixed dishes, protein from snacks and sweets; [3] Grains include (whole and refined): cooked grains, breads, rolls, tortillas, quick breads and bread products, ready-to-eat cereals, cooked cereals, baby food cereals, baby food grains, grains from mixed dishes, grains from snacks and sweets; [4] Total Fruits include: whole fruit, 100% fruit juice, baby food fruit, fruit from mixed dishes, fruit from snacks and sweets; [5] Vegetables include: vegetables excluding potatoes and legumes, white potatoes, 100% vegetables juice, baby food vegetables, vegetables from mixed dishes, vegetables from snacks and sweets; [6] Solid fats include: butter and animal fats, margarine, cream cheese, sour cream, whipped cream, cream and cream substitutes, mayonnaise, salad dressings and vegetable oils, solid fat from mixed dishes, solid fat from snacks and sweets; [7] Oils include: whipped cream, cream and cream substitutes, mayonnaise, salad dressings and vegetable oils, oils from mixed dishes, oils from snacks and sweets; [8] Added Sugars include: sugars and honey, sugar substitutes, jams, syrups, toppings, added sugars from mixed dishes, added sugar from snacks and sweets.

Large percentages of children from all ethnic groups consumed less dairy, protein foods, vegetables, and oil than the recommendations for their respective age groups (Table 4). The percent of children with intakes below recommendations increased with age for dairy, fruit, and vegetables. The proportion of children with intakes below the dietary recommendations varied by ethnicity. Across all age groups, NH-black children consistently had the greatest percentage of children not meeting the dairy food group recommendations. In contrast, this ethnic group also had the lowest prevalence of inadequate protein foods and oil intake. However, in general there were few significant ethnic differences in the percent of the population who had intakes below the recommendations for fruits or vegetables (Table 4).

Intakes of energy and macronutrients generally increased with age (Table 5). With a few exceptions, there were no differences in energy and macronutrient intakes when analyzed by ethnicity. NH-black children aged 12–23 months consumed significantly more energy (8%) than their Hispanic peers as well as significantly more carbohydrate (12%) than their Hispanic and NH-white peers. Hispanic children aged 2–3 years consumed significantly more protein than 2–3-years-old NH-white (8%) and NH-black (10%) children. Four to five-year-old NH-black children also consumed significantly more fat (14%) than 4–5-year-old Asian children (Table 5).

Table 4. Percent of children below the recommended intake of food groups by age and ethnicity, NHANES 2011–2014.

	12–23 Months * **Mean ± SE**	**2–3 Years **** **Mean ± SE**	**4–5 Years **** **Mean ± SE**
Total dairy [1] Recommended, (cup eq.)	1.57	2	2.5
All (%)	18.8 ± 2.9 [x]	44.3 ± 2.7 [y]	71.9 ± 3.6 [z]
Hispanic	13 ± 3.2 [a]	34.2 ± 4.4 [a]	63.5 ± 4.9 [a]
Non-Hispanic white	15.9 ± 5.3 [a]	39.4 ± 4.3 [a]	69.7 ± 6.9 [ab]
Non-Hispanic black	36.9 ± 5.5 [b]	70.4 ± 4.5 [b]	83.7 ± 3.1 [b]
Asian	20.3 ± 7.7 [ab]	49.5 ± 7.2 [a]	80.7 ± 5.0 [b]
Total Protein [2] Recommended, (oz. eq.)	2.1	2	4
All (%)	73.1 ± 3.6 [x]	41.3 ±3.5 [y]	93.9 ± 2.2 [z]
Hispanic	70.3 ± 6.6 [a]	31.8 ± 9.2 [a]	91.2 ± 3.1 [ab]
Non-Hispanic white	80.1 ± 6.0 [a]	53.5 ± 5.6 [b]	97.1 ± 2.5 [a]
Non-Hispanic black	54.2 ± 9.3 [b]	16.3 ± 5.1 [a]	79.5 ± 5.5 [b]
Asian	76.3 ± 10.2 [ab]	40.8 ± 15.6 [ab]	98.4 ± 2.9 [a]
Total grain [3] Recommended, (oz. eq.)	1.57	3	5
All (%)	3.5 ± 1.2 [x]	11.2 ± 2.4 [y]	38.3 ± 2.7 [z]
Hispanic	8.8 ± 2.8 [a]	17.0 ± 3.3 [a]	40.9 ± 3.8
Non-Hispanic white	2.3 ± 1.4 [b]	10.3 ± 3.1 [a]	39.8 ± 4.8
Non-Hispanic black	3.0 ± 1.6 [ab]	14.7 ± 4.1 [a]	39.3 ± 5.7
Asian	0.02 ± 0.5 [b]	0.01 ± 2.1 [b]	8.9 ± 21.3
Total fruits [4] Recommended, (cup eq.)	0.5	1	1
All (%)	6.1 ± 1.3 [x]	34.1 ± 3.4 [y]	38.3 ± 3.0 [y]
Hispanic	5.4 ± 2.0	34.0 ± 4.7	33.1 ± 5.3
Non-Hispanic white	6.7 ± 2.6	35.3 ± 6.2	39.8± 5.3
Non-Hispanic black	2.7 ± 1.9	33.3 ± 6.0	41.9 ± 5.7
Asian	11.3 ± 5.7	27.2 ± 7.9	39.7 ± 12.1
Total vegetables [5] Recommended, (cup eq.)	0.45	1	1.5
All (%)	45.4 ± 6.6 [x]	89.6 ± 1.8 [y]	98.1 ± 1.1 [z]
Hispanic	39.0 ± 7.6	79.1 ± 4.7 [a]	98.1 ± 1.0
Non-Hispanic white	48.5 ± 12.5	92.8 ± 3.9 [b]	98.6 ± 1.9
Non-Hispanic black	42.5 ± 12.3	90.5 ± 3.6 [ab]	98.3 ± 1.3
Asian	45.6 ± 10.9	89.2 ± 4.2 [ab]	97.0 ± 1.9

Table 4. *Cont.*

	12–23 Months * Mean ± SE	2–3 Years ** Mean ± SE	4–5 Years ** Mean ± SE
Oils [6] Recommended, (tsp)	-	4	4
All (%)	-	81.2 ± 2.7 [x]	66.5 ± 4.2 [y]
Hispanic	-	82.5 ± 4.4 [a]	79.6 ± 5.0 [a]
Non-Hispanic white	-	85.0 ± 3.8 [a]	68.0 ± 6.3 [a]
Non-Hispanic black	-	65.7 ± 6.4 [b]	43.2 ± 6.7 [b]
Asian	-	79.0 ± 8.1 [ab]	65.2 ± 9.7 [ab]

Weighted populations are 3,700,568, 8,374,256, and 7,928,277 for 12–13 month, 2–3 and 4–5 year groups, respectively. Means with different superscripts are significantly different by age ([x,y,z]) and by race/ethnicity within age groups ([a,b]), $p < 0.05$. SE, Standard Error; eq, equivalents. [1] Total Dairy include: Milk, flavored milk, dairy drinks and substitutes, total cheese, total yogurt, dairy from mixed dishes, dairy from snacks and sweets. For 12–23 months old children this food group only includes milk; [2] Protein include: meats, poultry, seafood, eggs, cured meats/poultry, plant-based protein foods, baby food meat, protein from mixed dishes, protein from snacks and sweets. For 12–23 months old children this food group only includes beef, poultry, and seafood; [3] Grains include (whole and refined): cooked grains, breads, rolls, tortillas, quick breads and bread products, ready-to-eat cereals, cooked cereals, baby food cereals, baby food grains, grains from mixed dishes, grains from snacks and sweets; [4] Total Fruits include: whole fruit, 100% fruit juice, baby food fruit, fruit from mixed dishes, fruit from snacks and sweets; [5] Vegetables include: 100% vegetables juice, baby food vegetables, vegetables from mixed dishes, vegetables from snacks and sweets. For 12–23 months old children, this food group (vegetables) excludes legumes; [6] Oils include: whipped cream, cream and cream substitutes, mayonnaise, salad dressings and vegetable oils, oils from mixed dishes, oils from snacks and sweets; * Recommended amounts of food groups for 12–23 months developed from [22]; ** Recommended amounts of food groups for 2–3 and 4–5 years were derived from [3], translated to serving sizes on www.choosemyplate.gov.

Table 5. Usual intake of total energy and macronutrient intake in children by age and ethnicity, NHANES 2011–2014.

	0–11 Months (Mean ± SE)	12–23 Months (Mean ± SE)	2–3 Years (Mean ± SE)	4–5 Years (Mean ± SE)
Energy (kcal)				
All	805 ± 16 [w]	1253 ± 31 [x]	1461 ± 19 [y]	1599 ± 31 [z]
Hispanic	800 ± 18	1238 ± 29 [a]	1503 ± 44	1587 ± 42
Non-Hispanic white	803 ± 21	1251 ± 48 [ab]	1431 ± 31	1599 ± 45
Non-Hispanic black	815 ± 44	1342 ± 38 [b]	1499 ± 48	1687 ± 60
Asian	803 ± 45	1179 ± 74 [ab]	1470 ± 57	1538 ± 43
Carbohydrate (g)				
All	102 ± 3 [w]	164 ± 4 [x]	199 ± 4 [y]	220 ± 4 [z]
Hispanic	102 ± 3	161 ± 5 [a]	201 ± 6	216 ± 6
Non-Hispanic white	103 ± 4	162 ± 7 [a]	195 ± 6	221 ± 5
Non-Hispanic black	102 ± 7	181 ± 6 [b]	203 ± 6	228 ± 7
Asian	102 ± 7	155 ± 12 [ab]	203 ± 9	211 ± 8
Protein (g)				
All	20.4 ± 0.6 [w]	47.2 ± 1.1 [x]	52.9 ± 0.8 [y]	55.8 ± 1.4 [y]
Hispanic	20.2 ± 0.8	47.7 ± 1.1	56.1 ± 1.6 [a]	58.0 ± 1.7
Non-Hispanic white	20.4 ± 0.8	46.6 ± 1.9	51.7 ± 1.0 [b]	54.9 ± 1.9
Non-Hispanic black	19.8 ± 1.4	46.7 ± 1.4	51.4 ± 1.8 [b]	56.6 ± 2.4
Asian	20.2 ± 1.5	47.1 ± 3.1	53.9 ± 2.8 [ab]	54.1 ± 2.1
Total fat (g)				
All	36.5 ± 0.7 [w]	47.3 ± 1.5 [x]	52.6 ± 0.9 [y]	57.4 ± 1.6 [z]
Hispanic	35.7 ± 0.9	46.2 ± 1.1	54.0 ± 2.0	56.5 ± 1.8 [ab]
Non-Hispanic white	36.3 ± 0.9	48.8 ± 2.7	51.8 ± 1.5	57.3 ± 2.3 [ab]
Non-Hispanic black	38.4 ± 1.5	48.4 ± 2.0	55.0 ± 2.4	63.1 ± 3.3 [a]
Asian	35.6 ± 1.8	42.6 ± 2.6	50.7 ± 2.4	55.3 ± 2.2 [b]

Means with different superscripts are significantly different by age ([w,x,y,z]) and by race/ethnicity within age groups ([a,b]), $p < 0.05$. SE, Standard Error; g, grams.

Table 6 shows the proportion of children who had inadequate intakes (i.e., intakes below EAR) for various micronutrients from foods by age and ethnicity. The proportion of children with inadequate micronutrient intakes was generally low (less than 10% of the population) except for calcium (NH-black aged 2–3 years, and all ethnicities aged 4–5 years), Vitamin D (all ages and ethnicities), and vitamin E (all ages and ethnicities). A significantly higher proportion of 4–5 years-old NH-black children had inadequate intakes of calcium compared to NH-white and Hispanic children. Vitamin D inadequacy was generally higher in NH-black children as compared to Hispanic and NH-white children, while the opposite was true for vitamin E (Table 6).

Table 6. Percent of children below the Estimated Average Requirement (EAR) by age and ethnicity, NHANES 2011–2014.

	12–23 Months (Mean ± SE)	**2–3 Years (Mean ± SE)**	**4–5 Years (Mean ± SE)**
Calcium (mg), EAR	500	500	800
All (%)	2.3 ± 0.75 [x]	3.2 ± 0.66 [x]	33 ± 3.1 [y]
Hispanic	1.5 ± 0.87 [ac]	<1 [a]	22 ± 5.0 [a]
Non-Hispanic white	1.3 ± 0.88 [ac]	2.5 ± 0.85 [a]	32 ± 4.6 [ac]
Non-Hispanic black	6.7 ± 2.62 [a]	12.0 ± 3.5 [b]	49 ± 5.9 [b]
Asian	1.0 ± 1.18 [bc]	2.04 ± 1.34 [a]	40 ± 6.9 [bc]
Iron (mg), EAR	3.0	3.0	4.1
All (%)	1.9 ± 0.55 [xy]	<1 [x]	2.3 ± 0.36 [y]
Hispanic	3.5 ± 1.00 [a]	<1 [a]	2.3 ± 0.52
Non-Hispanic white	1.6 ± 0.62 [ab]	1.2 ± 0.36 [a]	2.6 ± 0.57
Non-Hispanic black	<1 [ab]	<1 [ab]	1.5 ± 0.67
Asian	<1 [b]	<1 [b]	1.04 ± 0.96
Magnesium (mg), EAR	65	65	110
All (%)	<1 [x]	<1 [x]	1.18 ± 0.44 [y]
Hispanic	<1	<1	<1
Non-Hispanic white	<1	<1	<1
Non-Hispanic black	<1	<1	<1
Asian	<1	<1	<1
Phosphorus (mg), EAR	380	380	405
All (%)	<1	<1	<1
Hispanic	<1	<1	<1
Non-Hispanic white	<1	<1	<1
Non-Hispanic black	<1	<1	<1
Asian	<1	<1	<1
Vitamin A, RAE (mcg), EAR	210	210	275
All (%)	<1 [x]	<1 [x]	3.4 ± 1.09 [y]
Hispanic	<1	<1	1.3 ± 0.87
Non-Hispanic white	<1	<1	3.0 ± 1.43
Non-Hispanic black	2.2 ± 1.4	2.2 ± 1.7	8.1 ± 4.52
Asian	<1	<1	7.5 ± 3.76
Vitamin C (mg), EAR	13	13	22
All (%)	<1 [x]	<1 [x]	2.2 ± 0.70 [y]
Hispanic	<1	<1	0.71 ± 0.38
Non-Hispanic white	<1	<1	3.2 ± 1.7
Non-Hispanic black	<1	<1	0.54 ± 0.43
Asian	2.6 ± 1.5	<1	6.5 ± 3.8

Table 6. *Cont.*

	12–23 Months (Mean ± SE)	2–3 Years (Mean ± SE)	4–5 Years (Mean ± SE)
Vitamin D (D2 + D3) (mcg), EAR	10	10	10
All (%)	78 ± 3.4^{x}	90 ± 1.7^{y}	94 ± 1.6^{y}
Hispanic	74 ± 3.4^{a}	84 ± 2.8^{a}	90 ± 1.8^{a}
Non-Hispanic white	76 ± 5.3^{a}	91 ± 2.4^{a}	94 ± 2.9^{ac}
Non-Hispanic black	92 ± 4.3^{b}	97 ± 1.7^{b}	98 ± 1.0^{bc}
Asian	76 ± 7.9^{ab}	91 ± 5.1^{ab}	97 ± 2.3^{bc}
Vitamin E (α-tocopherol, mg), EAR	5	5	6
All (%)	66 ± 4.5^{x}	48 ± 3.1^{y}	59 ± 3.6^{x}
Hispanic	79 ± 4.2^{a}	53 ± 6.1	72 ± 4.2^{a}
Non-Hispanic white	61 ± 8.15^{bc}	51 ± 5.1	59 ± 5.9^{ac}
Non-Hispanic black	55 ± 7.5^{b}	46 ± 5.2	43 ± 4.7^{b}
Asian	81 ± 9.7^{ac}	40 ± 8.2	52 ± 8.3^{bc}
Zinc (mg), EAR	2.5	2.5	4.0
All (%)	<1	<1	<1
Hispanic	<1	<1	<1
Non-Hispanic white	<1	<1	<1
Non-Hispanic black	<1	<1	<1
Asian	<1	<1	<1

Weighted populations are 700,568, 8,374,256, and 7,928,277 for 12–13 month, 2–3 and 4–5 year groups, respectively. Nutrient intakes were determined from food intake only. Means with different superscripts are significantly different by age (^{x,y}) and by race/ethnicity within age groups (^{a,b,c}), $p < 0.05$. EAR, Estimated Average Requirement; SE, Standard Error; mg, milligrams; mcg, micrograms.

4. Discussion

This report, using the nationally representative NHANES 2011–2012 & 2013–2014 dietary data, explored the consumption patterns of American infants and children by age and ethnicity and compared the current intakes with the age appropriate dietary recommendations. The results indicate that intakes of all food groups were low among 0–11 month-old children. While there was an increase in overall food consumption with age, there was a substantial percentage of the population among all age and ethnic groups who did not consume the recommended amounts for each food group and had inadequate intakes of key nutrients, such as calcium, vitamin D, and vitamin E from foods.

The results show that the intake of various food groups was low during the first year of life and increased gradually with age, suggesting increased intake of complementary foods. Complementary feeding generally starts when human milk or formula is no longer nutritionally sufficient. It is a major step in the development of eating behavior and directly affects the infant's growth and health [27–29]. Single-grain fortified infant cereals are often the first complementary food introduced and our data supports this assertion by showing that the intake of grain foods increased from 0.85 oz. eq. during 0–11 months to more than three oz. eq. at 12–23 months of age. Data from the Infant Feeding Practices Study II indicated that by four months of age, 40% of infants had consumed cereal, 17% had consumed fruits or vegetables [30], and more than 40% of mothers reported having introduced solid foods before their infant was four months old [31]. Another study also reported that 62% of parents introduced solid foods within the recommended 4–6 months age window while about 19% introduced solid foods prior to 4 months of age and about 19% started at 7 months of age or later [32]. Early and late introduction of solid foods (outside the 4–6 months window) is not optimal for infant health and nutrition as it may lead to increased risk for the development of chronic diseases such as islet autoimmunity (the pre-clinical condition leading to type 1 diabetes), obesity, adult-onset celiac disease, and eczema [33–35].

The AAP states that there is no reason to introduce whole food groups one after the other, instead, they recommend a gradual introduction of foods from all groups as soon as the infant is developmentally ready. The goal of complementary feeding is to eventually have the child eat the same well-balanced, nutritious mixed diet of 'family foods'. With that in mind, the AAP recommends that by 7–8 months of age, infants should be consuming foods from all food groups, including a variety of foods each day that may include: human milk/formula, meats, cereal, vegetables, fruits, eggs, and fish [2]. While children may not accept new foods right away, parents should be encouraged to offer foods multiple times (>10 exposures) for infants and toddlers to become accepting of new foods [36].

Our data show that the intakes of added sugar and fat increased with age, and mixed dishes contributed significant amounts to food groups. Contribution of mixed dishes increased at age 12–23 months and made up 25% of total grains and protein intake while more than 50% of fats came from mixed dishes. As children got older, the contributions of mixed dishes increased for each food group. Total dairy intake decreased after age 12–23 months, but contribution of mixed dishes to dairy intake continued to increase with age. At 4–5 years, mixed dishes contributed about 16% of total dairy but contributed 52% of cheese intake (data not presented), likely due to pizza consumption. Interestingly, mixed dishes also contributed about 30% of grain, protein, and vegetable intake (other components of pizza) for 4–5 years old children. Young children have high nutrient needs and relatively low energy requirements, leaving little room for added sugar- and fat-dense foods [16]. The 2015–2020 DGA recommend that no more than 10% of daily calories come from added sugars [3]. While the AAP has recognized that limited amounts of added sugars may be used to increase palatability of nutritious food options [37], the AHA recommends that children younger than two years of age should avoid added sugar all together. Additionally, the AHA states that if added sugar is consumed after two years of age, children should consume no more than 6 teaspoons per day due to the association between added sugar and increased CVD risk [26]. Our data showed that, regardless of ethnicity, the mean intake of added sugar among 4–5 years-old slightly exceeded the AHA recommendation. Given the association between added sugar consumption and increased energy intake and adiposity [26], our data suggest that the persistent over-consumption of added sugars beginning early in life could partially contribute to childhood obesity. Ethnic differences did exist among the added sugar consumption rates for 4–5 years-old children. Hispanic children consumed 27–39% less sugar than their NH-black and NH-white peers. These results align with a recent study where NH-white children were reported to have a higher mean intake of added sugars compared to Mexican American children [38]. In a small population study, NH-black children preferred significantly higher concentrations of sucrose when compared to NH-white children, which the authors attributed to differences in demographic factors, cultural practices, and genetic variation [39].

Our data also show that while about 19% of 12–23-month old children did not meet recommendations for dairy, the prevalence of inadequate dairy consumption increased with age; over 70% of children aged 4–5 years and over 60% children 2–5 years consumed less dairy than recommended and this represents over five million children in each of these age groups with dairy intakes below recommended levels. NH-black children 1–5 years of age consistently consumed about 30% less dairy than their peers of other ethnicities. Similar findings among older children have been reported previously [40,41]. In a small cross-sectional study, NH-black preschool children were reported to consume less dairy that their Hispanic peers, and a greater proportion of NH-black children across all age groups, compared to their peers of other ethnicities, did not meet the dairy food group recommendations [42]. This finding may be explained by the perceived genetic predisposition of the NH-black population toward lactose intolerance, as well as cultural beliefs and perceptions about the consumption of dairy products [43]. Since a significantly greater proportion of 2–3 and 4–5 years-old NH-black children had inadequate intakes of calcium and vitamin D compared to their peers of other ethnicities, consuming adequate foods from the dairy food group, which provides both of these essential nutrients, could be a simple and affordable solution [44].

Our data showed that protein foods were consistently under-consumed; over 70% of all 12–23 months-old children did not meet the protein food group recommendations (over 2.5 million children). Older NH-black children (2–3 and 4–5 years-old) consumed about 30% more protein foods then their NH-white and Hispanic peers, which is consistent with previous studies where NH-black children consumed more meat than Hispanic children [42]. In an earlier analysis of NHANES 2001–2004, a smaller proportion of NH-white children age 2–16 years met the meat and beans recommendations compared to their NH-black and Mexican American counterparts [40]. Meat is the main dietary source of iron and zinc; however, our results did not find any ethnic difference in prevalence of inadequate intake of these minerals.

The use of a cross-sectional study design was a major limitation of this study, preventing any determination of cause and effect. Additionally, the estimates of dietary intakes among young children were based on self-reported 24-h dietary recalls, which primary rely on the memory of parents/caregivers and as such are subject to reporting bias and may not fully account for day-to-day variations. Further, supplement intake was not included in our analysis, which would impact nutrient adequacy. Major strengths of this study included the use of a large nationally representative sample achieved through combining several sets of NHANES data, including for the first time nationally representative data for the Asian population.

5. Conclusions

In conclusion, the results from this study suggest that a substantial population of American infants and children from 0–5 years of age and various ethnic groups did not meet food group recommendations and had inadequate intakes of key nutrients such as calcium, vitamin D, and vitamin E from foods. Consumption of more nutrient dense foods (e.g., milk, fortified cereals, high omega-3 fish, fruits, etc.) should be encouraged to increase intakes of these and other nutrients; if this cannot be accomplished then an addition of dietary supplements should be considered. Additionally, our data showed that ethnic disparities exist for food intake among the very young American population, with NH-black children particularly standing out as the group who consistently consumed the least amount of dairy from 1–5 years of age.

Author Contributions: The authors' responsibilities were as follows—E.D., C.J.C., J.A.H., V.L.F.: project conception, designed research, developed overall research plan, determined content for manuscript and collaborated on the writing; V.L.F.: analyzed data and performed statistical analysis; All authors read and approved the final manuscript.

Acknowledgments: The study and the writing of the manuscript were supported by National Dairy Council. The Authors would like to thank Sanjiv Agarwal, Ph.D. Principle at NutriScience LLC for assistance with manuscript preparation.

References

1. Birch, L.; Arbor, A.; Savage, J.S.; Ventura, A. Influences on the development of children's eating behaviours: From infancy to adolescence. *Can. J. Diet. Pract. Res.* **2009**, *68*, 1–11.
2. Kleinman, R.E. (Ed.) *Pediatric Nutrition*, 7th ed.; American Academy of Pediatrics: Elk Grove Village, IL, USA, 2014.
3. 2015–2020 Dietary Guidelines for Americans. 8th Edition [Internet]; 2015. Available online: https://health.gov/dietaryguidelines/2015/ (accessed on 14 June 2018).
4. Kumanyika, S.K. Environmental influences on childhood obesity: Ethnic and cultural influences in context. *Physiol. Behav.* **2008**, *94*, 61–70. [CrossRef] [PubMed]
5. Satia, J.A. Diet-related disparities: Understanding the problem and accelerating solutions. *J. Am. Diet. Assoc.* **2009**, *109*, 610–615. [CrossRef] [PubMed]

6. Federal Register. Dietary Guidelines for Americans: Request for Comments on Topics and Questions. In *Federal Register*; 28 February 2018; Volume 83, No. 40. Available online: https://www.federalregister.gov/documents/2018/02/28/2018-04058/dietary-guidelines-for-americans-request-for-comments-on-topics-and-questions (accessed on 25 June 2018).
7. H.R.2642—113th Congress (2013–2014): Agricultural Act of 2014. 2014. Available online: https://www.congress.gov/bill/113th-congress/house-bill/2642 (accessed on 25 June 2018).
8. USDA. Pregnancy and Birth to 24 Months Project. Available online: https://www.cnpp.usda.gov/birthto24months (accessed on 8 March 2018).
9. Gillman, M.W.; Kleinman, K.; Rich-Edwards, J.Q.; Rifas-Shiman, S.L. Racial/ethnic differences in early-life risk factors for childhood obesity. *Pediatrics* **2010**, *125*, 686–695.
10. Huh, S.Y.; Rifas-Shiman, S.L.; Taberas, E.M.; Oken, E.; Gillman, M.W. Timing of solid food introduction and risk of obesity in preschool-aged children. *Pediatrics* **2011**, *127*, e544–e551. [CrossRef] [PubMed]
11. Baker, J.L.; Michaelsen, K.F.; Rasmussen, K.M.; Sorensen, T.I. Maternal prepregnant-body mass index, duration of breastfeeding, and timing of commentary food indirection are associated with infant weigh gain. *Am. J. Clin. Nutr.* **2004**, *80*, 1579–1588. [CrossRef] [PubMed]
12. Stettler, N.; Lotova, V. Early growth patterns and long-term obesity risk. *Curr. Opin. Clin. Nutr. Metab. Care* **2010**, *13*, 294–299. [CrossRef] [PubMed]
13. Krebs, N.F.; Westcott, J.E.; Butler, N.; Robinson, C.; Bell, M.; Hambidge, K.M. Meat as a first complementary food for breastfed infants: Feasibility and impact on zinc intake and status. *J. Pediatr. Gastroenterol. Nutr.* **2006**, *42*, 207–214. [PubMed]
14. Briefel, R.R.; Reidy, K.; Karwe, V.; Jankowski, L.; Hendricks, K. Toddlers' transition to table foods: Impact on nutrient intakes and food patterns. *J. Am. Diet. Assoc.* **2004**, *104*, S38–S44. [CrossRef] [PubMed]
15. Butte, N.F.; Fox, M.K.; Briefel, R.R.; Siega-Riz, A.M.; Dwyer, J.T.; Deming, D.M.; Reidy, K.C. Nutrient intakes of US infants, toddlers, and preschoolers meet or exceed dietary reference intakes. *J. Am. Diet. Assoc.* **2010**, *110*, S27–S37. [CrossRef] [PubMed]
16. Daniels, S.R.; Greer, F.R. Lipid screening and cardiovascular health in childhood. *Pediatrics* **2008**, *122*, 198–208. [CrossRef] [PubMed]
17. Centers for Disease Control and Prevention (CDC); National Center for Health Statistics. *National Health and Nutrition Examination Survey*; National Center for Health Statistics: Hyattsville, MD, USA. Available online: http://www.cdc.gov/nchs/nhanes/about_nhanes.htm (accessed on 9 February 2018).
18. Forum on Child and Family Statistics. Available online: https://www.childstats.gov/americaschildren/tables/pop1.asp (accessed on 10 June 2018).
19. Blanton, C.A.; Moshfegh, A.J.; Baer, D.J.; Kretsch, M.J. The USDA Automated Multiple-Pass Method accurately estimates group total energy and nutrient intake. *J. Nutr.* **2006**, *136*, 2594–2599. [CrossRef] [PubMed]
20. U.S. Department of Agriculture, Agricultural Research Service. What We Eat in America Food Categories 2013–2014. 2016. Available online: www.ars.usda.gov/nea/bhnrc/fsrg (accessed on 9 February 2018).
21. U.S. Department of Agriculture, Agricultural Research Service. USDA Food and Nutrient Database for Dietary Studies 2013–2014. 2016; Food Surveys Research Group Home Page. Available online: http://www.ars.usda.gov/nea/bhnrc/fsrg (accessed on 9 February 2018).
22. U.S. Department of Agriculture, Agricultural Research Service. USDA Food and Nutrient Database for Dietary Studies 2011–2012. 2014; Food Surveys Research Group Home Page. Available online: http://www.ars.usda.gov/ba/bhnrc/fsrg (accessed on 9 February 2018).
23. U.S. Department of Agriculture, Agricultural Research Service. Food Patterns Equivalents Database (FPED). 2017. Available online: https://www.ars.usda.gov/northeast-area/beltsville-md/beltsville-human-nutrition-research-center/food-surveys-research-group/docs/fped-overview/ (accessed on 9 February 2018).
24. Tooze, J.A.; Kipnis, V.; Buckman, D.W.; Carroll, R.J.; Freedman, L.S.; Guenther, P.M.; Krebs-Smith, S.M.; Subar, A.F.; Dodd, K.W. A mixed-effects model approach for estimating the distribution of usual intake of nutrients: The NCI method. *Stat. Med.* **2010**, *29*, 2857–2868. [CrossRef] [PubMed]
25. U.S. Department of Agriculture. Child and Adult Care Food Program (CACFP). Available online: https://www.fns.usda.gov/cacfp/meals-and-snacks (accessed on 9 February 2018).

26. Vos, M.B.; Kaar, J.L.; Welsh, J.A.; van Horn, L.V.; Feig, D.I.; Anderson, C.A.M.; Patel, M.J.; Munos, J.C.; Krebs, N.F.; Xanthakos, S.A.; et al. Added sugars and cardiovascular disease risk in children: A scientific statement from the American Heart Association. *Circulation* **2017**, *135*, e1017–e1034. [CrossRef] [PubMed]
27. Greer, F.R.; Sicherer, S.H.; Burks, A.W. Committee on Nutrition and Section on Allergy and Immunology. Effects of early nutritional interventions on the development of atopic disease in infants and children: The role of maternal dietary restriction, breastfeeding, timing of introduction of complementary foods, and hydrolyzed formulas. *Pediatrics* **2008**, *121*, 183–191. [PubMed]
28. Zutavern, A.; Brockow, I.; Schaaf, B.; von Berg, A.; Diez, U.; Borte, M.; Kraemer, U.; Herbarth, O.; Behrendt, H.; Wichmann, H.E.; et al. Timing of solid food introduction in relation to eczema, asthma, allergic rhinitis, and food and inhalant sensitization at the age of 6 years: Results from the prospective birth cohort study LISA. *Pediatrics* **2008**, *121*, e44–e52. [CrossRef] [PubMed]
29. Sloan, S.; Gildea, A.; Stewart, M.; Sneddon, H.; Iwaniec, D. Early weaning is related to weight and rate of weight gain in infancy. *Child Care Health Dev.* **2008**, *34*, 59–64. [CrossRef] [PubMed]
30. Grummer-Strawn, L.M.; Scanlon, K.S.; Fein, S.B. Infant feeding and feeding transitions during the first year of life. *Pediatrics* **2008**, *122*, S36–S42. [CrossRef] [PubMed]
31. Clayton, H.B.; Li, R.; Perrine, C.G.; Scanlon, K.S. Prevalence and reasons for introducing infants early to solid foods: Variations by milk feeding type. *Pediatrics* **2013**, *131*, e1108–e1114. [CrossRef] [PubMed]
32. Kuo, A.A.; Inkelas, M.; Slusser, W.M.; Maidenberg, M.; Halfon, N. Introduction of solid food to young infants. *Matern. Child Health J.* **2011**, *15*, 1185–1194. [CrossRef] [PubMed]
33. Arenz, S.; Kries, R. Protective effect of breastfeeding against obesity in childhood: Can a meta-analysis of observational studies help to validate the hypothesis? *Adv. Exp. Med. Biol.* **2005**, *569*, 40–48. [PubMed]
34. Tarini, B.; Carroll, A.; Sox, C.; Christakis, D. Systematic review of the relationship between early introduction of solid foods to infants and the development of allergic disease. *Arch. Pediatr. Adolesc. Med.* **2006**, *160*, 502–507. [CrossRef] [PubMed]
35. Butte, N.F.; Lopez-Alarcon, M.G.; Garza, C. *Nutrient Adequacy of Exclusive Breastfeeding for the Term Infant during the Frist Six Months of Life*; WHO: Geneva, Switzerland, 2002.
36. Sullivan, S.A.; Birch, L.L. Infant dietary experience and acceptance of solid foods. *Pediatrics* **1994**, *93*, 271–277. [PubMed]
37. Council on School Health; Committee on Nutrition. Snacks, sweetened beverages, added sugars, and schools. *Pediatrics* **2015**, *135*, 575–583.
38. Eicher Miller, H.A.; Fulgoni, V.L.; Keast, D.R. Processed food contributions to energy and nutrient intake differ among US children by race/ethnicity. *Nutrients* **2015**, *7*, 10076–10088. [CrossRef] [PubMed]
39. Pepino, M.Y.; Mennella, J.A. Factors contributing to individual differences in sucrose preference. *Chem. Senses* **2005**, *30*, i319–i320. [CrossRef] [PubMed]
40. Kirkpatrick, S.I.; Dodd, K.W.; Reedy, J.; Krebs-Smith, S.M. Income and race/ethnicity are associated with adherence to food-based dietary guidance among US adults and children. *J. Acad. Nutr. Diet.* **2012**, *112*, 624–635. [CrossRef] [PubMed]
41. Storey, M.L.; Forshee, R.A.; Anderson, P.A. Beverage consumption in the US population. *J. Am. Diet. Assoc.* **2006**, *106*, 1992–2000. [CrossRef] [PubMed]
42. Salvo, D.; Frediani, J.K.; Ziegler, T.R.; Cole, C.R. Food group intake patterns and nutrient intake vary across low-income Hispanic and African American preschool children in Atlanta: A cross sectional study. *Nutr. J.* **2012**, *11*, 62. [CrossRef] [PubMed]
43. National Medical Association. Lactose intolerance and African Americans: Implications for the consumption of appropriate intake levels of key nutrients. *J. Natl. Med. Assoc.* **2009**, *101*, 5S–23S.
44. Drewnowski, A. Measures and metrics of sustainable diets with a focus on milk, yogurt, and dairy products. *Nutr. Rev.* **2018**, *76*, 21–28. [CrossRef] [PubMed]

2

Maternal Iodine Status is Associated with Offspring Language Skills in Infancy and Toddlerhood

Maria Wik Markhus [1,*], Lisbeth Dahl [1], Vibeke Moe [2], Marianne Hope Abel [3,4], Anne Lise Brantsæter [3], Jannike Øyen [1], Helle Margrete Meltzer [3], Kjell Morten Stormark [5], Ingvild Eide Graff [1], Lars Smith [2] and Marian Kjellevold [1]

1 Institute of Marine Research, P.O box 1870 Nordnes, 5817 Bergen, Norway; lisbeth.dahl@hi.no (L.D.); jannike.oyen@hi.no (J.Ø.); ingr@norceresearch.no (I.E.G.); marian.kjellevold@hi.no (M.K.)

2 Department of Psychology, University of Oslo, 0316 Oslo, Norway; vibeke.moe@psykologi.uio.no (V.M); lrssmth@gmail.com (L.S.)

3 Division of Infection Control and Environmental Health, Norwegian Institute of Public Health, 0456 Oslo, Norway; mariannehope.abel@fhi.no (M.H.A.); annelise.brantsaeter@fhi.no; (A.L.B); hellemargrete.meltzer@fhi.no (H.M.M.)

4 Department of Nutrition, TINE SA, 0902 Oslo, Norway

5 Regional Centre for Child and Youth Mental Health and Child Welfare, Uni Research Health, Uni Research, P.O box 7810, 5020 Bergen, Norway. kjst@norceresearch.no

* Correspondence: maria.wik.markhus@hi.no

Abstract: Inadequate iodine status affects the synthesis of the thyroid hormones and may impair brain development in fetal life. The aim of this study was to explore the association between maternal iodine status in pregnancy measured by urinary iodine concentration (UIC) and child neurodevelopment at age 6, 12 and 18 months in a population-based cohort. In total, 1036 families from nine locations in Norway were enrolled in the little in Norway cohort. The present study includes $n = 851$ mother-child pairs with singleton pregnancies, no use of thyroid medication in pregnancy, no severe genetic disorder, data on exposure (UIC) in pregnancy and developmental outcomes (Bayley Scales of Infant and Toddler Development, third edition). Data collection also included general information from questionnaires. We examined associations between UIC (and use of iodine-containing supplements) and repeated measures of developmental outcomes using multivariable mixed models. The median UIC in pregnancy was 78 μg/L (IQR 46–130), classified as insufficient iodine intake according to the WHO. Eighteen percent reported use of iodine-containing multisupplements. A UIC below ~100 was associated with reduced receptive ($p = 0.025$) and expressive language skills ($p = 0.002$), but not with reduced cognitive or fine- and gross motor skills. Maternal use of iodine-containing supplements was associated with lower gross motor skills (b = −0.18, 95% CI = −0.33, −0.03, $p = 0.02$), but not with the other outcome measures. In conclusion, an insufficient iodine intake in pregnancy, reflected in a UIC below ~100 μg/L, was associated with lower infant language skills up to 18 months. The use of iodine-containing supplements was not associated with beneficial effects.

Keywords: Bayley; cohort; pregnancy; iodine status; iodine supplementation; infants; ICP-MS; mild to moderate iodine deficiency; neurodevelopment; urinary iodine concentration

1. Introduction

Iodine deficiency (ID) is considered one of the most common nutritional disorders globally and is the world's largest single cause of preventable brain impairment [1]. Infants and pregnant women are particularly vulnerable population groups [2], as ID may impair normal growth and development of the child, especially affecting brain development [3].

Iodine is an essential nutrient for the synthesis of the thyroid hormones triiodothyronine (T_3) and thyroxine (T_4). Dietary iodine is rapidly absorbed and the thyroid gland is dependent on regular and adequate supply through the diet in order to produce these vital hormones [4]. In the fetal brain, inadequate thyroid hormone levels impair differentiation, maturation, cell migration, and myelination [3]. The iodine turnover during pregnancy is increased because the mother synthesizes approximately 50% more T_4 to maintain maternal euthyroidism and transfer thyroid hormones to the fetus, and because iodine needs to be transferred to the fetus for fetal thyroid hormone production. In addition, the renal iodine clearance increases during pregnancy [5,6]. Critically low levels of thyroid hormones, associated with severe ID, cause neurological damage to the brain, particularly during the fetal and neonatal period, which can result in delayed motor and mental development [7–10]. Mild to moderate ID may also result in impaired mental development [11–14].

The World Health Organization (WHO) estimates that women in 21 European countries have inadequate iodine intake in pregnancy (defined as a median UIC < 150 μg/L), while only women in 10 countries are considered to have sufficient intake. No data are available in the remaining 23 countries [15]. In Norway, the public health focus on iodine has moved from endemic ID in certain inland areas at the beginning of the 20th century to the assumption of iodine sufficiency since 1950 [16]. However, there has never been a systematic monitoring program in Norway to confirm this assumption. The estimated iodine intake in the Norwegian population among adults and children shows that the intake of milk, dairy products and seafood contributes with ~80% of the total iodine intake [17,18]. This indicates that certain groups of the population may be at risk of a low iodine intake, e.g., subjects with allergy to milk or fish, vegetarians who do not consume fish, milk and dairy products (vegans), and others with low consumption of milk and fish. Other vulnerable groups that might have low iodine intake are pregnant and lactating women since there is a higher recommended intake of iodine during this period of life [19–21]. Data from the Norwegian Mother and Child Cohort Study (MoBa) (n = 61,904) showed inadequate iodine intake in pregnant Norwegian women and the authors suggested that sub-optimal iodine intake is a health concern in Norwegian pregnant women [22]. Several recent publications have documented mild to moderate iodine deficiency in pregnant women in different parts of Norway, with a median UIC of 92 μg/L (n = 777) in the Oslo area [23] and a median UIC of 75 μg/L (n = 197) in the Tromsø area [24]. Additionally, published results from the Litle in Norway cohort showed a median UIC of 85 μg/L (n = 954) in pregnancy [25]. Further studies and a better understanding of the consequences of mild to moderate ID in pregnancy on subsequent neurodevelopment in infancy and toddlerhood are scarce. Therefore, with samples and data from the Little in Norway study (LiN), the primary aim of this study was to explore whether maternal iodine status in pregnancy, measured by a spot UIC, was associated with child neurodevelopment up to age 18 months. A secondary aim was to investigate the potential impact of maternal iodine supplement use in pregnancy on the same outcome measures.

2. Materials and Methods

2.1. Study Design, Participants and Enrolment

The LiN study is a population-based prospective cohort established to investigate pre- and postnatal risk factors influencing developmental plasticity from pregnancy to age 18 months. Pregnant women were enrolled at nine public health clinics for mothers and children across all four Norwegian health regions. The clinics were chosen after considering demographic characteristics and size of the population to include participants from both cities and rural districts with a wide distribution of socioeconomic conditions. From each site, one public health care nurse was trained as a research assistant. Enrolment started in September 2011 and ended October 2012. Midwives at the public health clinics approached pregnant women 16–26 weeks gestation with an invitation to participate; however, some women were asked as late as weeks 31–34. Data collection up to age 18 months ended in November 2014. Attrition analysis for the mothers in the LiN study is reported by Fredriksen et al. [26].

Inclusion criteria for analysis in the present study were available data on UIC and on child development, singleton pregnancy, no thyroid medication in pregnancy, and no severe genetic disorder (Figure 1).

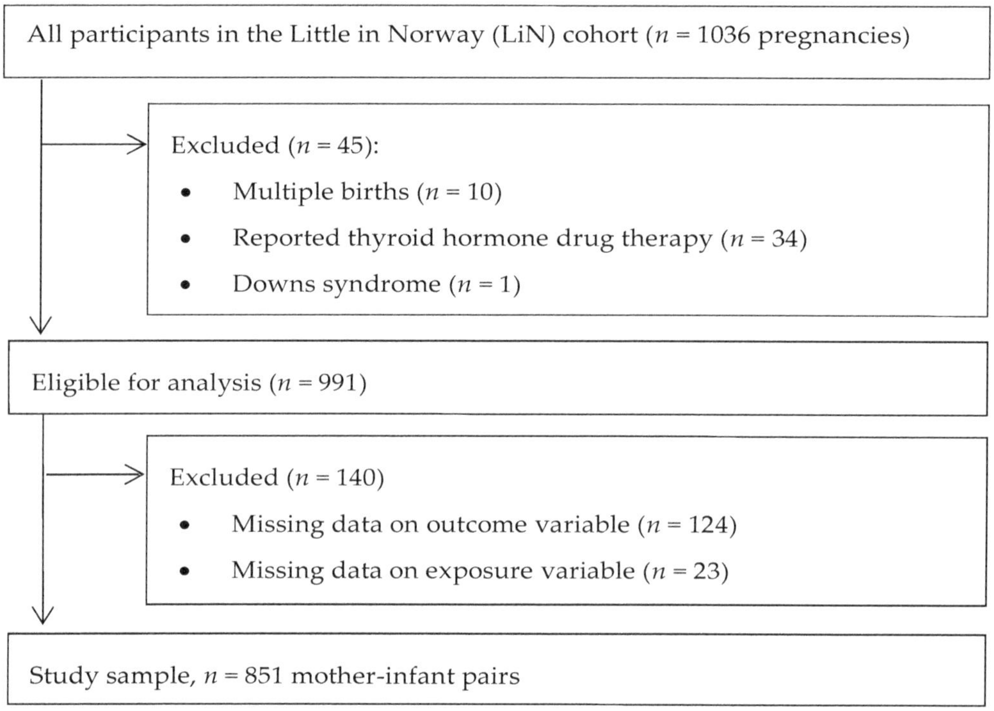

Figure 1. Flow chart showing the study population.

2.2. Data Collection

Participation entailed donating a spot urine sample for analysis of UIC, responding to questionnaires during pregnancy, and meeting with a research assistant after delivery for assessment of child neurodevelopment at 6, 12 and 18 months. The spot urine sample could be collected at home or on site, and be taken at any time. Details regarding time of sampling has been described elsewhere [25]. Data were collected by the research assistants based on interview of the parents, and by testing the child; through self-report questionnaires completed at the public health clinics; and self-report questionnaires completed at home. Details regarding data collection and the questionnaires have been described elsewhere [25,27]

2.3. Exposure Variables—Urinary Iodine Concentration and Use of Iodine Containing Supplements

Non-fasting spot-urine samples from the mothers were collected at the first (23.7 ± 5.0 gestational week) and the third (26.4 ± 1.6 gestational week) meeting with the research assistant at the public health clinic. The urine sample collected at the first meeting was preferably used in analysis (n = 851; if missing, urine sample collected at the third meeting was used (n = 7)). Urinary iodine is regarded as a good population biomarker of iodine intake because more than 92% of ingested iodine is excreted in the urine within 24–48 h [6]. Because it is impractical to collect 24-h samples in field studies, UIC were measured in spot urine collections [2]. Maternal hydration status affects spot-urine concentrations, and since creatinine is excreted in urine at a fairly constant rate, UIC per gram creatinine is often used with the aim to remove variation in UIC due to hydration. UIC in μg/L was used as the primary exposure since creatinine excretion varies in pregnancy with regards to gestational age, maternal age and body composition [6]. Additionally, as alternative exposure measures, we have included, in the online supplementary material, analyses of (1) UIC in μg/g creatinine and (2) residuals of UIC in μg/L after regressing log UIC on log urinary creatinine.

Questions on supplement use were embedded in a short web-based food frequency questionnaire explained elsewhere [25]. Iodine, ranging from 150 μg to 200 μg, was used in combination with other micronutrients, vitamins, with or without omega-3 fatty acids, by all users. Use of iodine supplement was coded yes or no employing compiled data from frequency questions ('never' was coded 'no', while '1–3 times per month', '1–3 times per week', '4–6 times per week', and 'daily' were coded 'yes').

2.4. Outcome Variables—Neurocognitive Development

The cognitive, language, and motor scales of the Bayley Scales of Infant and Toddler Development, third edition (Bayley-III) were used to assess the infants' developmental skills [28]. Bayley-III is an individually administered instrument designed to measure the developmental functioning of infants and toddlers, especially suited to detect developmental delays. The Bayley-III is commonly regarded as the gold standard in infant development assessment, provide good reliability and validity, and is often used as the instrument to validate other instruments [29,30]. At six and 12 months, the screening version of the test was used measuring all five domains: cognitive, receptive communication, expressive communication, gross motor and fine motor. At 18 months, the full-scale version was used measuring cognitive and language skills. The screening version is shorter than the full version comprising a selection of the test items employed in the full version. The two language scales are receptive communication, measuring verbal comprehension; and expressive communication, such as babbling, utterances, and gestures. Health care nurses, trained under supervision of clinical psychologists specialized in infant and child development, administered the test at the well-baby clinics. The parents were present in the room but instructed not to interfere with the testing.

2.5. Covariates

When recruited in pregnancy, participants completed a questionnaire onsite at their local public health clinic and a questionnaire at home including questions on age, pre-pregnancy weight and height, parity, education, marital status, use of iodine containing supplements, use of omega-3 supplements in pregnancy, and daily smoking in pregnancy [25]. When infants were born, public health care nurses recorded data including child gender.

2.6. Laboratory Analysis

Urine was collected at each site and stored at −18 °C pending analysis. Prior to analysis, the urine samples were defrosted in a refrigerator. UIC was determined by inductively coupled plasma mass-spectrometry (ICP-MS) after dilution with 1% tetrametylammonium hydroxid (TMAH). Prior to the analysis the samples were filtrated using a sterile membrane filter (0.45 μm pore size) and transferred to tubes appropriate for the analysis by the Agilent 7500 for ICP-MS at Institute of Marine Research, Bergen, Norway. Samples were analysed against a urine calibration curve (standard addition curve) to measure the unknown iodine concentration (127I) in the collected urine samples. Accuracy was verified with certified reference material; Seronorm Trace Elements Urine (Nycomed Pharma, Norway), iodine content: 84 μg/L (range, 72–96 μg/L) and 304 μg/L (range: 260–348 μg/L). In addition to UIC, I/Cr ratio and estimated 24 h UIE were determined. Determination of urinary creatinine concentration was analysed using the MAXMAT PL II multidisciplinary diagnostic platform with creatinine PAP kit [31].

2.7. Ethics

The trial complies with the Declaration of Helsinki and was commenced after approval by the Regional Committees for Medical and Health Research Ethics (2011/560 REK South-East). Written informed consent was obtained from the participants who could withdraw from the study at any time.

2.8. Statistical Analyses

Continuous variables are expressed as mean with SD for normally distributed data, as median with interquartile range (IQR) for non-normally distributed data, and categorical variables as numbers and percentages. ANOVA was used to compare numerical data and Pearson $\chi 2$ to compare categorical data in Table 1 on background characteristics.

Missing data on pre pregnancy body mass index (BMI) (n = 155 (18%)) were imputed by multiple imputation by chained equations in STATA, and 50 imputed datasets were generated for analyses. The imputation models included all variables included in the final analyses and was done separately for different exposures (UIC per liter, UIC per gram creatinine, UIC adjusted for creatinine by the residual method, and iodine supplement use in pregnancy). More details about the imputation models are provided in Method S1.

Multivariable mixed models were used to explore associations between exposures and repeated measures of cognitive score, receptive language skills, expressive language skills, fine motor skills, and gross motor skills. Associations between UIC and outcomes were modelled flexibly by use of restricted cubic splines (three knot positions, at percentiles 10, 50, and 90 of UIC). Potential time-varying effects were explored by testing interaction terms of exposure and time equal to zero. Outcome measures were standardized at each time point to obtain similar scales for the measurements. Since the mean and the variance at each time point by design were equal, generalized estimating equations were used to estimate the marginal effects, and an unstructured correlation matrix was specified to account for correlations between the repeated measurements. Results were reported as estimated mean across measurement occasions including 95% robust confidence intervals (CI). P-values for the overall associations of UIC and outcomes were calculated by testing all spline-coefficients equal to zero, and non-linearity by testing the second spline coefficient equal to zero.

We adjusted for potential confounding factors including maternal age, pre -pregnancy BMI, maternal education, marital status, parity, smoking in pregnancy, and included child gender, an important determinant of the outcomes, to increase the precision of the estimates. The sensitivity analysis on iodine containing supplement use also included use of omega-3 supplements as a covariate.

Two-tailed $p < 0.05$ was considered statistically significant. Statistical analyses of background characteristics were performed using Statistical Package for the Social Sciences (SPSS® Statistics Version 24). All remaining analyses were performed in STATA (version 15.0; Stata Corp., College Station, TX, USA). The package postrcspline for STATA was used for graphing of the flexible models [32].

3. Results

3.1. Background Characteristics

Mean gestational week for collection of urine sample used in the analyses was 23.7 ± 4.9. The median UIC in pregnancy was 78 μg/L (IQR 46–130, min 4, max 750). In total, 676 (79%) women had a UIC of less than 150 μg/L and 242 (28%) women had a UIC of less than 50 μg/L (Table 1). The ages (mean ± SD, (min-max)) in infancy and toddlerhood at the three time points for neurodevelopmental assessment were 6.1 ± 0.4 (4.4–8.2), 12.2 ± 0.6 (10.1–15.6), and 18.4 ± 0.8 (16.7–22.2) months, respectively. There was minimal loss to follow up (mean number of assessments were 2.7 of 3 for cognitive scores and language scores, and 1.9 of 2 for fine and gross motor scores).

In total, 155 (18%) women reported use of an iodine-containing supplement during the last three months before the spot-UIC was collected in pregnancy. Of the supplement users, daily use was reported by 69%, 4–6 days per week by 13.5%, 1–3 times per week by 12.3%, and, 1–3 times per month by 5.2%. The median (IQR) dose of iodine supplementation was 175 (25) μg. Considering the individual intake frequency this gives a median estimated daily intake of 150 (50) μg iodine from supplements. UIC was higher in supplement users (median 92 μg/L) compared to non-supplement users (median 77 μg/L), $p < 0.001$) (Table 1).

Table 1. Characteristics of the study population by UIC in pregnancy and by use of iodine-containing supplements.

Characteristic		UIC in Pregnancy (μg/L)					Iodine Supplement		
	n	All	<50	50–149	≥150	*p*-Value [1]	Non Users	Users	*p*-Value [2]
n	851	851	242	434	175		658	155	
UIC, μl/L [3,4],	851	78 (46,130)	33 (24,42)	83 (66,110)	200 (160,270)		77 (50,120)	92 (56,200)	<0.001
UIC, μg/g creatinine [3,4]	851	82 (53,124)	57 (38,86)	77 (53,110)	143 (105,222)		75 (44,120)	98 (59,190)	<0.001
UIC~Cr, μg/l [3,4]	851	81 (58,120)	63 (45,77)	80 (58,102)	178 (147,238)		78 (57,109)	110 (74,178)	<0.001
Age of mother (ys), mean ± SD	851	30.3 ± 4.7	30.2 ± 7.4	30.2 ± 4.5	30.7 ± 5.1	0.39	30.3 ± 4.6	30.2 ± 4.9	0.71
BMI, mean ± SD	696	23.4 ± 4.0	23.1 ± 3.7	23.6 ± 4.1	23.5 ± 4.3	0.40	23.4 ± 3.8	23.6 ± 4.8	0.60
Parity, %	851					0.15			0.38
Nulliparous	471	55	60	54	53		55	61	
Primiparous	275	32	26	35	34		33	28	
Multiparous	105	12	14	11	13		12	10	
Maternal education, %	851					0.39			0.37
Low (≤ 12 years)	182	21	24	22	16		21	17	
Medium (13–16 years)	323	38	38	37	41		38	43	
High (≥ 17 years)	346	41	39	41	43		41	41	
Maternal cohabitation, %	851					0.71			0.23
Yes	829	97	97	97	98		97	99	
No	22	2.6	2.9	2.8	1.7		3.0	1.3	
Iodine containing supplement, %	813								
Yes	155	19	12	18	31	<0.001	Na	Na	Na
No	658	81	88	82	69		Na	Na	
Daily smoking in pregnancy, %	851					0.30			0.76
Yes	24	2.8	4.1	2.1	2.9		97	97	
No	827	97	96	98	97		3.0	2.6	
Infant gender, %	851					0.60			0.69
Boys	433	51	50	52	49		52	50	
Girls	418	49	50	48	51		48	50	

[1] Comparison of numerical data with ANOVA and categories with pearson Χ2. [2] Comparison of numerical data with student's t-test (UIC-measures were log transformed) and categories with pearson Χ2. [3] Results reported as median (IQR) for all participants and UIC categories. [4] Values are log transformed and reported as mean ± SD. Abbreviations: UIC, Urinary iodine concentration; BMI, body mass index; Na, not applicable.

3.2. Urinary Iodine Concentration and Neurodevelopment

There was a positive correlation between UIC (μg/L) and UIC/creatinine (μg/g), rs = 0.54, $p < 0.001$, a strong positive correlation between UIC (μg/L) and UIC~creatinine (μg/L), rs = 0.73, $p < 0.001$, and even stronger positive correlation between UIC~creatinine (μg/L) and UIC/creatinine (μg/g), rs = 0.93, $p < 0.001$.

Having a low UIC (μg/L) in pregnancy (lower than ~100 μg/L) was significantly associated with poorer skills in language domains (receptive and expressive) in infancy and toddlerhood, but not with poorer cognitive score or fine- and gross motor skills (Figure 2A–E). The adjusted associations for both language outcomes displayed similar curve-shapes, but non-linearity was only significant for expressive language ($p = 0.003$) (Figure 2C).

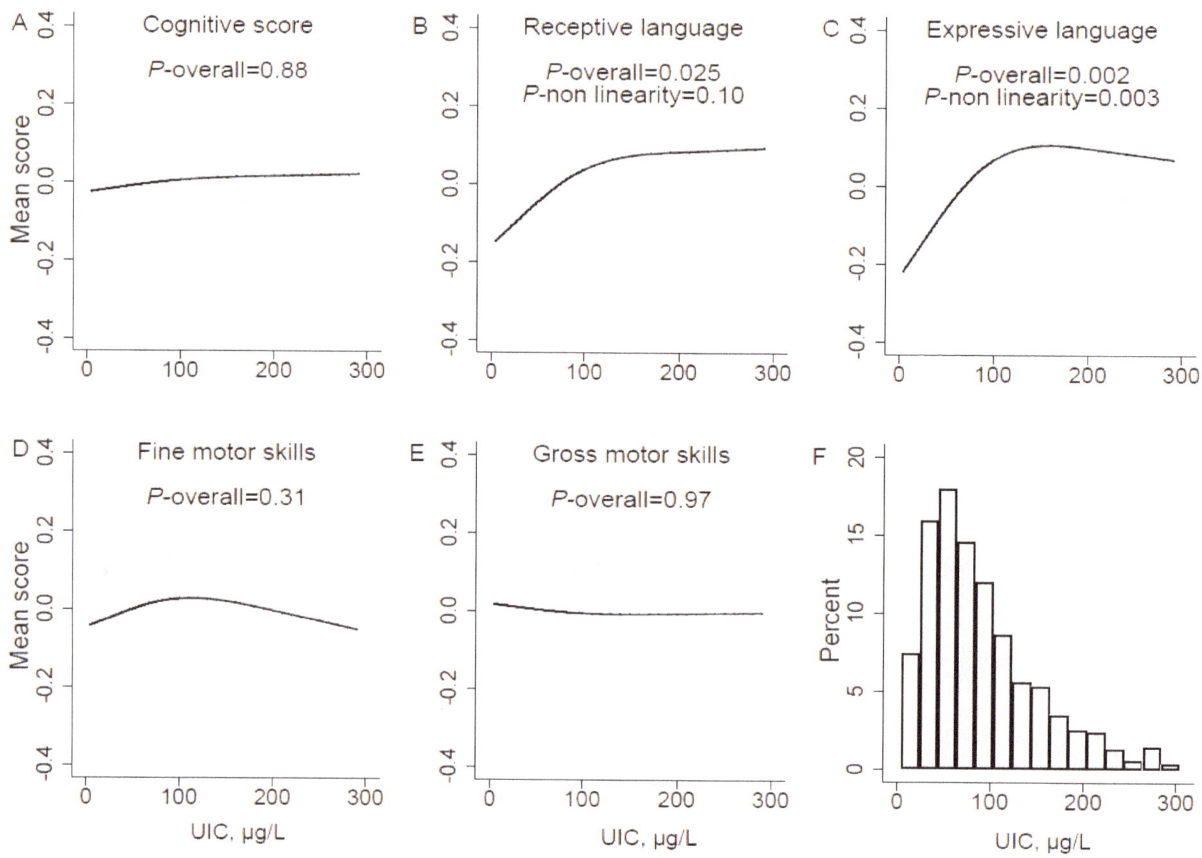

Figure 2. UIC μg/L in pregnancy and mean neurodevelopmental scores estimated in mixed models over sampling occasions at child age 6, 12, and 18 months. Panel A-E represent different neurodevelopmental domains, (**A**) Cognitive score; (**B**) Receptive language; (**C**) Expressive language; (**D**) Fine motor skills; (**E**) Gross motor skills. The histogram in panel (**F**) illustrates the distribution of urinary iodine concentration (μg/L) in the population. Associations were modelled flexibly by use of restricted cubic splines (three knot positions, at percentiles 10, 50, and 90 of UIC). Solid lines represent estimated means across measurement occasions, and the grey areas illustrate 95% robust confidence intervals (CI). P-values for the overall associations of UIC and outcomes were calculated by testing all spline-coefficients equal to zero, and non-linearity by testing the second spline coefficient equal to zero. Models are adjusted for maternal age, prepregnancy BMI, marital status, education, parity, daily smoking in pregnancy, and child sex.

The associations with both language outcomes were also significant in the unadjusted analysis (Figure S1). There was no evidence of interactions with time for any of the outcomes, meaning there was no evidence of differences in the effects at different ages in infancy and toddlerhood. The association curves looked similar for the alternative exposures of UIC adjusted for creatinine, but did not reach statistical significance (Figure S2 and Figure S3). All analyses were repeated including only complete cases, i.e., excluding $n = 117$ participants with missing information on pre-pregnancy BMI, and it did not change the results (Figure S4 and Table S1).

3.3. *Iodine Supplement use and Neurodevelopment*

Maternal use of iodine-containing supplements in pregnancy was associated with poorer gross motor skills, standardized beta = −0.18, 95% CI = −0.33, −0.03, $p = 0.02$ (Table 2).

Table 2. Longitudinal regressions of maternal use of iodine-containing supplement and the overall mean of standardized scores on child neurodevelopment. Non-users of iodine-containing supplements serve as reference group.

		Iodine Supplement					
Bayley III [1]	*n*	**Crude Models**			**Adjusted Models** [2]		
		B [3]	**95% CI**	*p*	**B** [3]	**95% CI**	*p*
Cognitive score	813	0.00	−0.13, 0.13	0.98	0.02	−0.11, 0.15	0.79
Receptive language	813	0.02	−0.10, 0.14	0.79	−0.02	−0.14, 0.11	0.81
Expressive language	813	0.07	−0.05, 0.20	0.26	0.05	−0.08, 0.18	0.44
Fine motor skills	810	−0.12	−0.25, 0.02	0.093	−0.10	−0.23, 0.03	0.15
Gross motor skills	810	−0.20	−0.35, −0.05	0.010	−0.18	−0.33, −0.03	0.020

[1] Bayley Scales of Infant and Toddler Development, third edition. [2] Models were adjusted for maternal age, prepregnancy BMI, marital status, education, parity, daily smoking in pregnancy, use of supplements containing omega-3 fatty acid in pregnancy, and child sex. [3] Standardized beta coefficient. B represents the standardized beta, i.e., the estimated difference in mean outcome score (in standard deviations) between the exposed and the non-exposed (to iodine supplement use).

4. Discussion

The main finding of this study is that mild to moderate ID during pregnancy may adversely affect neurodevelopment in infancy and toddlerhood. The study population was sufficiently large to conclude that the median UIC indicates insufficient iodine intake in this population of pregnant women in Norway [33]. This is to our knowledge the largest and most complete assessment to date of maternal iodine urinary status during pregnancy and its relation to repeated measures of infant and toddler neurodevelopment.

4.1. *Urinary Iodine Concentration and Neurodevelopment*

We found that an insufficient iodine intake in pregnancy, reflected in a UIC below ~100 μg/L, was associated with lower infant language skills up to 18 months. This accords with studies in older children and suggests that inadequate iodine intake in pregnancy has consequences already in early in life. In the ALSPAC study, Bath et al. [12] found that children of mothers with UIC < 150 μg/g creatinine were more likely to score within the lowest quartile on verbal IQ, reading accuracy, and reading comprehension at age 8-9 years than children of mothers with UIC ≥ 150 μg/g creatinine. In a similar study in Australia, mild ID (i.e., UIC < 150 μg/L) in pregnancy was associated with lower educational outcomes in children at age 9 years [34]. A prospective study from The Netherlands reported that low maternal UIC during pregnancy (< 10th percentile) was associated with impaired executive function in children at age four years [35]. In MoBa, Abel et al. [36] concluded that maternal iodine intake below the Estimated Average Requirement during pregnancy (160 μg/day) was associated with increased risk of child language delay, more behavior problems, and reduced fine motor skills at age 3. In a recent publication from The UK Robinson et al. found a positive association between iodine status before conception (I/Cr 108 μg/g) and child IQ [14]. The results from our study support these findings and expand current knowledge by indicating that adverse effects on inadequate iodine intake on neurodevelopment is detectable already in infancy.

Why we see an effect on language skills but not cognition is unclear, and further data are needed. A substantial body of research points to many interrelations between language development and cognition [37]. It may be speculated that poor language skills are more easily detected at this early age than cognitive impairment, or that language and cognition are undifferentiated at this age [30]. The fact that iodine status was found not to be significantly associated with cognition in this study could be due to lack of power in the study (too few participants and a high degree of measurement error on outcomes at such a young age). One can see that the cognition graph has the same shape as the language skill graphs, but the association was not significant. Nevertheless, our findings are in line with previous research, including Hynes et al. [38], who found that a group of adolescents had poorer performance and continued to lag behind their peers with respect to language and literacy development 15 years after being exposed to mild ID in pregnancy.

The associations we explored in this study were similar, but no longer statistically significant when UIC was adjusted for creatinine. Creatinine adjustment is commonly used to remove variation in UIC due to hydration status. However, including creatinine in the estimation of the exposure variable might also introduce bias since creatinine excretion is not constant between individuals, but vary with e.g., age, BMI, muscle mass/fitness level, and gestational age [6]. Consequently, creatinine-adjusted UIC is associated with maternal characteristics that are potential predictors of the outcomes.

4.2. Iodine Supplement Use and Neurodevelopment

We did not find evidence of a protective effect of iodine supplement use in pregnancy. On the contrary, maternal iodine supplement use was associated with lower infant gross motor skills. This finding may be due to chance since we did not control for multiple comparisons. Since only 18% of the participants reported use of iodine-containing supplements, there was limited power to detect differences between the groups. We assessed iodine supplement use over the past three months before the first UIC and it covered primarily the second trimester. Ideally, we should have had data from before pregnancy and in the first trimester. Consequently, it cannot be ruled out that iodine supplement use was initiated too late to counteract the detrimental impact of inadequate maternal iodine status in the most critical time of fetal brain development. Results from studies of iodine supplement use in pregnancy in areas of mild- to moderate ID show conflicting results, and more research is needed [39]. Our findings of no benefit are supported by recent results from in MoBa [36,40] where it was found that the use of iodine supplements during pregnancy had no beneficial effect on the children's neurodevelopment. Also, in a recently published RCT from India and Thailand, daily iodine supplementation in mildly iodine-deficient pregnant women (median UIC: 131 μg/L) had no effect on child neurodevelopment at age 5–6 years [41]. Altogether, this suggests a superior effect of habitual/long-term iodine intake from food, and that poor iodine intake and status before pregnancy cannot be compensated for by iodine-containing supplements in pregnancy.

4.3. Strengths and Limitations

A major strength of this study is the relatively large study population with data on UIC, the repeated measures of individually administered assessment of infant neurodevelopmental outcomes, and the minimal loss to follow up. An important limitation to the study is the use of a single spot-UIC which is not regarded as a good measure of iodine status at an individual level and thus it limits the statistical power when exploring associations to outcomes [6,42–44]. Observational studies tend to have a larger proportion of participants from higher socioeconomic status, introducing selection bias. However, associations between exposures and outcomes are not necessarily biased [45]. In this study population, however, there was a considerable proportion also of low-income mothers. Interestingly, we did not find any associations between UIC and education level or income. However, the observational design means we cannot rule out the possibility of residual confounding.

4.4. Implications of Findings

This study provides supporting evidence that mild to moderate ID in pregnancy impairs brain development and should be prevented. Reduced communication skills can influence the child's possibilities to obtain information about the environment and is an early predictor of later school performance and IQ [46]. Consequently, poorer communication skills may reduce the capacity for the child to reach its developmental potential. Insufficient iodine status in pregnancy is a public health concern and actions are urgently needed. It could be questioned whether the cut-off for median UIC defining adequate iodine intake in pregnancy by the WHO of 150 μg/L (corresponding to an intake of 250 μg/day) is too high [1]. Our results, and also results from MoBa [36,40], suggests that a cutoff of UIC ~100 μg/L (or intake of ~160 μg/day) would be adequate. Recommendations for pregnant women should not be higher than necessary since securing an adequate iodine intake for pregnant women by food fortification may put other population groups at risk of iodine excess [47].

5. Conclusions

This study provides further evidence for a potential negative impact of insufficient iodine status in pregnancy on child neurodevelopment. The results showed that the tipping point for adverse developmental outcomes was UIC ~100 μg/L. Furthermore, we found no indication of a protective effect of iodine-containing supplements used in pregnancy, however, RCTs are needed to elucidate the impact of iodine supplement use. Preventing mild- to moderate ID in pregnant women by securing adequate iodine status before conception is an optimal strategy, since use of iodine containing supplements in pregnancy may be too late to counteract the detrimental effects of inadequate iodine intake.

Supplementary Materials

Method S1: Imputation; Table S1: Longitudinal regressions of maternal use of iodine-containing supplement and the overall mean of standardized scores on child neurodevelopment. Non-users of iodine-containing supplements serve as reference group. Complete case analysis; Figure S1: UIC μg/L in pregnancy and the overall mean of standardized neurodevelopmental scores in infancy and toddlerhood. Panel A-E represent different neurodevelopmental domains, A: Cognitive score; B: Receptive language; C: Expressive language; D: Fine motor skills; E Gross motor skills. The histogram in panel F illustrates the distribution of urinary iodine concentration (μg/L) in the population. Associations were modelled flexibly by use of restricted cubic splines (three knot positions, at percentiles 10, 50, and 90 of UIC). Solid lines represent estimated means across measurement occasions, and the grey areas illustrate 95% robust confidence intervals (CI). P-values for the overall associations of UIC and outcomes were calculated by testing all spline-coefficients equal to zero, and non-linearity by testing the second spline coefficient equal to zero. Models are crude; Figure S2: UIC~Cr, μg/l in pregnancy and the overall mean of standardized neurodevelopmental scores in infancy and toddlerhood. Panel A-E represent different neurodevelopmental domains, A: Cognitive score; B: Receptive language; C: Expressive language; D: Fine motor skills; E Gross motor skills. The histogram in panel F illustrates the distribution of urinary iodine concentration (μg/L) in the population. Associations were modelled flexibly by use of restricted cubic splines (three knot positions, at percentiles 10, 50, and 90 of UIC). Solid lines represent estimated means across measurement occasions, and the grey areas illustrate 95% robust confidence intervals (CI). P-values for the overall associations of UIC and outcomes were calculated by testing all spline-coefficients equal to zero, and non-linearity by testing the second spline coefficient equal to zero. Models are crude; Figure S3: UIC, μg/g creatinine and the overall mean of standardized neurodevelopmental scores in infancy and toddlerhood. Panel A-E represent different neurodevelopmental domains, A: Cognitive score; B: Receptive language; C: Expressive language; D: Fine motor skills; E Gross motor skills. The histogram in panel F illustrates the distribution of UIC (μg/g) in the population. Associations were modelled flexibly by use of restricted cubic splines (three knot positions, at percentiles 10, 50, and 90 of UIC). Solid lines represent estimated means across measurement occasions, and the grey areas illustrate 95% robust confidence intervals (CI). P-values for the overall associations of UIC and outcomes were calculated by testing all spline-coefficients equal to zero, and non-linearity by testing the second spline coefficient equal to zero. Models are adjusted for maternal age, prepregnancy BMI, marital status, education, parity, daily smoking in pregnancy, and child sex. The solid line is the dose–response curve; the grey area represents the 95% confidence interval; Figure S4: UIC μg/L in pregnancy and mean neurodevelopmental scores estimated in mixed models over sampling occasions at child age 6, 12, and 18 months. Panel A-E represent different neurodevelopmental domains, **A**: Cognitive score; **B**: Receptive language; **C**: Expressive language; **D**: Fine motor skills; **E:** Gross motor skills. The histogram in panel **F** illustrates the distribution of urinary iodine concentration (μg/L) in the population. Associations were modelled flexibly by use of restricted cubic splines (three knot positions, at percentiles 10, 50, and 90 of UIC). Solid lines represent estimated means across measurement occasions, and the grey areas illustrate 95% robust confidence intervals (CI). P-values for the overall associations of UIC and outcomes were calculated by testing all spline-coefficients equal to zero, and non-linearity by testing the second spline coefficient equal to zero. Models are adjusted for maternal age, prepregnancy BMI, marital status, education, parity, daily smoking in pregnancy, and child sex. Complete case analysis

Author Contributions: V.M., L.S., M.K., L.D., M.W.M., I.E.G., K.M.S., and H.M.M. designed research; M.K., L.D. and, M.W.M. conducted research; L.S. provided essential data necessary for the research; M.H.A., M.W.M., A.L.B., and J.Ø. analyzed data or performed statistical analysis; M.W.M. and M.H.A. wrote the paper; M.W.M. and M.K. had primary responsibility for final content; All authors read and approved the final manuscript.

Acknowledgments: We are grateful to all the families that participated in the LiN-study and to the LiN-project workers for the acquisition of data.

References

1. WHO; UNICEF; ICCIDD. *Assessment of Iodine Deficiency Disorders and Monitoring Their Elimination*; World Health Organization: Geneva, Switzerland, 2007.
2. Ma, Z.F.; Skeaff, S.A. Assessment of Population Iodine Status. In *Iodine Deficiency Disorders and Their Elimination*; Springer: Berlin, Germany, 2017; pp. 15–28.
3. Zimmermann, M.B. The role of iodine in human growth and development. *Semin. Cell Dev. Biol.* **2011**, *22*, 645–652. [CrossRef] [PubMed]
4. Zimmermann, M.B. Iodine deficiency in pregnancy and the effects of maternal iodine supplementation on the offspring: A review. *Am. J. Clin. Nutr.* **2009**, *89*, 668S–672S. [CrossRef] [PubMed]
5. Andersen, S.; Karmisholt, J.; Pedersen, K.M.; Laurberg, P. Reliability of studies of iodine intake and recommendations for number of samples in groups and in individuals. *Br. J. Nutr.* **2008**, *99*, 813–818. [CrossRef] [PubMed]
6. Zimmermann, M.B.; Andersson, M. Assessment of iodine nutrition in populations: Past, present, and future. *Nutr. Rev.* **2012**, *70*, 553–570. [CrossRef] [PubMed]
7. DeLong, G.R.; Stanbury, J.B.; Fierro-Benitez, R. Nerological signs in congenital iodine deficiency disorder (endemic cretinism). *Dev. Med. Child Neurol.* **1985**, *27*, 317–324. [CrossRef] [PubMed]
8. Pharoah, P.; Buttfield, I.; Hetzel, B. Neurological damage to the fetus resulting from severe iodine deficiency during pregnancy. *Lancet* **1971**, *297*, 308–310. [CrossRef]
9. Hetzel, B. Iodine deficiency disorders (idd) and their eradication. *Lancet* **1983**, *322*, 1126–1129. [CrossRef]
10. Delange, F. The disorders induced by iodine deficiency. *Thyroid* **1994**, *4*, 107–128. [CrossRef] [PubMed]
11. Zimmermann, M.B. The adverse effects of mild-to-moderate iodine deficiency during pregnancy and childhood: A review. *Thyroid* **2007**, *17*, 829–835. [CrossRef] [PubMed]
12. Bath, S.; Steer, C.; Golding, J.; Emmett, P.; Rayman, M. Effect of inadequate iodine status in UK pregnant women on cognitive outcomes in their children: Results from the avon longitudinal study of parents and children (alspac). *Lancet* **2013**, *382*, 331–337. [CrossRef]
13. Bougma, K.; Aboud, F.; Harding, K.; Marquis, G. Iodine and mental development of children 5 years old and under: A systematic review and meta-analysis. *Nutrients* **2013**, *5*, 1384–1416. [CrossRef] [PubMed]
14. Robinson, S.M.; Crozier, S.R.; Miles, E.A.; Gale, C.R.; Calder, P.C.; Cooper, C.; Inskip, H.M.; Godfrey, K.M. Preconception maternal iodine status is positively associated with iq but not with measures of executive function in childhood. *J. Nutr.* **2018**, *148*, 959–966. [CrossRef] [PubMed]
15. Zimmermann, M.B.; Gizak, M.; Abbott, K.; Andersson, M.; Lazarus, J.H. Iodine deficiency in pregnant women in europe. *Lancet Diabetes Endocrinol.* **2015**, *3*, 672–674. [CrossRef]
16. Dahl, L.; Meltzer, H.M. The Iodine Content of Foods and Diets. In *Norwegian perspectives*; Elsevier Inc.: Amsterdan, The Netherlands, 2009; pp. 345–352.

17. Brantsaeter, A.L.; Knutsen, H.K.; Johansen, N.C.; Nyheim, K.A.; Erlund, I.; Meltzer, H.M.; Henjum, S. Inadequate iodine intake in population groups defined by age, life stage and vegetarian dietary practice in a norwegian convenience sample. *Nutrients* **2018**, *10*, 230. [CrossRef] [PubMed]
18. Nystrom, H.F.; Brantsaeter, A.L.; Erlund, I.; Gunnarsdottir, I.; Hulthen, L.; Laurberg, P.; Mattisson, I.; Rasmussen, L.B.; Virtanen, S.; Meltzer, H.M. Iodine status in the nordic countries—Past and present. *Food Nutr. Res.* **2016**, *60*, 31969. [CrossRef] [PubMed]
19. The Norwegian Directorate of Health. Norwegian Recommendations for Nutrition and Physical Activity (*in Norwegian*). 2005. Available online: https://helsedirektoratet.no/publikasjoner/anbefalinger-om-kosthold-ernering-og-fysisk-aktivitet (accessed on 20 January 2018).
20. World Health Organization, Unicef. *Reaching Optimal Iodine Nutrition in Pregnant and Lactating Women and Young Children*; World Health Organization: Geneva, Switzerland, 2007.
21. Untoro, J.; Mangasaryan, N.; de Benoist, B.; Darnton-Hill, I. Reaching optimal iodine nutrition in pregnant and lactating women and young children: Programmatic recommendations. *Public Health Nutr.* **2007**, *10*, 1527–1529. [CrossRef] [PubMed]
22. Brantsaeter, A.L.; Abel, M.H.; Haugen, M.; Meltzer, H.M. Risk of suboptimal iodine intake in pregnant norwegian women. *Nutrients* **2013**, *5*, 424–440. [CrossRef] [PubMed]
23. Henjum, S.; Aakre, I.; Lilleengen, A.M.; Garnweidner-Holme, L.; Borthne, S.; Pajalic, Z.; Blix, E.; Gjengedal, E.L.F.; Brantsaeter, A.L. Suboptimal iodine status among pregnant women in the oslo area, norway. *Nutrients* **2018**, *10*, 280. [CrossRef] [PubMed]
24. Berg, V.; Nøst, T.H.; Skeie, G.; Thomassen, Y.; Berlinger, B.; Veyhe, A.S.; Jorde, R.; Odland, J.Ø.; Hansen, S. Thyroid homeostasis in mother–child pairs in relation to maternal iodine status: The misa study. *Eur. J. Clin. Nutr.* **2017**, *71*, 1002. [CrossRef] [PubMed]
25. Dahl, L.; Wik Markhus, M.; Sanchez, P.V.R.; Moe, V.; Smith, L.; Meltzer, H.M.; Kjellevold, M. Iodine deficiency in a study population of norwegian pregnant women-results from the little in norway study (lin). *Nutrients* **2018**, *10*, 513. [CrossRef] [PubMed]
26. Fredriksen, E.; von Soest, T.; Smith, L.; Moe, V. Patterns of pregnancy and postpartum depressive symptoms: Latent class trajectories and predictors. *J. Abnorm. Psychol.* **2017**, *126*, 173–183. [CrossRef] [PubMed]
27. Fredriksen, E.; von Soest, T.; Smith, L.; Moe, V. Parenting stress plays a mediating role in the prediction of early child development from both parents' perinatal depressive symptoms. *J. Abnorm. Child. Psychol.* **2018**, 1–16. [CrossRef] [PubMed]
28. Bayley, N. Bayley Scales of Infant and Toddler Development® (bayley-iii®). The United States of America, 2006. Available online: https://www.pearsonclinical.com/childhood/products/100000108/bayley-scales-of-infant-and-toddler-development-third-edition-bayley-iii-screening-test.html (accessed on 20 January 2017).
29. Lung, F.W.; Shu, B.C.; Chiang, T.L.; Chen, P.F.; Lin, L.L. Predictive validity of bayley scale in language development of children at 6–36 months. *Pediatr. Int.* **2009**, *51*, 666–669. [CrossRef] [PubMed]
30. Albers, C.A.; Grieve, A.J. Bayley scales of infant and toddler development, third edition. *J Psychoeduc. Assess* **2007**, *25*, 180–190. [CrossRef]
31. ERBA Diagnostics France. Maxmat Creatinine Pap Reag. ERBA Diagnostics France: Montpellier, France. Available online: file:///C:/Users/mwi/AppData/Local/Microsoft/Windows/INetCache/IE/MMZGL9RY/PI-e-CREA_PAP-18.pdf (accessed on 8 September 2018).
32. Buis, M. Postrcspline:Stata Module Containing Post-Estimation Commands for Models Using a Restricted Cubic Spline. Available online: https://ideas.repec.org/c/boc/bocode/s456928.html (accessed on 1 November 2017).
33. Vejbjerg, P.; Knudsen, N.; Perrild, H.; Laurberg, P.; Andersen, S.; Rasmussen, L.B.; Ovesen, L.; Jorgensen, T. Estimation of iodine intake from various urinary iodine measurements in population studies. *Thyroid* **2009**, *19*, 1281–1286. [CrossRef] [PubMed]
34. Hynes, K.L.; Otahal, P.; Hay, I.; Burgess, J.R. Mild iodine deficiency during pregnancy is associated with reduced educational outcomes in the offspring: 9-year follow-up of the gestational iodine cohort. *J. Clin. Endocrinol. Metab.* **2013**, *98*, 1954–1962. [CrossRef] [PubMed]
35. Van Mil, N.H.; Tiemeier, H.; Bongers-Schokking, J.J.; Ghassabian, A.; Hofman, A.; Hooijkaas, H.; Jaddoe, V.W.; de Muinck Keizer-Schrama, S.M.; Steegers, E.A.; Visser, T.J.; et al. Low urinary iodine excretion during early

pregnancy is associated with alterations in executive functioning in children. *J. Nutr.* **2012**, *142*, 2167–2174. [CrossRef] [PubMed]
36. Abel, M.H.; Caspersen, I.H.; Meltzer, H.M.; Haugen, M.; Brandlistuen, R.E.; Aase, H.; Alexander, J.; Torheim, L.E.; Brantsaeter, A.L. Suboptimal maternal iodine intake is associated with impaired child neurodevelopment at 3 years of age in the norwegian mother and child cohort study. *J. Nutr.* **2017**, *147*, 1314–1324. [CrossRef] [PubMed]
37. Interrelations of Language and Cognitive Development. Available online: https://www.researchgate.net/publication/265905729_Interrelations_of_language_and_cognitive_development (accessed on 8 September 2018).
38. Hynes, K.L.; Otahal, P.; Burgess, J.R.; Oddy, W.H.; Hay, I. Reduced educational outcomes persist into adolescence following mild iodine deficiency in utero, despite adequacy in childhood: 15-year follow-up of the gestational iodine cohort investigating auditory processing speed and working memory. *Nutrients* **2017**, *9*, 1354. [CrossRef] [PubMed]
39. Harding, K.B.; Pena-Rosas, J.P.; Webster, A.C.; Yap, C.M.; Payne, B.A.; Ota, E.; De-Regil, L.M. Iodine supplementation for women during the preconception, pregnancy and postpartum period. *Cochrane Database Syst. Rev.* **2017**, *3*, CD011761. [CrossRef] [PubMed]
40. Abel, M.; Ystrom, E.; Caspersen, I.; Meltzer, H.; Aase, H.; Torheim, L.; Askeland, R.; Reichborn-Kjennerud, T.; Brantsæter, A. Maternal iodine intake and offspring attention-deficit/hyperactivity disorder: Results from a large prospective cohort study. *Nutrients* **2017**, *9*, 1239. [CrossRef] [PubMed]
41. Gowachirapant, S.; Jaiswal, N.; Melse-Boonstra, A.; Galetti, V.; Stinca, S.; Mackenzie, I.; Thomas, S.; Thomas, T.; Winichagoon, P.; Srinivasan, K.; et al. Effect of iodine supplementation in pregnant women on child neurodevelopment: A randomised, double-blind, placebo-controlled trial. *Lancet Diabetes Endocrinol.* **2017**, *5*, 853–863. [CrossRef]
42. Pearce, E.N.; Caldwell, K.L. Urinary iodine, thyroid function, and thyroglobulin as biomarkers of iodine status. *Am. J. Clin. Nutr.* **2016**, *104*, 898S–901S. [CrossRef] [PubMed]
43. Konig, F.; Andersson, M.; Hotz, K.; Aeberli, I.; Zimmermann, M.B. Ten repeat collections for urinary iodine from spot samples or 24-hour samples are needed to reliably estimate individual iodine status in women. *J. Nutr.* **2011**, *141*, 2049–2054. [CrossRef] [PubMed]
44. Ma, Z.F.; Venn, B.J.; Manning, P.J.; Cameron, C.M.; Skeaff, S.A. The sensitivity and specificity of thyroglobulin concentration using repeated measures of urinary iodine excretion. *Eur. J. Nutr.* **2018**, *57*, 1313–1320. [CrossRef] [PubMed]
45. Nilsen, R.M.; Vollset, S.E.; Gjessing, H.K.; Skjaerven, R.; Melve, K.K.; Schreuder, P.; Alsaker, E.R.; Haug, K.; Daltveit, A.K.; Magnus, P. Self-selection and bias in a large prospective pregnancy cohort in norway. *Paediatr. Perinat. Epidemiol.* **2009**, *23*, 597–608. [CrossRef] [PubMed]
46. Newman, R.; Ratner, N.B.; Jusczyk, A.M.; Jusczyk, P.W.; Dow, K.A. Infants' early ability to segment the conversational speech signal predicts later language development: A retrospective analysis. *Dev. Psychol.* **2006**, *42*, 643–655. [CrossRef] [PubMed]
47. Sun, D.; Codling, K.; Chang, S.; Zhang, S.; Shen, H.; Su, X.; Chen, Z.; Scherpbier, R.W.; Yan, J. Eliminating iodine deficiency in china: Achievements, challenges and global implications. *Nutrients* **2017**, *9*, 361. [CrossRef] [PubMed]

3

Dairy Consumption at Snack Meal Occasions and the Overall Quality of Diet during Childhood: Prospective and Cross-Sectional Analyses from the IDEFICS/I.Family Cohort

Iris Iglesia [1,2,3,4], Timm Intemann [5,6], Pilar De Miguel-Etayo [1,2,3,7,*], Valeria Pala [8], Antje Hebestreit [5], Maike Wolters [5], Paola Russo [9], Toomas Veidebaum [10], Stalo Papoutsou [11], Peter Nagy [12], Gabriele Eiben [13,14], Patrizia Rise [15], Stefaan De Henauw [16], Luis A Moreno [1,2,3,7] and on behalf of the IDEFICS/I.Family consortia

1 Growth, Exercise, Nutrition and Development (GENUD) Research Group, University of Zaragoza, 50009 Zaragoza, Spain; iglesia@unizar.es (I.I.); lmoreno@unizar.es (L.A.M.)
2 Instituto Agroalimentario de Aragón (IA2), 50013, Zaragoza, Spain
3 Instituto de Investigación Sanitaria Aragón (IIS Aragón); 50009 Zaragoza, Spain
4 Red de Salud Materno-infantil y del Desarrollo (SAMID), Instituto de Salud Carlos III, Madrid, 50009 Zaragoza, Spain
5 Leibniz Institute for Prevention Research and Epidemiology—BIPS, 28359 Bremen, Germany; intemann@bips.uni-bremen.de (T.I.); hebestr@leibniz-bips.de (A.H.); wolters@bips.uni-bremen.de (M.W.)
6 Institute of Statistics, Bremen University, 28359 Bremen, Germany
7 Centro de Investigación Biomédica en Red de Fisiopatología de la Obesidad y Nutrición (CIBERObn), Instituto de Salud Carlos III, 28029 Madrid, Spain
8 Epidemiology and Prevention Unit, Department of Preventive & Predictive Medicine, Fondazione IRCCS Istituto Nazionale dei Tumori, 20133 Milan, Italy; valeria.pala@istitutotumori.mi.it
9 Epidemology & Population Genetics, Institute of Food Sciences, National Research Council, 83100 Avellino, Italy; prusso@isa.cnr.it
10 Department of Chronic Diseases, National Institute for Health Development, 11619 Tallinn, Estonia; toomas.veidebaum@tai.ee
11 Research and Education Institute of Child Health, 2018 Strovolos, Cyprus; stalo.papoutsou@gmail.com
12 Department of Pediatrics, University of Pécs, 7622 Pécs, Hungary; peter.nagy@kk.pte.hu
13 Department of Public Health and Community Medicine, University of Gothenburg, 405 30 Gothenburg, Sweden; gabriele.eiben@medfak.gu.se
14 Department of Biomedicine and Public Health, School of Health and Education, University of Skövde, 541 28 Skövde, Sweden
15 Department of Pharmacological Sciences, University of Milan, 20122 Milan, Italy; patrizia.rise@unimi.it
16 Department of Public Health, Ghent University, 9000 Ghent, Belgium; Stefaan.DeHenauw@UGent.be
* Correspondence: pilardm@unizar.es

Abstract: There is scarce information on the influence of dairy consumption between main meals on the overall diet quality through childhood, constituting the main aim of this research. From the Identification and prevention of Dietary- and lifestyle induced health EFfects In Children and infantS (IDEFICS) study, and based on the data availability in each period due to drop outs, 8807 children aged 2 to 9.9 years from eight European countries at baseline (T0: 2007–2008); 5085 children after two years (T1); and 1991 after four years (T3), were included in these analyses. Dietary intake and the Diet Quality Index (DQI) were assessed by two 24 hours dietary recalls (24-HDR) and food frequency questionnaire. Consumption of milk and yogurt ($p = 0.04$) and cheese ($p < 0.001$) at snack meal occasions was associated with higher DQI scores in T0; milk and yogurt ($p < 0.001$), and cheese ($p < 0.001$) in T1; and cheese ($p = 0.05$) in T3. Consumers of milk ($p = 0.02$), yogurt ($p < 0.001$), or cheese ($p < 0.001$) throughout T0 and T1 at all snack moments had significantly higher scores of

DQI compared to non-consumers. This was also observed with the consumption of cheese between T1 and T3 ($p = 0.03$). Consumption of dairy products at snack moments through childhood is associated with a better overall diet quality, being a good strategy to improve it in this period.

Keywords: dairy; snack; diet quality; children

---

1. Introduction

Dietary factors in relation with obesity at different life stages from early childhood to adolescence are barely understood [1]. Recently, some eating patterns such as eating frequency, snacking, or skipping meals have been suggested to influence energy intake regulation [2].

In fact, for this specific age target, the consumption of at least four meal occasions per day is recommended, whereas the effect of eating five or more meals per day remains to be elucidated [3]. However, composition of snack meal occasions and their association with total dietary intake or body composition have not been investigated in depth during childhood [4].

The main dairy products consumed are (1) yogurt, which is defined as a food in the form of a thick, slightly sour liquid that is made by adding bacteria to milk and (2) cheese. Other dairy products consumed were included in milky desserts, which are a pooled group of foods that contain a lot of milk, and sweetened milk, which has an added sugar portion inside. Dairy products are good sources of calcium, which helps maintain bone mineral content and could reduce the risk of fractures later in life [5].

Some studies have also suggested that dairy consumption may have a protective effect against the development of obesity and cardiovascular diseases (CVD) [6]. Yet, the literature in children and adolescents in this sense is scant; in general, studies indicate either a beneficial or a neutral effect of dairy foods or calcium consumption on body weight or body composition [6,7].

Besides, an understanding of the tracking of dietary intake appears to be relevant for formulating policies focused on nutrition related health outcomes such as obesity. In dietary survey, tracking is defined as similar levels of dietary intake over time [8]. Despite childhood and adolescence being critical periods for physical development, not many studies have investigated the tracking of dietary intake during these periods.

In order to facilitate the appraisal of adequate dietary intake, diet quality indices (DQIs) have been used in various studies. DQIs have shown to provide an adequate overview of an individual's dietary intake and consequently to assess the compliance with food-based dietary guidelines (FBDG). A number of diet quality indicators have arisen, but their associations with health-related outcomes are still debated [9]. For instance, Vyncke et al. [10] showed good validity of the DQI for adolescents when comparing food and nutrient intakes and biomarkers in European adolescents using that index. Nevertheless, up to date, there is no study assessing the association of the consumption of dairy products with these DQIs and likewise none considering specific occasions of consumption as snack meal occasions considering the childhood period so widely.

Therefore, the objective of this study is to describe food consumption focusing on dairy products at snack meal occasions (mid-morning, mid-afternoon, after-dinner) during childhood and to investigate their relationship with the overall diet quality (cross-sectionally and longitudinally).

2. Material and Methods

2.1. Study Subjects

This study is based on the "Pan-European IDEFICS/I.Family children cohort", which can be found at the ISRCTN registry under the ID ISRCTN62310987. The "Identification and prevention of Dietary- and lifestyle induced health EFfects In Children and infantS" (IDEFICS) cohort comprised a total of

16,228 children aged between 2 and 9.9 years (y) old at baseline (T0) [11–13]. They were examined from autumn 2007 to spring 2008 in a community based baseline survey (T0) in eight European countries and also in a follow-up performed in 2009–2010 (T1) and from 2013 to 2014 in the "Investigating the determinants of food choice, lifestyle and health in European children, adolescents and their parents" (I.Family) (T3) study. Final included samples in the follow-ups comprised 11,041 and 6055 children of the original IDEFICS cohort in T1 and T3, respectively [11–13]. The design of the study was not thought to provide a representative sample for each country but constituted the starting point of the largest European children's prospective cohort study established up to date, involving Sweden, Germany, Hungary, Italy, Cyprus, Spain, Belgium, and Estonia. In each country, two separated cities or regions were involved in the study to have an intervention and a control region. This community intervention was carried out between autumn 2008 and spring 2009.

Children from 2 to 9.9 y who lived in the specific regions and who belonged to the selected pre-schools, kindergartens, or primary schools were eligible for recruitment. Children were approached via schools and kindergartens. In addition to the informed consent signed by parents, each child was asked to give verbal approval immediately before examination (or proper informed consent if they were older than 12 y in T3). In each country, participating centers obtained ethical approval from the local responsible authorities in accordance with the ethical standards laid down in the 1964 Declaration of Helsinki and its later amendments [14].

The general purpose of both studies IDEFICS and I.Family was to understand the mechanisms of childhood obesity and how to prevent it and to identify determinants of eating habits, lifestyles, and health in European children and their families. The attrition rate was defined by Langeheine et al. [14]. Children's age and weight status was positively associated with attrition; however, mother's age, migrant background, and educational level were associated with lower attrition. Taking into consideration the availability of the variables for this study [age, sex, BMI z-scores, education of the families, region, valid data on the two dietary assessment methods 24-HDR and food frequency questionnaire (FFQ)], total samples in each of the surveys were 8807 in T0, 5085 in T1, and 1991 children in T3 for cross-sectional analyses. In relation to longitudinal analyses, we finally included: 3838 children for tracking between T0 and T1; 974 children for tracking between T1 and T3; and 977 children with available data to assess the tracking between T0 and T3. In Figure 1, the flow chart of the selection process is provided.

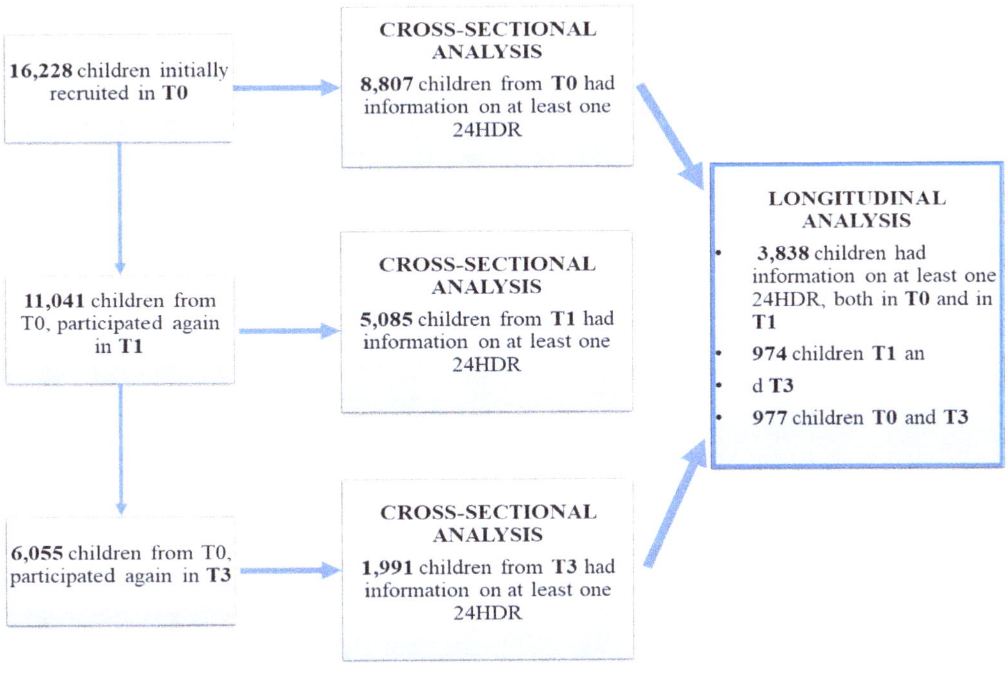

Figure 1. Flow chart of the sampling.

2.2. Dietary Assessment

For the purpose of this study, dietary intake was assessed using the computer-assisted 24-h dietary recall (24-HDR), called SACINA ("Self-Administered Children and Infant Nutrition Assessment") in T0 and T1 and SACANA ("Self-Administered Children, Adolescents, and Adult Nutrition Assessment") in T3. SACANA was the revised and extended web-based version of the SACINA off-line 24-HDR. SACINA was based on the previous HELENA-DIAT ("HELENA-DIetary Assessment Tool") software [15] developed within the HELENA Study (http://www.helenastudy.com) for adolescents. The absolute validity of proxy-reported energy intakes from SACINA [16] was investigated based on comparison with total energy expenditure measured using the doubly labeled water technique. SACANA was validated twice. In IDEFICS, both at T0 and T1, parents or caregivers were those who reported the information on amount and type of all foods and drinks that were consumed by the children during the previous weekday. In T3, this was done by the children themselves with the help of a parent from the age of 8 y. Estimation of portion size was assisted using standardized photographs. For children who had lunch in the canteen, school meals were assessed using a standardized observer sheet, completed by trained staff. Country-specific food composition tables (FCT) were used to match simple foods or recipes [17]. All nutrients and energy values were expressed per 100 g edible portion. Standard units were taken from McCance and Widdowson's [18] food composition tables (FCT). As the Italian FCT provided nutrient data only for raw foods, a raw/cooked coefficient was applied when large raw/cooked deviations were expected after preparation by boiling or steaming [16].

In a subsample, in T0 and T1, two 24-HDR were recorded, but to not lose participants in this study, only the first 24-HDR was considered in each child (also in T3).

SACINA instrument offered food and beverage reporting during six meal occasions: breakfast, mid-morning snack (everything recalled from breakfast to lunch), lunch, afternoon snack (everything recalled from lunch to dinner), evening meal, and evening snack (everything recalled after dinner) [16]. It was also possible to add more snack occasions.

Missing or implausible values that could not be corrected were imputed by country, food group, and age-specific median intakes (this represented 0.01% of the entries for SACINA and 0.14% for SACANA). Incomplete 24-HDR and those with four or more imputed values were excluded from the analysis.

For the cross-sectional analyses in all periods, intake (in grams per day) of the food items that belongs to the food group of dairy products consumed at mid-morning-snack, mid-afternoon snack, after dinner, and during the day, and the total energy intake (TEI) in kcal per day were provided. In the category "milk", whole milk, skimmed, and semi-skimmed milk were included; in "yogurt", all types of yogurt; in "cheese", all types of cheese; in "milky desserts" were products such as junket or rice pudding; and in "sweetened milk", there were products such as milk-shakes. "Milky desserts + sweetened milk" considered together as a category, and cheese, were only described for main meal occasions and considering all snack occasions together due to their low consumption.

The food frequency questionnaire (FFQ), which was part of the Children's Eating Habits Questionnaire (CEHQ) in the IDEFICS study [19], was also used in the cohort to calculate the Diet Quality Index (DQI) in each survey. The FFQ was found to provide reproducible and valid data [19,20]. In T0 and T1, the CEHQ included 43 food items clustered into 36 according to their nutritional profiles, as it was previously described [19], and also to make them comparable to the food categories of the 24-HDR. Similarly, in T3, the FFQ included the food items from T0 and added 17 food items due to older children and adolescents usually eating a wider range of food groups than the youngest. All food items were also re-arranged with the same nutritional profile purpose in 43 categories.

2.3. Diet Quality Index

The Diet Quality Index (DQI) was used in this study to account for the overall diet quality of the children´s diet. This index was originally developed for preschool children [21] and was later adapted and validated for its use in adolescents [10]. It consists of three components: dietary quality, dietary diversity, and dietary equilibrium. The basis to compute it was described previously in Vyncke´s and in Huybrechts et al.'s research [10,21]. This index was previously used as an indicator of compliance with the Flemish Food Based Dietary Guidelines (FBDG), which are similar to the dietary guidelines in other countries and in the World Health Organization CINDI (Countrywide Integrated Non-communicable Disease Intervention program) pyramid [10].

Dietary quality component expressed whether the food consumption of the child was of optimal quality within a food group. It was represented by a "preference group", an "intermediate group" and a "low-nutrient, energy-dense group". This classification can be observed in Appendix A Table A1. To calculate this dietary quality component, the amount of food groups consumed was considered. As we used a qualitative FFQ, sex-, age-, and country-specific medians of the portion sizes of the corresponding food groups were derived based on the 24-HDR. Portion sizes were multiplied by the derived frequencies from the FFQ to get the amount of food groups consumed daily, according to Bel-Serrat et al., Koster-Rasmussen et al., and Marcinkevage et al. [19,22,23].

Dietary diversity expressed the degree of variation in the diet by giving points ranging from 0 to 9 for each different serving of food consumed from the recommended food group (those from the list of preferable groups in Appendix A Table A1).

Finally, dietary equilibrium was calculated from the difference between the adequacy component (which is the percentage of the minimum recommended intake for each of the main food groups) and the excess component (which is the percentage of intake exceeding the upper level of the recommendation) [10]. The actual recommendations to calculate the adequacy and the excess of each food group are based on the Flemish Food Based Dietary Guidelines (FBDG) [24] for the different age ranges: <10 y and ≥ 10 y.

These three components of the DQI are presented in percentages. The dietary quality component ranged from −100 to 100%, while dietary diversity and dietary equilibrium ranged from 0 to 100%. To compute the DQI, the mean of these components was calculated. As such, the DQI ranged from 33 to 100%, with higher scores reflecting higher diet compliance. The score was calculated at baseline, T1, and T3 surveys. DQI scores for an individual provide an estimate of diet quality relative to dietary guidelines.

2.4. Body Mass Index

All measurements followed standard and validated procedures in T0, T1, and T3 surveys. Children were weighted in fasting status, without shoes and with light clothing on a body composition analyzer (Tanita BC 420 MA specifically adapted for children's feet in T0 and T1, and TANITA BC 418 MA in T3), recorded to the nearest 0.1 kg. Height was measured with a stadiometer (SECA 225 in T0 and T1, and SECA 213 in T3, Birmingham, UK) and recorded to the nearest 0.1 cm. Body mass index (BMI) was calculated by dividing body weight in kilograms by squared body height in meters and transformed to an age- and sex-specific z–score according to Cole et al. [25].

2.5. Sociodemographic Factors

Highest educational level of the parents according to International Standard Classification of Education (ISCED) was used as proxy indicator for socio-economic status of the family [26].

2.6. Intervention

Intervention was designed to address key obesity-related behaviors (diet, physical activity, and stress) in 4 levels: individual (children), family (parents), schools, and community. Briefly, six messages related to these behaviors were delivered through 10 modules targeted across all the levels: (1) increase water consumption; (2) increase the consumption of fruits and vegetables; (3) reduce daily screen time; (4) increase daily physical activity; (5) improve the time of family quality; (6) ensure adequate sleep duration. More information in this respect can be found elsewhere [27]. As this intervention took part between T0 and T1, we used a covariate to avoid the possible effect this might have in our analyses.

2.7. Statistical Analysis

The distribution of the sample regarding the categories of parents' education at baseline (T0) and in the two follow-up examinations (T1 and T3) as well as per country and per region (intervention or control) were presented stratified by sex and age group. Similarly, descriptive data of the study sample for the BMI z-score, diet quality, total energy intake, total dairy intake, and the food items eaten at snack meals and main meals occasions were presented as means and standard deviations for each survey and age group and sex.

Multiple linear regression analyses adjusted by BMI z-score, total energy intake, education of parents (the category of the one with highest education level) in the last survey of the tracking (T1 or T3), and region (control vs. intervention) were used to determine the differences in DQI between those who had consumed dairy products at snack occasions and those who did not. Similarly, for the prospective analysis, the dairy consumption at snack occasions was categorized in several groups of "consumers" at T0 and T1: dairy consumers at T0 and T1, non-consumers either in T0 and T1, dairy consumers in T0 but not in T1, and finally, non-dairy consumers in T0 but consumers in T1. After the creation of these groups, multiple linear regression analyses were again applied to investigate the differences in DQI between the healthy (consumers in both surveys and non-consumers in the first survey but consumers in the final survey, apart from the case for milky desserts and sweetened milk, for which it was the opposite) and unhealthy (non-consumers in both surveys, consumers in the first survey but non-consumers in the final survey, apart from the case for milky desserts and sweetened milk, for which it was the opposite) tracking groups after adjustment by the already mentioned variables. The same was done for T0–T3 and T1–T3 tracking surveys. The Statistical Package for Social Sciences version 22.0 (SPSS Inc., Chicago, IL, USA) was used for analyses. All statistical tests were stratified by sex and age group (<6 y and 6–9.9 y for T0 and T1, and <10 y and ≥10 y for T3), and corresponding p values were two-sided, considering $p < 0.05$ as statistically significant.

3. Results

Figures 2–4 are presented in order to easily observe the mean amounts of main groups of dairy products consumed during all snack occasions per country in T0, T1, and T3, respectively. In general, the main obtained observation is the drop out of the consumption of dairy products at these occasions. In T0 (Figure 2), milk and yogurt are the categories more consumed in snack occasions. However, in Cyprus and Spain, sweetened milks are more consumed than yogurt, while in Hungary and Germany, sweetened milk is the most consumed category of dairy products.

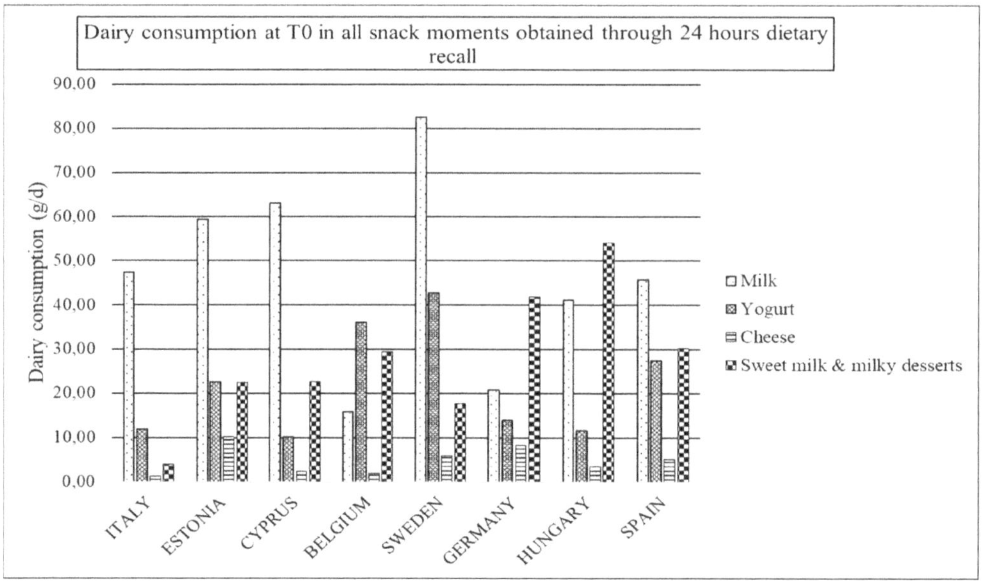

Figure 2. Dairy consumption at T0 in all snack moments obtained through 24 HDR.

In T1 (Figure 3), milk is the most consumed dairy product at snack occasions for Italy, Estonia, Cyprus, and Sweden, while yogurt is for Belgium and Spain. In Cyprus, sweetened milk is more consumed than yogurt, while again in Hungary and Germany, sweetened milk is the category of dairy product with the highest consumption with regards T3 in Figure 4.

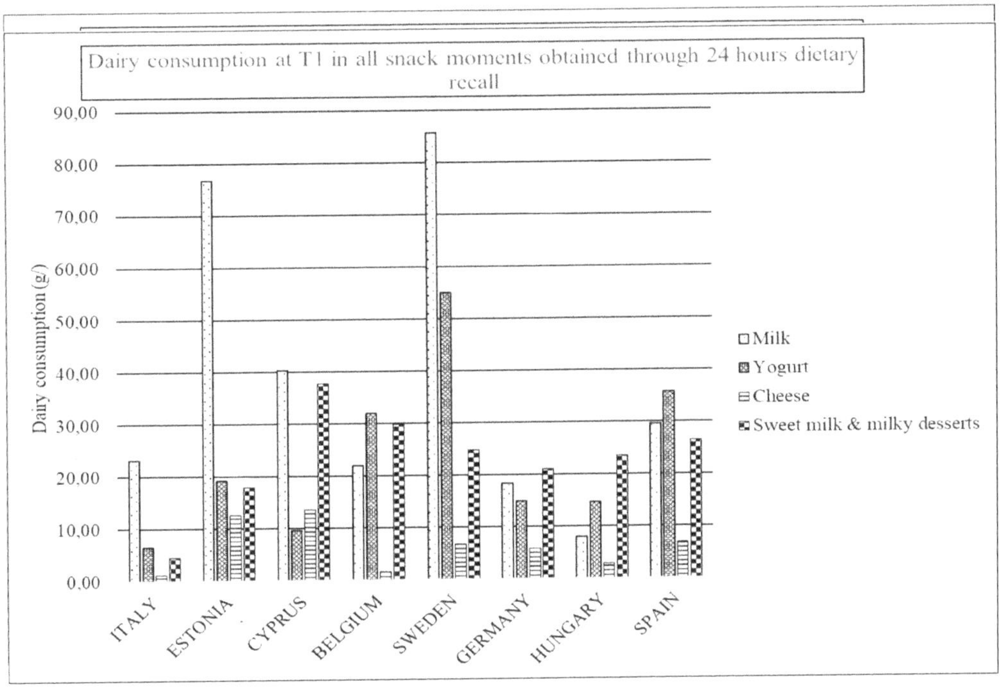

Figure 3. Dairy consumption at T1 in all snack moments obtained through 24 HDR.

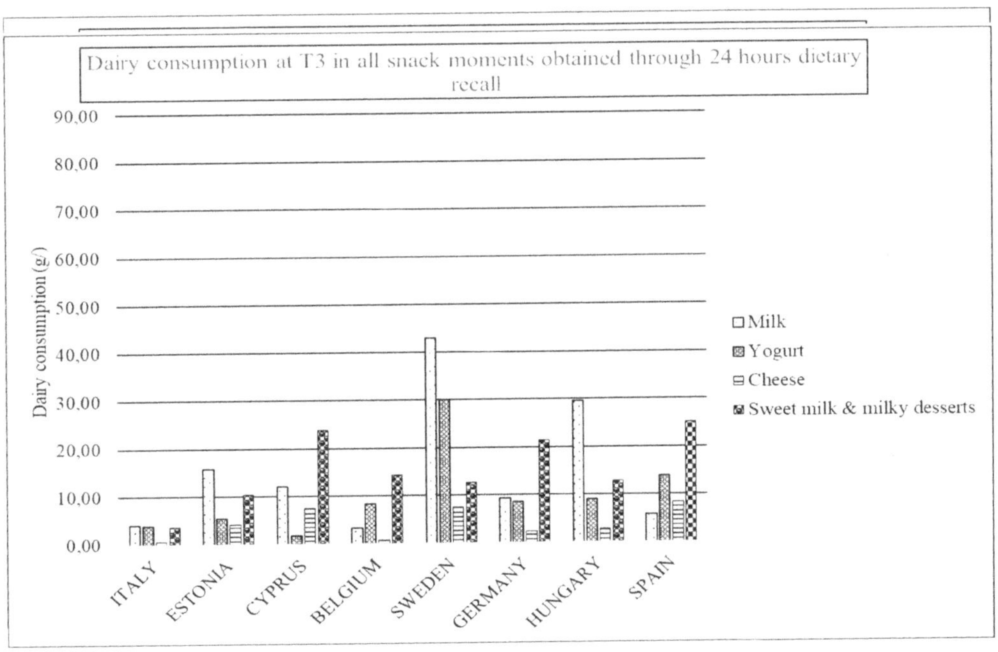

Figure 4. Dairy consumption at T3 in all snack moments obtained through 24 HDR.

Descriptive characteristics of the sample are shown in Tables 1 and 2 in terms of distribution of the samples per surveys for age and sex categories, BMI z-scores, total energy consumption, total dairy intake, and DQI. Besides, in Tables 2 and 3, the consumption of dairy products at main meals and snack occasions by sex and age categories and by survey, respectively, are shown.

The percentage of energy contribution of dairy products (obtained throughout the 24-HDR) during snack occasions decreased over time (decreased 3% from T0 to T1 and from T1 to T3; from T0 to T3, a 6% energy contribution of dairy products decreased; data not shown).

Boys showed higher energy intakes and total dairy intake at any main meal compared to girls, while they had lower scores of DQI in any survey or age category (Table 2). In Table 3, dairy intakes for total and each snack meal occasions are described for the three survey periods. In general, in T0, the consumption of dairy products at snack occasions was higher than in T1 and even higher than in T3, both in terms of absolute values in grams per day (Table 3) and in terms of relative energy contribution at snack occasions (data not shown). Consumption of milk was higher than yogurt at any snack moment of the day in any survey and in any age or sex category. Besides, the mid-afternoon snack moment was the one in which the children or adolescents consumed higher amounts of dairy products.

Table 1. Descriptive characteristics of the children participating in the different surveys T0, T1, and T3.

	T0				T1				T3			
	Boys		Girls		Boys		Girls		Boys		Girls	
	2–6 y	6–10 y	2–6 y	6–10 y	2–6 y	6–12 y	2–6 y	6–12 y	<10 y	≥10 y	<10 y	≥10 y
N	1961	2504	1814	2528	501	2076	445	2063	450	575	418	548
BMI z-score *	0.18 (1.18)	0.54 (1.25)	0.21 (1.11)	0.54 (1.17)	0.24 (1.20)	0.61 (1.22)	0.27 (1.19)	0.60 (1.17)	0.50 (1.24)	0.57 (1.28)	0.29 (1.21)	0.34 (1.21)
Education of the Families (ISCED 2011) T0												
High education	888	1064	832	1122	253	987	249	991	241	310	260	278
Medium education	905	1220	847	1204	214	931	175	927	188	245	144	241
Low education	168	220	135	202	34	158	21	145	21	20	14	29
Country												
Italy	483	558	388	553	129	657	101	612	64	112	50	107
Estonia	131	215	138	254	148	351	131	390	109	95	85	84
Cyprus	168	263	163	273	6	149	9	159	11	30	11	35
Belgium	116	83	105	76	34	166	35	148	28	34	24	38
Sweden	296	326	272	320	70	207	60	204	57	87	74	67
Germany	372	528	369	513	31	206	38	203	38	96	48	66
Hungary	224	392	247	395	17	90	18	87	29	25	20	30
Spain	171	139	132	144	66	250	53	260	45	45	46	40
Region												
Control	918	1146	821	1201	250	1088	226	1065	224	241	186	231
Intervention	1043	1358	993	1327	251	988	219	998	226	334	232	317

* This row corresponds to mean and (standard deviations), while the rest of the rows are number of participants (N).

Table 2. Description of dietary information (diet quality, energy, and dairy intakes) at main meals for boys and girls in the different age categories for each survey period.

	T0 (2007–2008)				T1 (2009–2010)				T3 (2013–2014)			
	Boys		Girls		Boys		Girls		Boys		Girls	
	2–6 y	6–10 y	2–6 y	6–10 y	2–6 y	6–12 y	2–6 y	6–12 y	<10 y	≥10 y	<10 y	≥10 y
Diet Quality Index (DQI)	79.97 (16.03)	80.7 (18.04)	80.62 (16.12)	83.22 (17.36)	85.69 (19.09)	85.22 (18.98)	87.75 (18.02)	87.90 (19.32)	99.76 (16.82)	97.86 (18.43)	101.26 (18.56)	100.85 (18.54)
Total energy intake (kcal/day)	1460.25 (509.69)	1675.2 (568.23)	1374.55 (502.57)	1529.91 (512.75)	1634.04 (512.72)	1774.23 (571.07)	1503.72 (516.58)	1619.30 (546.67)	1648.12 (688.47)	1611.99 (650.67)	1485.81 (624.40)	1482.05 (570.48)
Total Dairy intake (g/day)	334.98 (241.84)	318.52 (259.12)	303.78 (232.57)	270.34 (227.84)	368.29 (240.99)	322.90 (258.65)	326.51 (235.56)	282.67 (217.55)	254.35 (234.82)	233.52 (211.30)	239.90 (218.76)	209.64 (218.83)
Breakfast												
Milk (g/day)	91.65 (108.40)	81.99 (102.58)	81.50 (109.20)	68.42 (95.64)	93.01 (105.67)	101.01 (109.21)	83.77 (101.28)	85.54 (98.19)	82.39 (105.70)	90.42 (109.42)	74.75 (97.52)	60.73 (86.92)
Yogurt (g/day)	15.88 (54.35)	13.95 (53.02)	13.38 (47.33)	12.01 (47.72)	17.09 (54.97)	14.52 (52.88)	14.71 (46.42)	15.41 (53.01)	13.82 (50.98)	12.81 (51.47)	14.31 (47,47)	12.84 (45.03)
Milk + yogurt (g/day)	107.52 (114.57)	95.93 (109.33)	94.87 (113.38)	80.43 (101.39)	110.10 (112.07)	115.53 (112.43)	98.48 (101.12)	100.95 (102.19)	96.21 (111.50)	103.23 (113.29)	89.06 (104.68)	73.57 (92.78)
Cheese (g/day)	2.81 (14.91)	2.10 (10.87)	2.75 (16.77)	2.01 (10.72)	2.42 (17.89)	2.20 (13.56)	2.22 (13.23)	2.45 (12.74)	2.93 (18.51)	2.91 (11.78)	4.33 (15.82)	2.92 (14.88)
Milky desserts + sweetened milk (g/day)	18.43 (59.55)	18.85 (60.80)	15.0 (55.25)	18.0 (57.38)	9.91 (39.58)	13.27 (50.81)	14.38 (51.88)	14.70 (52.09)	19.11 (62.77)	16.27 (61.13)	17.86 (59.63)	19.53 (60.09)
Lunch												
Milk (g/day)	17.94 (54.56)	21.06 (66.53)	16.55 (49.79)	15.57 (56.80)	28.76 (68.95)	20.57 (63.58)	23.03 (63.68)	16.52 (54.93)	19.89 (59.72)	17.22 (60.40)	20.45 (62.79)	13.60 (55.78)
Yogurt (g/day)	7.93 (34.60)	6.80 (32.38)	5.31 (27.95)	6.53 (31.57)	6.12 (30.47)	9.29 (37.73)	7.48 (36.98)	7.89 (33.81)	6.08 (31.51)	6.95 (33.40)	4.95 (26.53)	5.20 (28.56)
Milk + yogurt (g/day)	25.86 (63.77)	27.85 (72.77)	21.86 (56.56)	22.10 (63.71)	34.88 (73.83)	29.86 (72.11)	30.51 (71.31)	24.41 (62.64)	25.97 (67.12)	24.17 (68.12)	25.40 (68.52)	18.80 (61.52)
Cheese (g/day)	4.76 (26.32)	5.14 (21.89)	5.57 (22.08)	6.05 (26.21)	8.93 (27.65)	6.19 (24.24)	7.01 (25.01)	6.0 (23.03)	5.15 (22.16)	3.14 (16.42)	3.29 (16.71)	4.06 (22.16)
Milky desserts + sweetened milk (g/day)	4.76 (26.32)	6.63 (37.93)	4.53 (32.40)	6.04 (29.57)	9.3343 (40.37)	8.91 (39.96)	8.87 (36.58)	8.92 (38.27)	19.11 (62.77)	16.27 (61.13)	17.86 (59.63)	19.53 (60.09)

Table 2. *Cont.*

	T0 (2007–2008)				T1 (2009–2010)				T3 (2013–2014)			
	Boys		Girls		Boys		Girls		Boys		Girls	
	2–6 y	6–10 y	2–6 y	6–10 y	2–6 y	6–12 y	2–6 y	6–12 y	<10 y	≥10 y	<10 y	≥10 y
Dinner												
Milk (g/day)	31.82 (77.85)	37.53 (88.72)	29.60 (71.51)	27.85 (74.04)	46.62 (86.76)	33.59 (81.77)	39.13 (82.87)	28.67 (74.64)	29.21 (83.20)	20.52 (63.42)	24.16 (66.39)	23.57 (72.32)
Yogurt (g/day)	11.16 (43.63)	8.33 (37.91)	8.75 (37.16)	6.57 (31.09)	9.56 (39.47)	8.57 (37.95)	9.94 (35.80)	9.60 (38.29)	7.08 (37.16)	7.24 (41.46)	8.06 (37.65)	7.24 (35.13)
Milk + yogurt (g/day)	42.98 (88.38)	45.86 (94.60)	38.35 (78.99)	34.43 (78.51)	56.18 (93.29)	42.16 (87.77)	49.08 (88.711)	38.27 (81.77)	36.29 (89.57)	27.76 (74.37)	32.22 (74.44)	30.80 (80.52)
Cheese (g/day)	5.57 (20.68)	6.35 (23.29)	6.22 (23.95)	6.07 (24.40)	7.39(25.55)	7.80 (27.85)	7.93 (30.45)	6.91 (24.30)	5.54 (19.36)	5.04 (20.79)	5.47 (21.27)	5.06 (21.46)
Milky desserts + sweetened milk (g/day)	10.99 (43.65)	14.01 (52.42)	9.83 (42.30)	9.29 (41.32)	8.27 (34.45)	7.52 (34.48)	6.20 (28.03)	6.99 (31.20)	19.11 (62.77)	16.27 (61.13)	17.86 (59.63)	19.53 (60.09)

All the data in cells correspond to means and (standard deviations).

Table 3. Description of the dietary information at snack meal occasions for boys and girls in the different age categories per survey (in g/day, SD).

	T0 (2007–2008)				T1 (2009–2010)				T3 (2013–2014)			
	Boys		Girls		Boys		Girls		Boys		Girls	
	2–6 y	6–10 y	2–6 y	6–10 y	2–6 y	6–12 y	2–6 y	6–12 y	<10 y	≥10 y	<10 y	≥10 y
All Snacks												
Milk	56.19 (107.24)	44.21 (96.46)	53.25 (98.03)	38.27 (85.70)	65.18 (105.80)	41.95 (104.65)	55.3 (100.27)	31.86 (82.24)	20.08 (67.87)	15.30 (60.70)	13.90 (49.47)	12.50 (50.40)
Yogurt	22.82 (64.18)	18.60 (64.27)	20.49 (58.75)	16.25 (53.78)	31.75 (71.75)	21.57 (65.00)	24.79 (61.20)	17.17 (53.32)	11.15 (43.62)	9.10 (43.11)	12.73 (47.15)	9.35 (46.02)
Milk + yogurt	79.0 (123.33)	62.81 (117.68)	73.74 (110.84)	54.52 (101.14)	96.93 (120.76)	63.52 (121.63)	80.09 (114.39)	49.03 (96.46)	31.23 (81.24)	24.39 (73.17)	26.63 (68.95)	21.85 (71.41)
Cheese	4.66 (17.82)	5.19 (19.14)	4.89 (17.53)	4.54 (14.52)	6.11 (24.35)	6.19 (20.82)	6.17 (24.38)	6.07 (20.00)	3.52 (20.47)	3.30 (21.74)	4.39 (28.20)	3.27 (17.63)
Milky desserts + sweetened milk	26.71 (76.55)	27.81 (78.17)	26.06 (73.29)	26.77 (79.95)	17.84 (54.88)	19.74 (64.80)	15.57 (53.75)	17.96 (61.27)	12.18 (50.76)	10.16 (51.12)	14.76 (56.62)	14.70 (54.13)
Mid-Morning Snack												
Milk	5.62 (37.97)	7.06 (37.31)	6.74 (31.62)	8.92 (40.37)	15.52 (57.68)	5.22 (31.39)	12.02 (46.36)	3.38 (25.80)	2.65 (25.46)	1.85 (20.79)	1.84 (17.11)	2.53 (25.68)
Yogurt	4.97 (28.56)	3.98 (36.07)	4.28 (24.83)	2.98 (20.92)	5.24 (28.92)	4.63 (27.20)	5.45 (28.57)	3.56 (22.38)	2.61 (20.23)	0.96 (11.86)	1.68 (13.42)	0.55 (7.39)
Milk + yogurt	10.59 (47.47)	11.04 (52.94)	11.01 (39.82)	11.90 (44.88)	20.76 (64.58)	9.85 (41.12)	17.47 (53.23)	6.94 (33.80)	5.26 (32.30)	2.80 (23.86)	3.52 (21.60)	3.078 (26.67)
Mid-Afternoon Snack												
Milk	20.0 (59.83)	18.90 (64.26)	19.04 (56.46)	14.66 (53.59)	27.18 (66.59)	20.03 (66.15)	29.70 (70.63)	18.34 (61.91)	10.21 (46.01)	8.62 (46.96)	8.97 (41.74)	6.03 (33.35)
Yogurt	12.74 (45.01)	8.90 (40.01)	12.04 (43.94)	8.43 (37.76)	15.45 (49.04)	10.24 (42.81)	14.25 (46.07)	9.23 (38.52)	5.54 (30.16)	3.73 (26.79)	5.35 (35.12)	5.622 (32.71)
Milk + yogurt	32.74 (74.24)	27.80 (76.23)	31.08 (70.06)	23.10 (65.54)	42.65 (78.59)	30.27 (77.86)	43.96 (83.28)	27.58 (72.05)	15.75 (56.64)	12.35 (54.30)	14.32 (54.10)	11.66 (49.43)
After-Dinner Snack												
Milk	30.57 (76.31)	18.25 (58.92)	27.48 (70.75)	14.68 (51.15)	22.46 (67.60)	16.69 (59.16)	13.573 (52.99)	10.14 (45.60)	7.22 (41.18)	4.83 (31.98)	3.09 (22.65)	3.93 (24.63)
Yogurt	5.11 (32.82)	5.72 (34.34)	4.17 (28.85)	4.84 (31.36)	11.05 (46.01)	6.71 (39.05)	5.09 (29.69)	4.38 (29.39)	3.0 (25.17)	4.41 (29.35)	5.70 (30.13)	3.18 (28.98)
Milk + yogurt	35.67 (81.69)	23.98 (67.58)	31.65 (75.45)	19.53 (59.05)	33.52 (80.93)	23.40 (70.36)	18.66 (60.16)	14.52 (54.14)	10.22 (48.25)	9.24 (42.92)	8.78 (37.62)	7.12 (37.70)

All the data in cells correspond to means and (standard deviations).

In Table 4, children who consumed dairy products at snack occasions had, in general, higher adjusted means of DQI scores apart from those consuming sweetened milk or milky desserts. Specifically, the consumption of the sum of milk and yogurt ($p = 0.04$) and cheese ($p < 0.001$) determined higher DQI scores in T0; yogurt ($p < 0.001$), the sum of milk and yogurt ($p < 0.001$), and cheese ($p < 0.001$) in T1, and only cheese in T3 ($p = 0.052$). In contrary, those consuming sweetened milk in T0 had significantly lower DQI scores ($p = 0.03$).

When analyzing longitudinally the consumption of dairy products at snack occasions and their tracking for each survey (Table 5), results pointed to the same direction. The adjusted tracking of the DQI mean values by groups of dairy consumers and non-consumers throughout T0 and T1 in all snack occasions showed that those who consumed either milk ($p = 0.02$), yogurt ($p < 0.001$), or cheese ($p < 0.001$) determined significantly higher scores of DQI. The same result was observed between the tracking of T1 and T3 for cheese ($p = 0.03$) and for the combined category of milky desserts and sweetened milk with only borderline significance ($p = 0.054$).

Table 4. DQI by non-consumers and consumers of the different dairy products considering all snack meal occasions, cross-sectional analyses in T0 and T1.

		T0		T1		T3	
		Means	(CI 95%) *p*-Values	Means	(CI 95%) *p*-Values	Means	(CI 95%) *p*-Values
All Snacks							
Milk (g/day)	NON CONSUMERS (N)	85.91 (6640)	(−0.06, 1.71)	86.17 (4082)	(−0.24, 2.39)	99.73 (1831)	(−2.46, 3.40)
	CONSUMERS (N)	87.21 (2160)	0.06	88.22 (1002)	0.11	100.88 (160)	0.75
Yogurt (g/day)	NON CONSUMERS (N)	86.06 (7754)	(−0.43, 1.92)	85.92 (4429)	(2.66, 5.73)	99.68 (1867)	(−1.68, 4.88)
	CONSUMERS (N)	87.41 (1042)	0.22	90.96 (654)	<0.001	101.96 (124)	0.34
Milk + yogurt (g/day)	NON CONSUMERS (N)	85.74 (5843)	(0.06, 1.68)	85.47 (3538)	(1.44, 3.71)	99.60 (1720)	(−1.32, 3.34)
	CONSUMERS (N)	87.18 (2957)	0.04	89.09 (1546)	<0.001	101.27 (271)	0.40
Cheese (g/day)	NON CONSUMERS (N)	85.34 (7453)	(1.02, 3.13)	85.92 (4262)	(1.39, 4.21)	99.56 (1845)	(−0.03, 6.06)
	CONSUMERS (N)	88.35 (1346)	<0.001	89.95 (821)	<0.001	103.16 (146)	0.052
Milky desserts (g/day)	NON CONSUMERS (N)	86.25 (8203)	(−2.69, 0.35)	86.50 (4709)	(−1.56, 2.39)	99.93 (1869)	(−5.32, 1.28)
	CONSUMERS (N)	85.81 (593)	0.13	87.40 (374)	0.68	98.18 (122)	0.23
Sweetened milk (g/day)	NON CONSUMERS (N)	86.32 (7405)	(−2.21, −0.12)	86.38 (4442)	(−0.87, 2.25)	99.75 (1930)	(−2.95, 6.25)
	CONSUMERS (N)	85.71 (1392)	0.03	87.90 (641)	0.39	102.33 (61)	0.48

95% confidence intervals and *p*-values correspond to linear regression analyses adjusted by BMI z-score (age and sex adjusted), energy intake, higher education of the parents, and type of region only for T1 and T3 (control or intervention).

Table 5. Diet Quality Index by groups according to tracking of dairy products consumption at snack meal occasions between T0 and T1, T1 and T3, T0 and T3.

		T0–T1		T1–T3		T0–T3	
		Mean DQI (n)	(CI 95%) p-Values	Mean DQI (n)	(CI 95%) p-Values	Mean DQI (n)	(CI 95%) p-Values
All Snacks							
Milk	UNHEALTHY TRACKING	85.46 (3039)	(0.26, 3.20)	98.85 (908)	(−2.35, 6.88)	98.74 (914)	(−3.12, 5.20)
	HEALTHY TRACKING	88.11 (799)	0.02	101.27 (66)	0.34	100.71 (77)	0.62
Yogurt	UNHEALTHY TRACKING	85.49 (3388)	(1.70, 5.36)	98.86 (921)	(−3.14, 7.05)	98.79 (928)	(−4.06, 5.0)
	HEALTHY TRACKING	89.91 (450)	<0.001	101.73 (53)	0.45	100.47 (63)	0.84
Milk + yogurt	UNHEALTHY TRACKING	84.90 (2675)	(1.36, 3.96)	98.65 (860)	(−0.95, 6.26)	98.59 (859)	(−2.09, 4.48)
	HEALTHY TRACKING	88.56 (1163)	<0.001	101.75 (114)	0.15	100.85 (132)	0.48
Cheese	UNHEALTHY TRACKING	85.14 (3235)	(1.74, 5.0)	98.63 (913)	(0.43, 9.95)	-	-
	HEALTHY TRACKING	89.59 (603)	<0.001	104.85 (61)	0.03		
Milky desserts + sweetened milk*	HEALTHY TRACKING	86.34 (450)	(−1.36, 2.31)	96.81 (120)	(−0.07, 6.96)	98.11 (85)	(−2.61, 5.27)
	UNHEALTHY TRACKING	85.97 (3388)	0.61	99.33 (854)	0.054	98.97 (906)	0.51

95% confidence intervals and p-values correspond to linear regression analyses adjusted by BMI z-score (age and sex adjusted), energy intake, higher education of the parents in the final survey (T1 or T3 accordingly), and type of region only for T1 and T3 (control or intervention). Healthy tracking: consumers in both surveys, non-consumers in the first survey but consumers in the final survey (apart from the case for milky desserts and sweetened milk, for which it was the opposite). Unhealthy tracking: non-consumers in both surveys, consumers in the first survey but non-consumers in the final survey (apart from the case for milky desserts and sweetened milk, for which it was the opposite). There are no data for cheese in T0–T3 because the unhealthy tracking group was empty.

4. Discussion

The main outcome of the present study showed that children who consumed dairy products at snack meal occasions had a higher diet quality than their non-consumers counterparts, both in the cross-sectional and the prospective analysis. To the best of our knowledge, this is the first study showing such association in such a large sample of children in a prospective cohort. These results seem relevant due to their influence on growth and development in children and adolescents.

There are several definitions of eating occasions in between meals. There is evidence that eating three main meals and two or three snacks per day (nibbling, frequent small intakes) is considered better for health than eating fewer but larger meals (gorging, infrequent large meals) [3,28]. Therefore, a standard definition is required to facilitate comparisons and further research. At the same time, these differences could influence the direction and the magnitude of the associations with diet quality and other health outcomes [29]. Eating occasions in between meals (snacking) can help to control hunger, but snacking should not replace proper meals [28]. Indeed, the snacking habit is commonly associated with poor health outcomes and dietary patterns [30], mainly when the snacks are high-energy dense foods, which might contribute as a factor in the development of childhood overweight and obesity. Although eating at least four meals per day is recommended for children older than 2 years of age [3], some studies have investigated the association between snacking and body mass index and have shown mixed results [31]. The reason could be that their food composition is often poorly described [4]. In this perspective, our study brings some elements showing that dairy products consumption during snack meal occasions might positively affect the overall diet quality.

Our results showed that, in European children, milk and yogurt are generally the dairy most consumed at snack occasions apart from Germany and Hungary, where sweetened milk and milky desserts are mainly consumed, in agreement with previous results [32]. Assessment of children's diet is of considerable interest because food habits and behavior acquired during childhood and adolescence are used to track until adulthood [33]. In our study, the percentage of energy corresponding to dairy products in relation to the total energy intake consumed at snack occasions decreased over time, as did the absolute values of dairy consumption, except for younger boys between T0 and T1, which may be related to a decrease in the parental influence on children's dietary patterns [34].

Previous studies in adults suggested that the beneficial effect of dairy products may be dependent on the type of dairy products consumed [35–37]. Therefore, given the low dairy products consumption along the day observed in the studied children and adolescents, snack time could be a good opportunity to increase daily intakes of milk and yogurt, specifically among girls who have shown lower consumption of dairy products both in main meals and at snack meal occasions.

Tracking of milk and/or yogurt and/or cheese consumption is also associated with high DQI scores. Other authors have also shown that dairy consumption is linked to healthy dietary patterns and lifestyle factors in adults [38]. This is confirmed in our study.

Children who consumed milk and yogurt had a positive relationship with a combination of high physical activity and low sedentary behaviors over the years [39]. The most likely reason is the clustering of different lifestyle behaviors, such as physical activity, smoking, or dietary behavior [40]. Moreover, the consumption of yogurt and other dairy products has been shown to be associated with a high diet quality, a decreased risk of weight gain and obesity, as well as decreased risk of cardiovascular diseases [41], and it may contribute to a healthier insulin profile in adults [42].

Some studies have suggested that dairy intake and its contribution to calcium intake could have a protective effect on the development of type 2 diabetes, as an inverse association with the incidence of insulin resistance, independently of age and family history of diabetes, was shown [43,44]. A recent review suggests a neutral effect of dairy intake on adiposity during early and middle childhood and a modestly protective effect in adolescence [45]. Dairy intake also contributes to dietary fat consumption; however, there is recent evidence showing the positive health effects of dairy fat [41,46]. There is only one recent cross-sectional study showing that a frequent consumption of yogurt was associated with a better healthy eating index in US children [47]. However, information on the association between dairy consumption and diet quality in children is scarce; for this reason, we are providing further evidence showing that those children consuming higher amounts of dairy products (specifically yogurt and milk) had also higher values of diet quality index and that this association is maintained after two years.

During the last years, an obesogenic environment has been developed [48], leading to an increase of unhealthy eating habits [49], among other lifestyle behaviors components. For instance, a recent review also found an association between watching TV during meals and a high consumption of energy-dense high-fat, high-sugar foods such as savory snacks in children [50]. Therefore, our results show an agreement with available guidelines suggesting a benefit in the replacement of energy-dense foods by dairy products at snack time in terms of diet quality [28].

The present study is subject to a number of limitations. For instance, the fact that the number of participants on each survey decreased progressively may affect our results as, normally, those who are healthier and with higher social position are less likely to drop out. However, in our cohorts, drop-outs showed to slightly distort the distribution of children's BMI for those above the 99% percentile, affecting marginally exposure-outcome associations [14]. Besides, food consumption was obtained using only a single 24-HDR. Although the use of multiple 24-HDRs may have provided more reliable data, this method is still considered as a valid tool for the estimation of population means, as random errors cancel out on a group level [51]. The diet quality index was obtained from the combination of FFQ and 24-HDR, as it was previously done by other authors [20,21]. In addition, the DQI, based on the FFQ, was previously shown to be a good approach when compared with a 3 days record in Flemish pre-schoolers [21]. Moreover, the sample size was reduced for the prospective analysis, although a considerable sample size was achieved. Regarding the moment of consumption and specifically snacking, our study included any food or beverage intake outside of the usual main meals (breakfast, lunch, and dinner) without the possibility to discriminate structured snacks from nibbling behavior.

The standardized dietary assessment and linkage to country-specific food composition tables using validated 24-HDR software as well as the cooperation with schools, which enabled the assessment of school meal information, are the main strengths of this study. The assessment period covered almost an entire year, taking into account seasonal variations in the diet. Moreover, the large sample size comprises data from eight European countries; the strictly standardized data assessment, documentation, and data cleaning processing guarantee the highest possible data quality.

In conclusion, higher consumption of milk, yogurt, and cheese at snack meal occasions throughout childhood is related to a higher diet quality. Inclusion of dairy products outside the main meals could be a good strategy to decrease the consumption of energy-dense foods in children and adolescents.

Author Contributions: Conceptualization—I.I., P.D.M.-E. and L.A.M.; Formal analysis, T.I.; Methodology, V.P., A.H. and M.W.; Supervision—P.R. (Paola Russo), T.V., S.P., P.N., G.E., P.R. (Patrizia Rise), S.D.H. and L.A.M.; Writing—original draft, I.I., P.D.M.-E. and L.A.M.; Writing–review & editing—I.I., P.D.M.-E. and L.A.M. All authors have read and agreed to the published version of the manuscript.

Acknowledgments: We thank all members of the study teams and particularly the children and their parents for their participation in the study. The information in this document reflects the authors' view and is provided as it.

Abbreviations

BMI	body mass index
CVD	cardiovascular diseases
CEHQ	Children's Eating Habits Questionnaire
CINDI	Countrywide Integrated Non-communicable Disease Intervention program
DQI	dietary quality index; FBDG: food-based dietary guidelines
FCT	food composition tables
FFQ	food frequency questionnaire
HDR	hours dietary recall
HELENA-DIAT	HELENA-DIetary Assessment Tool
HELENA	Healthy Lifestyle in Europe by Nutrition in Adolescence
IDEFICS	Identification and prevention of Dietary- and lifestyle induced health EFfects In Children and infantS
ISCED	International Standard Classification of Education
SACANA	Self-Administered Children, Adolescents, and Adult Nutrition Assessment
SACINA	Self-Administered Children and Infant Nutrition Assessment
SPSS	Statistical Package for Social Sciences
TEI	total energy intake
UK	United Kingdom

Appendix A

Table A1. Categorization of the food groups among 'preferable consumption', 'intermediate consumption', or 'low consumtion' groups *n* [10].

Preferable	IDEFICS (T0/T1): Water, wholemeal bread, wholemeal cereals, unsweetened breakfast cereals, raw vegetables, fresh fruit, cooked meat, eggs, fresh fish, plain yogurt I.Family (T3) additionally: replacement foods (e.g., tofu), poultry boiled, canned fish, vegetable oils
Intermediate	IDEFICS (T0/T1): light soft drinks, fruit juices, milk, white bread, cereals (pasta and rice ...), sweetened breakfast cereals, cooked vegetables, sweetened fruit, nuts, ketchup, fried meat, cold cults, fried eggs, fried fish, sweetened yogurt, cheese, butter and margarine I.Family (T3) additioanlly: coffee and tea, dried fruits
Low	IDEFICS (T0/T1): Soft drinks, chocolates, salty snacks, ice-creams, biscuits, candies, chocolate/nut-based spread, fried potatoes, mayonnaise I.Family (T3) additionally: poultry fried

References

1. Howarth, N.C.; Huang, T.T.; Roberts, S.B.; Lin, B.H.; McCrory, M.A. Eating patterns and dietary composition in relation to BMI in younger and older adults. *Int. J. Obes.* **2007**, *31*, 675–684. [CrossRef] [PubMed]
2. Kirk, R.R. 2nd plenary session of 'body weight balance and regulation'. Role of dietary carbohydrate and frequent eating in body-weight control. *Proc. Nutr. Soc.* **2000**, *59*, 349–358. [CrossRef] [PubMed]
3. Agostoni, C.; Braegger, C.; Decsi, T.; Kolacek, S.; Koletzko, B.; Mihatsch, W.; Moreno, L.A.; Puntis, J.; Shamir, R.; Szajewska, H.; et al. Role of dietary factors and food habits in the development of childhood obesity: A commentary by the ESPGHAN Committee on Nutrition. *J. Pediatr. Gastroenterol. Nutr.* **2011**, *52*, 662–669. [CrossRef] [PubMed]
4. *EUropean Food Information Council (EUFIC) (2007) Is Eating between Meals Good for Our Health?* EUFIC: Brussels, Belgium, 2007.
5. van den Heuvel, E.G.H.M.; Steijns, J.M.J.M. Dairy products and bone health: how strong is the 444 scientific evidence? *Nutr. Res. Rev.* **2018**, *31*, 164–178. [CrossRef]
6. Moreno, L.A.; Bel-Serrat, S.; Santaliestra-Pasias, A.; Bueno, G. Dairy products, yogurt consumption, and cardiometabolic risk in children and adolescents. *Nutr. Rev.* **2015**, *73*, 8–14. [CrossRef]

7. Spence, L.A.; Cifelli, C.J.; Miller, G.D. The Role of Dairy Products in Healthy Weight and Body Composition in Children and Adolescents. *Curr. Nutr. Food Sci.* **2011**, *7*, 40–49. [CrossRef]
8. Ambrosini, G.L.; Emmett, P.M.; Northstone, K.; Jebb, S.A. Tracking a dietary pattern associated with increased adiposity in childhood and adolescence. *Obesity* **2014**, *22*, 458–465. [CrossRef]
9. Marshall, S.; Burrows, T.; Collins, C.E. Systematic review of diet quality indices and their associations with health-related outcomes in children and adolescents. *J. Hum. Nutr. Diet.* **2014**, *27*, 577–598. [CrossRef]
10. Vyncke, K.; Cruz Fernandez, E.; Fajo-Pascual, M.; Cuenca-Garcia, M.; De Keyzer, W.; Gonzalez-Gross, M.; Moreno, L.A.; Beghin, L.; Breidenassel, C.; Kersting, M.; et al. Validation of the Diet Quality Index for Adolescents by comparison with biomarkers, nutrient and food intakes: The HELENA study. *Br. J. Nutr.* **2012**, *109*, 2067–2078. [CrossRef]
11. Ahrens, W.; Bammann, K.; de Henauw, S.; Halford, J.; Palou, A.; Pigeot, I.; Siani, A.; Sjostrom, M. Understanding and preventing childhood obesity and related disorders–IDEFICS: A European multilevel epidemiological approach. *Nutr. Metab. Cardiovasc. Dis.* **2006**, *16*, 302–308. [CrossRef]
12. Ahrens, W.; Bammann, K.; Siani, A.; Buchecker, K.; De Henauw, S.; Iacoviello, L.; Hebestreit, A.; Krogh, V.; Lissner, L.; Marild, S.; et al. The IDEFICS cohort: design, characteristics and participation in the baseline survey. *Int. J. Obes* **2011**, *35*, S3–S15. [CrossRef] [PubMed]
13. Ahrens, W.; Siani, A.; Adan, R.; De Henauw, S.; Eiben, G.; Gwozdz, W.; Hebestreit, A.; Hunsberger, M.; Kaprio, J.; Krogh, V.; et al. Cohort Profile: The transition from childhood to adolescence in European children-how I.Family extends the IDEFICS cohort. *Int. J. Epidemiol.* **2016**. [CrossRef] [PubMed]
14. Langeheine, M.; Pohlabeln, H.; Lauria, F.; Veidebaum, T.; Tornaritis, M.; Molnar, D.; Eiben, G.; de Henauw, S.; Moreno, L.A.; Williams, G.; et al. Attrition in the European Child Cohort IDEFICS/I.Family: Exploring Associations Between Attrition and Body Mass Index. *Front Pediatr.* **2018**, *6*, 212. [CrossRef] [PubMed]
15. Vereecken, C.A.; Covents, M.; Sichert-Hellert, W.; Alvira, J.M.; Le Donne, C.; De Henauw, S.; De Vriendt, T.; Phillipp, M.K.; Beghin, L.; Manios, Y.; et al. Development and evaluation of a self-administered computerized 24-h dietary recall method for adolescents in Europe. *Int. J. Obes.* **2008**, *32*, S26–S34. [CrossRef] [PubMed]
16. Hebestreit, A.; Bornhorst, C.; Pala, V.; Barba, G.; Eiben, G.; Veidebaum, T.; Hadjigergiou, C.; Molnar, D.; Claessens, M.; Fernandez-Alvira, J.M.; et al. Dietary energy density in young children across Europe. *Int. J. Obes.* **2014**, *38*, S124–S134. [CrossRef] [PubMed]
17. Hebestreit, A.; Barba, G.; De Henauw, S.; Eiben, G.; Hadjigeorgiou, C.; Kovacs, E.; Krogh, V.; Moreno, L.A.; Pala, V.; Veidebaum, T.; et al. Cross-sectional and longitudinal associations between energy intake and BMI z-score in European children. *Int. J. Behav. Nutr. Phys. Act.* **2016**, *13*, 23. [CrossRef]
18. McCance, W. *The Composition of Foods*, 6th ed.; The Royal Society of Chemistry and the Food Standards Agency: London, UK, 2002.
19. Bel-Serrat, S.; Mouratidou, T.; Pala, V.; Huybrechts, I.; Bornhorst, C.; Fernandez-Alvira, J.M.; Hadjigeorgiou, C.; Eiben, G.; Hebestreit, A.; Lissner, L.; et al. Relative validity of the Children's Eating Habits Questionnaire-food frequency section among young European children: The IDEFICS Study. *Public Health Nutr.* **2013**, *17*, 266–276. [CrossRef]
20. Lanfer, A.; Hebestreit, A.; Ahrens, W.; Krogh, V.; Sieri, S.; Lissner, L.; Eiben, G.; Siani, A.; Huybrechts, I.; Loit, H.M.; et al. Reproducibility of food consumption frequencies derived from the Children's Eating Habits Questionnaire used in the IDEFICS study. *Int. J. Obes.* **2011**, *35*, S61–S68. [CrossRef]
21. Huybrechts, I.; Vereecken, C.; De Bacquer, D.; Vandevijvere, S.; Van Oyen, H.; Maes, L.; Vanhauwaert, E.; Temme, L.; De Backer, G.; De Henauw, S. Reproducibility and validity of a diet quality index for children assessed using a FFQ. *Br. J. Nutr.* **2010**, *104*, 135–144. [CrossRef]
22. Koster-Rasmussen, R.; Siersma, V.; Halldorsson, T.I.; de Fine Olivarius, N.; Henriksen, J.E.; Heitmann, B.L. Missing portion sizes in FFQ–alternatives to use of standard portions. *Public Health Nutr.* **2014**, *18*, 1914–1921. [CrossRef]
23. Marcinkevage, J.; Mayen, A.L.; Zuleta, C.; DiGirolamo, A.M.; Stein, A.D.; Ramirez-Zea, M. Relative Validity of Three Food Frequency Questionnaires for Assessing Dietary Intakes of Guatemalan Schoolchildren. *PLoS ONE* **2015**, *10*, e0139125. [CrossRef] [PubMed]
24. Belgian Health Council. *De actieve voedingsdriehoekeen praktische voedingsen beweeggids (Nutritional Recommendations for Belgium. Revised version 2012)*; Belgian Health Council: Brussels, Belgium, 2012.

25. Cole, T.J.; Freeman, J.V.; Preece, M.A. British 1990 growth reference centiles for weight, height, body mass index and head circumference fitted by maximum penalized likelihood. *Stat. Med.* **1998**, *17*, 407–429. [CrossRef]
26. UNESCO Institute for Statistics. *International Standard Classification of Education ISCED 2011*; UNESCO: Montreal, QC, CA, 2012; ISBN 978-92-9189-123-8.
27. De Henauw, S.; Baranowski, T.; Pigeot, I. Special Issue: Prevention of childhood obesity: Results from the IDEFICS study. *Obes. Rev.* **2015**, *16*, 1–174.
28. EUFIC. The European Food Information Council.10 Healthy Lifestyle Tips for Adults. Last Revision: 7 June 2017 [14 June 2017]. Available online: http://www.eufic.org/en/healthy-living/article/10-healthy-lifestyle-tips-for-adults (accessed on 4 February 2020).
29. Leech, R.M.; Worsley, A.; Timperio, A.; McNaughton, S.A. Characterizing eating patterns: A comparison of eating occasion definitions. *Am. J. Clin. Nutr.* **2015**, *102*, 1229–1237. [CrossRef]
30. Bellisle, F. Meals and snacking, diet quality and energy balance. *Physiol. Behav.* **2014**, *134*, 38–43. [CrossRef]
31. Nicklas, T.A.; Yang, S.J.; Baranowski, T.; Zakeri, I.; Berenson, G. Eating patterns and obesity in children. The Bogalusa Heart Study. *Am. J. Prev. Med.* **2003**, *25*, 9–16. [CrossRef]
32. Julián, C.; Santaliestra-Pasías, A.; Miguel-Berges, M.; Moreno, L. Frequency and quality of mid-afternoon snack among Spanish children. *Nutr. Hosp.* **2017**, *34*, 827–833. [CrossRef]
33. Kelder, S.H.; Perry, C.L.; Klepp, K.I.; Lytle, L.L. Longitudinal tracking of adolescent smoking, physical activity, and food choice behaviors. *Am. J. Public Health* **1994**, *84*, 1121–1126. [CrossRef]
34. Verloigne, M.; Van Lippevelde, W.; Maes, L.; Brug, J.; De Bourdeaudhuij, I. Family- and school-based correlates of energy balance-related behaviours in 10-12-year-old children: A systematic review within the ENERGY (EuropeaN Energy balance Research to prevent excessive weight Gain among Youth) project. *Public Health Nutr.* **2012**, *15*, 1380–1395. [CrossRef]
35. Rosell, M.; Hakansson, N.N.; Wolk, A. Association between dairy food consumption and weight change over 9 y in 19,352 perimenopausal women. *Am. J. Clin. Nutr.* **2006**, *84*, 1481–1488. [CrossRef]
36. Wang, H.; Troy, L.M.; Rogers, G.T.; Fox, C.S.; McKeown, N.M.; Meigs, J.B.; Jacques, P.F. Longitudinal association between dairy consumption and changes of body weight and waist circumference: The Framingham Heart Study. *Int. J. Obes.* **2014**, *38*, 299–305. [CrossRef] [PubMed]
37. Mozaffarian, D.; Hao, T.; Rimm, E.B.; Willett, W.C.; Hu, F.B. Changes in diet and lifestyle and long-term weight gain in women and men. *N. Engl. J. Med.* **2011**, *364*, 2392–2404. [CrossRef] [PubMed]
38. Martinez-Gonzalez, M.A.; Sayon-Orea, C.; Ruiz-Canela, M.; de la Fuente, C., Gea, A.; Bes-Rastrollo, M. Yogurt consumption, weight change and risk of overweight/obesity: The SUN cohort study. *Nutr. Metab. Cardiovasc. Dis.* **2014**, *24*, 1189–1196. [CrossRef] [PubMed]
39. Santaliestra-Pasias, A.M.; González-Gil, E.M.; Pala, V.; Intemann, T.; Hebestreit, A.; Russo, P.; Van Aart, C.; Galli, C.; Veidebaum, T.; Molnar, D.; et al. Prospective associations between lifestyle behaviors and dairy consumption: The IDEFICS study. *Nutr. Metab. Cardiovasc. Dis.* **2020**, *30*, 514–522. [CrossRef] [PubMed]
40. Panahi, S.; Fernandez, M.A.; Marette, A.; Tremblay, A. Yogurt, diet quality and lifestyle factors. *Eur. J. Clin. Nutr.* **2016**, *71*, 573–579. [CrossRef]
41. Astrup, A. Yogurt and dairy product consumption to prevent cardiometabolic diseases: Epidemiologic and experimental studies. *Am. J. Clin. Nutr.* **2014**, *99*, 1235S–1242S. [CrossRef]
42. Wang, H.; Livingston, K.A.; Fox, C.S.; Meigs, J.B.; Jacques, P.F. Yogurt consumption is associated with better diet quality and metabolic profile in American men and women. *Nutr. Res.* **2013**, *33*, 18–26. [CrossRef]
43. Rosell, M.; Johansson, G.; Berglund, L.; Vessby, B.; de Faire, U.; Hellenius, M.L. Associations between the intake of dairy fat and calcium and abdominal obesity. *Int. J. Obes. Relat. Metab. Disord.* **2004**, *28*, 1427–1434. [CrossRef]
44. Yerlikaya, O.; Acu, M.; Kinik, O. Importance of dairy products in cardiovascular diseases and type 2 diabetes. *Crit. Rev. Food Sci. Nutr.* **2013**, *53*, 902–908. [CrossRef]
45. Dror, D.K. Dairy consumption and pre-school, school-age and adolescent obesity in developed countries: A systematic review and meta-analysis. *Obes. Rev.* **2014**, *15*, 516–527. [CrossRef]
46. Kratz, M.; Baars, T.; Guyenet, S. The relationship between high-fat dairy consumption and obesity, cardiovascular, and metabolic disease. *Eur. J. Nutr.* **2013**, *52*, 1–24. [CrossRef] [PubMed]
47. Zhu, Y.; Wang, H.; Hollis, J.H.; Jacques, P.F. The associations between yogurt consumption, diet quality, and metabolic profiles in children in the USA. *Eur. J. Nutr.* **2015**, *54*, 543–550. [CrossRef] [PubMed]

48. Popkin, B.M. Technology, transport, globalization and the nutrition transition food policy. *Food Policy* **2006**, *31*, 554–569. [CrossRef]
49. Popkin, B.M. Global nutrition dynamics: The world is shifting rapidly toward a diet linked with noncommunicable diseases. *Am. J. Clin. Nutr.* **2006**, *84*, 289–298. [CrossRef]
50. Avery, A.; Anderson, C.; McCullough, F. Associations between children's diet quality and watching television during meal or snack consumption: A systematic review. *Matern. Child Nutr.* **2017**. [CrossRef]
51. Rutishauser, I.H. Dietary intake measurements. *Public Health Nutr.* **2005**, *8*, 1100–1107. [CrossRef]

4

Colostrum and Mature Human Milk of Women from London, Moscow, and Verona: Determinants of Immune Composition

Daniel Munblit [1,2,3,*], Marina Treneva [2,4], Diego G. Peroni [2,5], Silvia Colicino [6], LiYan Chow [1], Shobana Dissanayeke [7], Priya Abrol [1], Shreya Sheth [1], Alexander Pampura [2,4], Attilio L. Boner [8], Donna T. Geddes [2,9], Robert J. Boyle [1,2,†] and John O. Warner [1,2,†]

1 Department of Paediatrics, Imperial College London, London W2 1NY, UK; lychow8@gmail.com (L.C.); p.abrol@doctors.org.uk (P.A.); shreya.sheth10@imperial.ac.uk (S.S.); r.boyle@nhs.net (R.J.B.); j.o.warner@imperial.ac.uk (J.O.W.)

2 International Inflammation (in-FLAME) Network of the World Universities Network, Sydney 2006, NSW, Australia; trenevamarina@mail.ru (M.T.); diego.peroni@unipi.it (D.G.P.); apampura1@mail.ru (A.P.); donna.geddes@uwa.edu.au (D.T.G.)

3 Faculty of Pediatrics, I. M. Sechenov First Moscow State Medical University, Moscow 119991, Russia

4 Allergy Department, Veltischev Clinical Pediatric Research Institute of Pirogov Russian National Research Medical University, Moscow 125412, Russia

5 Department of Clinical and Experimental Medicine, Section of Paediatrics, University of Pisa, 56126 Pisa, Italy

6 National Heart and Lung Institute, Imperial College London, London SW3 6NP, UK; s.colicino@imperial.ac.uk

7 Royal Holloway University of London School of Biological Sciences, Biomedical Sciences, London TW20 0EX, UK; shobanadis@hotmail.com

8 Department of Life and Reproduction Sciences, Section of Paediatrics, University of Verona, 37124 Verona, Italy; attilio.boner@univr.it

9 School of Chemistry and Biochemistry, The University of Western Australia, Perth 6009, WA, Australia

* Correspondence: daniel.munblit08@imperial.ac.uk

† These authors contributed equally to this work.

Abstract: Cytokines and growth factors in colostrum and mature milk may play an important role in infant immune maturation, and may vary significantly between populations. We aimed to examine associations between environmental and maternal factors, and human milk (HM) cytokine and growth factor levels. We recruited 398 pregnant/lactating women in the United Kingdom, Russia, and Italy. Participants underwent skin prick testing, questionnaire interview, and colostrum and mature milk sampling. HM cytokine and growth factor levels were quantified by electro-chemiluminescence. We found significant geographical variation in growth factor levels, but no evidence of variation between sites in cytokine detectability. There was an inverse correlation between time of milk sampling and growth factor levels in colostrum for Hepatocyte Growth Factor (HGF) and TGFβ1 and TGFβ3, but not TGFβ2, and levels were significantly higher in colostrum than mature milk for all growth factors. The kinetics of decline were different for each growth factor. Cytokines were present at much lower levels than growth factors, and the decline over time was less consistent. HM growth factors and cytokine levels vary between populations for unknown reasons. Levels of HM mediators decline at different rates postpartum, and these findings suggest specific biological roles for HM growth factors and cytokines in early postnatal development.

Keywords: colostrum; human milk; immune modulators; immunologically active molecules; cytokines; growth factors; environmental influence

1. Introduction

Human milk (HM) is usually the first source of nutrition for a newborn, and an important factor assisting infants in the first months of life, not only as a nutrition source but also as a manner of adapting infants to their extra-uterine environment. Breastfeeding is known to have positive short- and long-term effects on child health, although its influence on allergy development is still debatable [1]. There have been few attempts to investigate relationships between maternal and environmental factors and immune active profiles of HM. Data from a variety of studies suggest that factors such as country of maternal origin, diet, exercise, and exposure to smoke or farming environment in early life may influence colostrum and HM constituents [2–22].

It has been shown that Hepatocyte Growth Factor (HGF) is known to regulate vascular endothelial growth factor (VEGF) production from endothelial cells [23] and complements VEGF biological activity in the infant gut [24]. HGF levels in maternal serum change throughout pregnancy, peaking at 30 to 40 weeks of gestation and then decreasing upon delivery [25]. As levels of HGF are 20 to 30 times higher in colostrum than in maternal serum [26] it is reasonable to propose that HGF is actively excreted into HM in order to support infant's gut immunity maturation and growth.

Inverse relationships between the risk of atopic diseases, associated with T-helper lymphocyte type 2 (TH2) immune response, and indicators of early-life exposure to infections, such as high birth order or sibship size, early attendance at day care, and early exposure to pets or other animals are well described [27]. The "hygiene hypothesis" remains one of the most popular current hypotheses on early-life exposures and allergy risk [28]. It has been suggested that farming environment [6], higher bacterial exposure [7], or maternal country of origin [5] may have significant impacts on HM immune composition, and such effects on HM composition may be an important pathway through which early variations in microbial exposures influence risk of allergy development.

Our study aimed to prospectively investigate the relationship between maternal and environmental factors and levels of HGF, Transforming Growth Factor beta (TGFβ)1,2,3 and detectability of TH1 and TH2 cytokines using colostrum and HM samples collected from birth cohorts in three regions; the UK, eastern Europe, and continental Europe.

2. Materials and Methods

2.1. Study Setting, Eligibility Criteria, and Ethics

The investigations and sample collection have been conducted following ethical approval by Ethics committee in three countries participating in the study: West London Rec 3 (UK) (Ref. number 10/H0706/32) and all paperwork has been completed according to the hospital R&D Joint Research Office (UK) (JROSM0072) policy; Ethical Committee of the Azienda Ospedaliera di Verona (Italy) (approval No. 1288), and Moscow Institute of Paediatrics and Child Health of Ministry of Health of Russian Federation (Russia) (approval No. 1-MS/11). All women provided written informed consent.

Women were enrolled at antenatal and postnatal units of three participating centres—St. Mary's Hospital, London, UK; Maternity Hospital No. 1, Moscow, Russia; G.B. Rossi Hospital, Verona, Italy. Inclusion criteria for the study were: healthy term infants and their mothers intending to breastfeed and willing to comply with the study procedures.

Exclusion criteria were: maternal immunosuppressive treatment during lactation, or severe illness; infants with a major birth defect, admitted to neonatal intensive care, other severe illness, born prematurely (<37 weeks gestation), or with low birth weight (<2nd centile).

2.2. Medical Records and Interview

Following enrolment, participants underwent allergy skin prick testing (SPT) and answered a 10 min interview-based questionnaire regarding their medical history. Exposure variables recorded were selected based on a detailed review of known determinants of HM composition [29].

Information collected from the recruited women included parity; age; mode of delivery; details of residence environment, such as mould presence at home, regular contact with animals and/or pets at home; exposure to tobacco smoke (smoker or living in household with smoker or self-reported passive smoker); any reports of infections during pregnancy. We also obtained information on maternal dietary preferences—fish, fresh fruit, and probiotic intake. Participant medical records were reviewed by study personnel to extract relevant health information which was not available from questionnaires, prior to breast milk analysis. SPT was undertaken using the following solutions: Histamine 1% Positive Control, Glycerol Negative Control, House Dust Mite (*Dermatophagoides pteronyssinus*), Cat (*Felix domesticus*), Grass Pollen, Birch pollen, Peanut, Hazelnut, Egg (all from Stallergenes, SA 92160 Anthony, France), and Cow's milk (ALK-Abello, Hørsholm, Denmark). SPT was performed by standard technique using 1 mm lancets (ALK-Abello, Hórsholm, Denmark), and were read at 15 min. Allergic sensitization was defined as a wheal $\geq$3 mm to at least one allergen, in the context of a wheal $\geq$3 mm to histamine and no wheal to the negative control.

2.3. *Human Milk Sampling*

Participants were given sterile tubes to collect their own colostrum (once in the first 6 days of life) and mature HM (once at 4–6 weeks postpartum). Local site investigators and participating mothers were asked to collect colostrum or milk at the first morning breastfeed, by manual expression (colostrum) or collecting the drip (mature milk) from the contra-lateral breast during feeding [15]. Colostrum samples were frozen at −50 °C to −80 °C within 12 h of collection. HM samples were collected at home, stored in the fridge for not longer than 4 h, and transported to participating units by study staff, and frozen at 50 °C to −80 °C within 12 h of collection. It has been previously demonstrated that storage for 6 months at either −20 °C or −80 °C did not influence the concentration of immune active factors in human milk [30]. After thawing, samples were centrifuged at 1500× *g* for 15 min at 4 °C. The lipid layer was removed with a pipette and aqueous fraction was analysed for immune modulators [31]. All milk samples were transported to London at −70 °C where the samples were stored at −80 °C until analysis.

2.4. *Electro-Chemiluminescence*

We used electro-chemiluminescence to measure immune mediators in colostrum and breast milk samples for Th1 and Th2 cytokines, HGF, and TGFβ1-3 (MesoScale Discovery, Rockville, MD, USA). Laboratory experiments were run according to manufacturer's protocol, using an eight-point standard curve. No dilution was used for Th1 and Th2 cytokines and HGF, and 1:2 dilution for TGFβ assays, following pilot experiments which showed that TGFβ2 levels in undiluted milk samples were often greater than the upper limit of detection. Assays were run in duplicate, and mediator levels were excluded where the CV was >25%—Median (IQR) levels and assay detection limits for each immune mediator studied are shown in Table A1.

2.5. *Protein Analysis*

We used turbidimetry to assess total protein concentration in colostrum samples (Abbott Architect Analyser C8000, Abbott, Abbott Park, IL, USA). For turbidimetry colostrum, proteins were denatured by benzethonium chloride, then measured at 404 nm. Pilot experiments determined that a 1:30 onboard dilution was needed to bring the colostrum protein concentration to within the linear measurement range of the Architect Analyser (3–60 g/L). Prior to protein analysis samples were thawed and centrifuged at 3000× *g* for 15 min at 4 °C. Next, 300 μL of supernatant were carefully transferred to the tubes and loaded into the Architect device for the analysis.

2.6. *Statistical Analysis*

Maternal factors and levels/detection of cytokines and growth factors were summarized using standard descriptive statistics. As outcome variables were not normally distributed, non-parametric tests such as the Mann–Whitney *U*-test, were used to compare independent observations of different populations for unadjusted analyses. All growth factors have been presented as a continuous variable (pg/mL), whilst data on cytokines were transformed into a binary variable (detectable versus undetectable). Since concentration of growth factors and cytokines were assayed twice (in both colostrum and breast milk) for many participants, we used a mixed-effect regression model to account for the absence of independence between those two measures and to evaluate a broad range of variables. Continuous data with non-parametric distribution were log-transformed for inclusion in regression models.

Model selection was based on major approaches such as Akaike and Bayesian information criteria. Difference between groups effects (maternal and environmental factors) as well as within subject effects were evaluated using multilevel mixed-effect regression model. Factors and covariates included in the models were: parity, maternal sensitisation, maternal age, site of collection, mode of delivery—vaginal birth/caesarean section, mould presence at home, pets at home or regular contact; exposure to tobacco smoke (i.e., maternal active smoking or living in household with smoker or self-reported passive smoker) at recruitment; at least one self-reported maternal infection during pregnancy; maternal diet—fish intake at least once per week versus less often; daily fresh fruit versus less often; daily probiotic versus none/less often.

As models were used for the statistical analysis, the sample size reduced slightly, due to incomplete data for one or more variables included in the multivariate model in 56 individuals. This explains discrepancy in colostrum numbers. Reduced numbers were included in analysis of human milk samples, due to missing samples. Milk samples were missing due to cessation of breastfeeding before this time, due to mother's not supplying a sample within the four to six week time window for sampling, and due to loss to follow up/not contactable women.

Outcomes assessed were levels of HGF, TGFβ1, TGFβ2, TGFβ3, and cytokine detectability. Relationship between corrected growth factor levels and time (measured as HGF/Protein, TGFβ1/Protein, TGFβ2/Protein, and TGFβ3/Protein in pg/g) was assessed using the Spearman rank correlation coefficient. Results were considered significant when p-values were reported at a level less than 0.05. Bonferroni correction was used in mixed models analyses to control for false discovery.

3. Results

3.1. Study Population

Total of 481 mothers were recruited into the study from June 2011 to March 2012 from the birth centres and antenatal and postnatal units of secondary and tertiary hospitals from three countries, located in Northern Europe, Eastern Europe, and the Mediterranean area. Of 481 women, 398 (UK $n = 101$, Russia $n = 221$, Italy $n = 76$) provided samples and were included in this study. The 83 mothers unwilling or unable to provide colostrum samples postnatally were not evaluated further.

Demographic data of the participants is presented in Table 1. Significant differences between groups were seen for most variables recorded. Maternal age (highest in Italy), maternal allergic sensitization (highest in UK), rate of Caesarean section (highest in UK), tobacco smoke exposure (highest in Russia), antenatal infections (highest in Italy), and time of colostrum collection (earlier in Russia than other sites) all differed significantly. There was also weak evidence for differences in parity and birth weight across centres). Infant sex did not significantly differ across sites.

3.2. Association between Collection Time and Colostrum/Breast Milk Composition

Among the environmental and maternal factors analysed we found time of milk sample collection postpartum to have the most significant influence on growth factor levels, and a mixed effect on cytokine detectability. A significant decline over time in colostrum was seen for HGF, TGFβ1 and TGFβ3, IL2, IL5, IL10, and IFNγ. No significant influence but similar trends were seen for most of the other mediators (Table 2 and Figure 1). Differences between colostrum and mature milk showed similar findings for growth factors, which were all statistically significant. For cytokine detectability in breast milk versus colostrum, findings were mixed and not entirely consistent with the changes seen over time in colostrum. IL10 was more commonly detected in colostrum than in HM, but IL4 and IFNγ were more commonly detected in HM, despite no change or a decline in detectability over time in colostrum samples. Other cytokines showed no significant difference between colostrum and HM (Table 2).

Table 1. Characteristics of study participants.

	UK	Russia	Italy	*p*-Value (Three Countries)
Maternal allergic sensitisation *	35/94 (37)	22/156 (14)	9/40 (23)	<0.01 [a]
Maternal Age (years)	32.8 (4.78)	29.8 (4.45)	37.4 (5.38)	<0.01 [b]
Vaginal Delivery	70/101 (69)	188/219 (86)	62/76 (82)	<0.01 [a]
Male sex	54/101 (53)	118/216 (55)	41/76 (54)	0.98 [a]
Birth Weight (grams)	3527 (535.37)	3526 (438.97)	3328 (476.95)	0.05 [b]
Primiparous women	55/100 (55)	93/216 (43)	29/75 (39)	0.06 [a]
Household tobacco smoke exposure	30/99 (30)	135/218 (62)	25/76 (33)	<0.01 [a]
Antenatal Infections †	16/100 (16)	61/211 (29)	29/76 (38)	<0.01 [a]
Time of colostrum collection (hours)	58.61 (33.2)	50.03 (14.34)	57.84 (26.52)	<0.01 [b]

[a] Pearson χ^2 test has been used; [b] ANOVA test has been used. Data shown are (*n*/(%)) for binary variables, and (mean (S.D.)) for continuous variables; * Defined as skin prick test wheal ≥3 mm to at least one of a panel of common allergens; † Antenatal infection is defined as at least one self-reported maternal infection during pregnancy.

Table 2. Relationship between time of sample collection and milk composition.

Immune Modulator	Colostrum Composition			Paired Differences between HM and Colostrum of Colostrum and Breast Milk Composition		
	Change over Time	β	*p*-Value	Difference between Colostrum and HM over Time	β	*p*-Value
HGF	Lower	−0.01	<0.001 **	Higher in colostrum	−1.35	<0.001 **
TGFβ1	Lower	−0.003	0.01 *	Higher in colostrum	−0.93	<0.001 **
TGFβ2	No change	−0.003	0.12	Higher in colostrum	−1.12	<0.001 **
TGFβ3	Lower	−0.01	<0.001 **	Higher in colostrum	−2.03	<0.001 **
IL2	Lower	−0.02	0.02 *	No difference	0.32	0.30
IL4	No change	−0.01	0.22	Higher in HM	0.72	0.04 *
IL5	Lower	−0.03	<0.001 **	No difference	−0.54	0.09
IL10	Lower	−0.02	<0.001 **	Higher in colostrum	−1.66	<0.001 **
IFNγ	Lower	−0.01	0.04 *	Higher in HM	1.20	<0.001 **
IL12	No change	−0.01	0.12	No difference	−0.11	0.73
IL13	No change	−0.01	0.09	No difference	0.09	0.72

Data shown are concentration (pg/mL) for growth factors, and detectable versus not detectable for cytokines. A multilevel mixed-effect regression model was used for all analyses, which were adjusted to the following factors: Parity, Maternal Atopy, Maternal age, Site of collection, Mode of delivery, Mould presence at home, Pets at home or regular contact; Exposure to tobacco smoke; At least one self-reported maternal infection during pregnancy; Maternal diet. HM, human milk; HGF, Hepatocyte Growth Factor. * p value < 0.05; ** p value < 0.01.

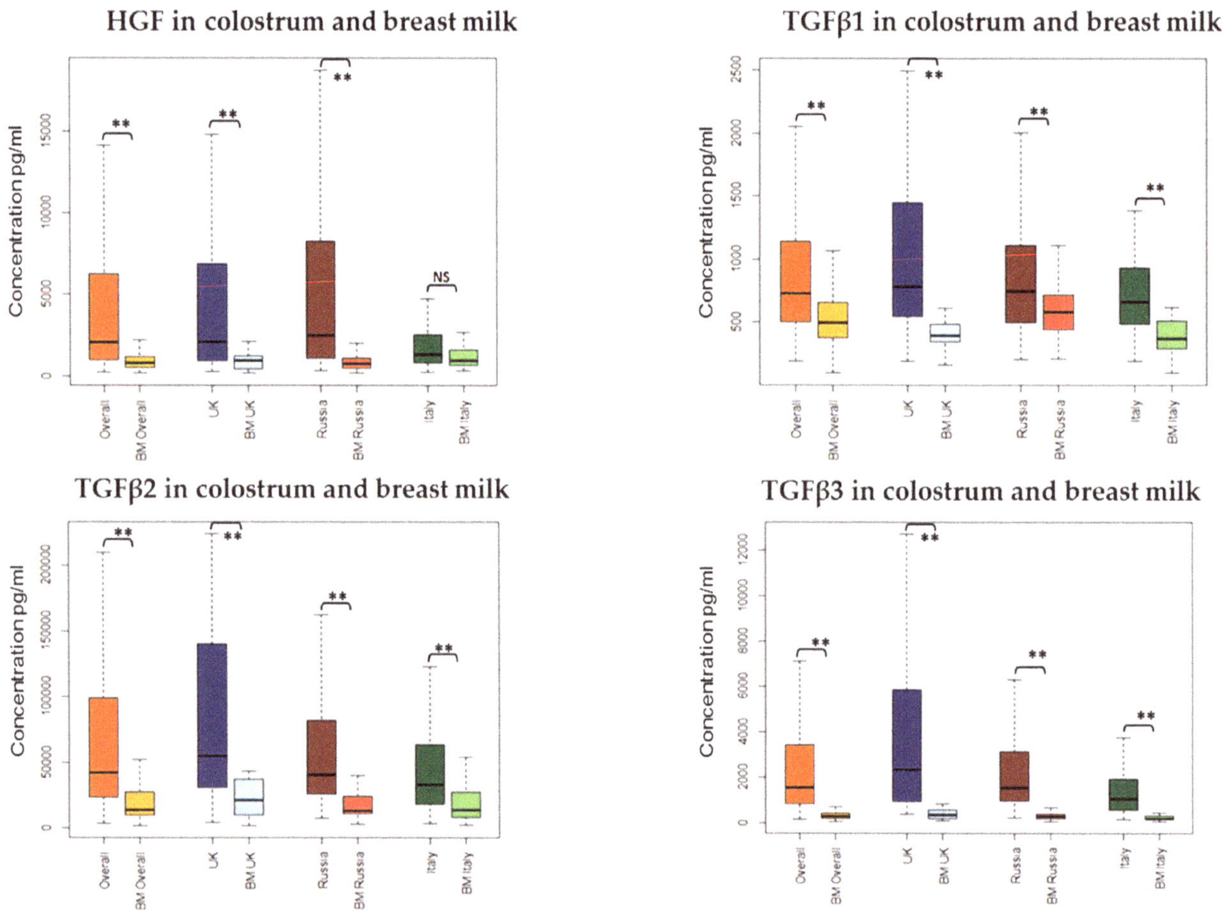

Figure 1. Unadjusted growth factors concentration (pg/mL) in colostrum and breast milk across all sites (overall) and at each site of collection (London, Moscow, and Verona). ** p value < 0.01.

3.3. Association between Collection Site and Colostrum/Breast Milk Composition

3.3.1. Growth Factors

We found a significant influence of country of residence on some growth factor concentrations (Table 3 and Figure 2). TGFβ2 and TGFβ3 showed consistent findings in colostrum and HM samples—levels of both factors were higher in UK and lower in Italy, with intermediate levels in Russian women. HGF was lowest in the colostrum, but not HM, of mothers in Italy (mean log HGF 7.38, SE 0.12 in Italy; 7.98 (0.11) UK; 7.99 (0.10) Russia). TGFβ1 did not show consistent differences between sites in colostrum and HM analyses, with higher levels in UK colostrum samples compared with Italy (mean log TGFβ1 6.80 (0.07) in the UK; 6.53 (0.08) Italy); and high levels in Russian HM samples (6.36 (0.08)) compared with Italy (5.86 (0.11)) or the UK (5.96 (0.11)). We evaluated a number of other maternal factors for association with growth factor concentrations, and found weak evidence of an association between fish consumption less than once a week and higher levels of TGFβ1 (mean log TGFβ1 6.72 (0.06) for less than once a week; 6.57 (0.05) for more than once a week); and primiparity with higher levels of HGF in colostrum (7.87 (0.08) for primiparous; 7.69 (0.08) for multiparous) and HM (6.92 (0.11) for primiparous; 6.75 (0.11) for multiparous).

Table 3. Concentration (pg/mL) of growth factors in colostrum and breast milk and exposures associated with the levels.

	Median (IQR) pg/mL	Important Growth Factor Level Difference between the Groups	
		Colostrum	
HGF	2055.31 (964–6239)	UK and Russia higher than in Italy	$p < 0.001$
		Primipara higher than Multipara	$p = 0.05$
TGFβ1	731.534 (505–1142)	UK higher than Italy	$p = 0.01$
		Fish consumption Less than once a week higher than At least once a week	$p = 0.04$
TGFβ2	42,209.88 (23,847–98,597)	UK higher than Russia and Italy	$p < 0.05$
TGFβ3	1535.081 (847–3395)	UK higher than Russia higher than Italy	$p < 0.05$
		Breast Milk	
HGF	784.041 (508–1189)	Primiparous higher than Multigravida	$p = 0.05$
TGFβ1	493.514 (375–653)	Russia higher than UK and Italy	$p < 0.05$
TGFβ2	14,040.62 (10,080–27,262)	UK higher than Russia and Italy	$p < 0.05$
TGFβ3	279.41 (183–395)	UK higher than Russia higher than Italy	$p < 0.05$

A multilevel mixed-effect regression model was used for all analyses, which was adjusted using Bonferroni correction, to the following factors: Parity, Maternal Atopy, Maternal age, Site (Country) of collection, Mode of delivery—labour versus no labour, Mould presence at home, Pets at home or regular contact; Exposure to tobacco smoke (i.e., smoker or living in household with smoker or self-reported passive smoker) at recruitment; At least one self-reported maternal infection during pregnancy; Maternal diet—fish intake at least once per week versus less often; daily fresh fruit versus less often; daily probiotic versus none/less often.

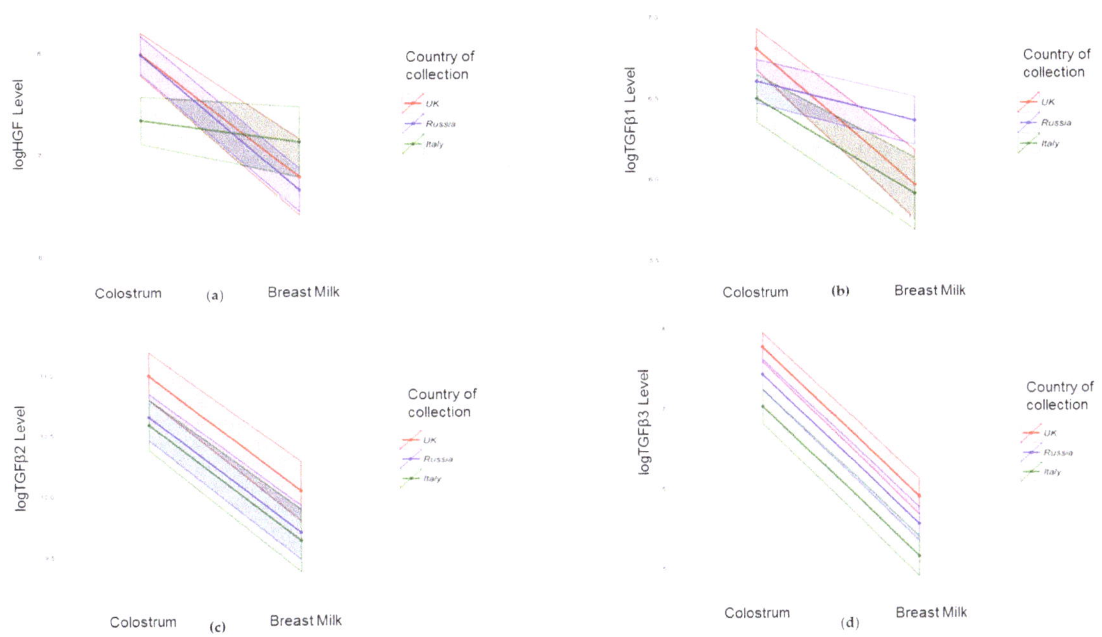

Figure 2. Association between site of collection and growth factor concentrations in colostrum and breast milk. Data shown are mean (bold line) and 95% CI (shaded area) for log transformed concentrations of HGF (**a**); TGFβ1 (**b**); TGFβ2 (**c**); and TGFβ3 (**d**) in the UK (**red**), Russia (**blue**), and Italy (**green**). A multilevel mixed-effect regression model was used for all analyses which were adjusted to the following factors: Parity, Maternal Atopy, Maternal age, Site (Country) of collection, Mode of delivery, Mould presence at home, Pets at home or regular contact; Exposure to tobacco smoke, at recruitment; At least one self-reported maternal infection during pregnancy; Maternal diet.

3.3.2. Cytokines

Women reporting infections during pregnancy had detectable levels of IL5 less often in comparison to mothers reporting no antenatal infections (Table 4). Smoking, type of delivery, and antenatal infections were not related to detection of cytokines in HM or colostrum.

Table 4. Detectability of Th1 and Th2 Cytokines in Colostrum and Human Milk.

	Colostrum Detectable	Human Milk Detectable	Factors Associated with Cytokines Detectability
IL2	49/342 (14%)	38/190 (20%)	NA
IL4	35/342 (10%)	30/190 (16%)	NA
IL5	77/342 (23%)	27/190 (14%)	Antenatal infections OR 0.49 (95% CI 0.25–0.98)
IL10	225/342 (66%)	69/190 (36%)	NA
IFNγ	66/342 (19%)	92/190 (48%)	NA
IL12	63/342 (18%)	31/190 (16%)	NA
IL13	86/342 (25%)	58/190 (31%)	NA

NA—no association. A multilevel mixed-effect regression model was used for all analyses which were adjusted to the following factors: Parity, Maternal Atopy, Maternal age, Site (Country) of collection, Mode of delivery, Mould presence at home, Pets at home or regular contact; Exposure to tobacco smoke, at recruitment; At least one self-reported maternal infection during pregnancy; Maternal diet.

3.3.3. Protein and Sodium in Colostrum

Protein in human colostrum declines over time ($r = -0.42$; $p < 0.001$) with all growth factor levels demonstrating a significant and marked decline over time, although the slope of decline varied between growth factors. When corrected for protein, the correlation between growth factor levels and time of collection was inconsistent between factors, with a significant decline seen for HGF/Protein, an increase over time seen for TGFβ1/Protein and TGFβ2/Protein, and no change over time seen for TGFβ3/Protein. The relationship between time of colostrum collection and growth factor or growth factor/Protein level for the four growth factors measured is shown in Table A2 and Figure 3.

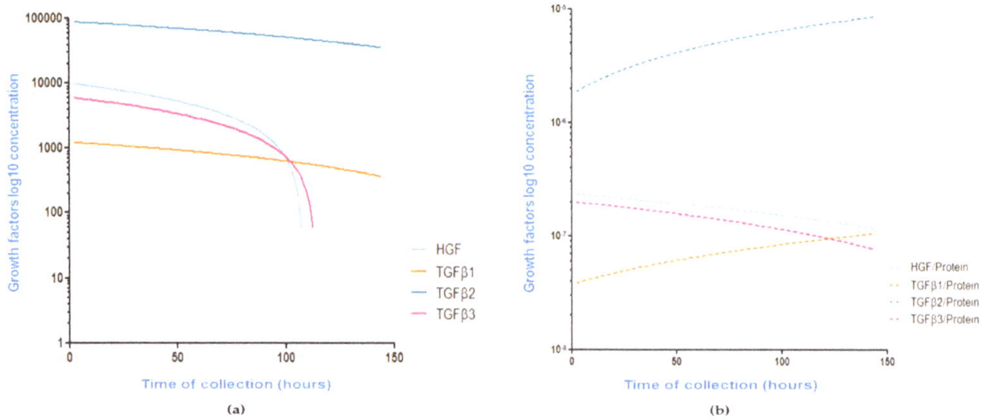

Figure 3. Effect of correcting growth factor concentrations for total protein level on the relationship between concentration and time. Data show nonlinear curves for unadjusted concentrations (pg/mL) of HGF (**blue**), TGFβ1 (**orange**), TGFβ2 (**green**), and TGFβ3 (**pink**) in colostrum in relation to time of sampling. Correlations were explored using raw data (**a**); and the ratio of growth factor concentration to protein concentration in the same sample (**b**). Trends in absolute and relative growth factors concentration in colostrum change over time. All correlation coefficients were statistically significant apart from the TGFβ3/Protein ratio in Figure 3b.

4. Discussion

In this large prospective cohort study, we have confirmed earlier findings of significant differences in milk composition between sites, but were not able to explain these differences through maternal or environmental factors. We identified important differences between mediators in kinetics of decline postpartum and these data suggest specific mechanisms controlling HM immune composition, and support important biological roles for HM immune factors in the developing infant.

Data from a variety of studies suggest that colostrum and HM constituents may be influenced by the country of origin and a number of environmental conditions which may differ significantly from one location to another [3–7,32], but the cause of this difference is still unclear. Our data suggest that HGF levels were lower in the colostrum/milk of Italian mothers and TGFβ2 and TGFβ3 were higher in colostrum/milk of UK mothers with the same significant difference for colostral TGFβ1 (Figure 2). Amoudruz showed that Mali women have higher levels of TGF-β1 in comparison with women born in Sweden [5]. Peroni reported higher HM TGF-β1 in a farming compared with urban environment [6]. Tomicic found Estonian mothers have lower HM TGFβ2 than Swedish mothers [7] which the authors suggested may be due to differences in microbial exposure. Orivuori et al. assessed HM samples collected in four countries of continental Europe and Finland and showed TGFβ1 levels to be highest in Finland and sIgA lowest in Germany [32]. We explored a number of maternal and demographic variables including markers of microbial load such as maternal report of probiotic, pet, and mould exposure, but we were not able to confirm these previous findings.

At present, we do not possess strong evidence of maternal allergic status influences on qualitative and quantitative immunological constituents in HM. We did not find any relationship between the levels of growth factors and/or detectability of cytokines and maternal allergy; this is in agreement with data from other studies which found no obvious trend in HM composition of allergic mothers compared to non-allergic [32–34].

Our data show some evidence for higher levels of HGF and TGFβ3 in the colostrum of primiparous women. Data from some studies suggest that parity does not influence HM composition. This borderline trend can be seen in some (but not all [3,35]) other studies [4,36,37], suggesting that higher levels of certain immune active markers can be found in the HM of primiparous mothers, which may be an additional mechanism to explain decreased allergy risk with an increase of birth order.

We found some evidence that fish intake during pregnancy can influence HM composition [3]—we found higher colostrum TGFβ1 in women eating fish less than once a week. This adds to a confusing picture, with Urwin reporting TGF-β1 levels to be highest in the colostrum of women residing in the river and lake region of China [3], well known for high fish consumption and Hawkes not finding any relationship between fish oil intervention and TGFβ1 levels [38]. Thus, the reasons behind differences in the HM immunological profile between countries remain unclear. Further work should consider genetic and gene/environment influences, as well as detailed dietary assessments, in addition to the factors evaluated in this study. Data from So-Yeon Lee and co-authors show that breastfeeding was found to be associated with a reduced risk of allergic sensitisation in children with CT/CC geno-type, suggesting gene-environment interaction between the CD14C-159T polymorphism and breastfeeding in relation to aeroallergen sensitisation [39].

It is well established that colostrum is particularly rich in immunologically active molecules and that levels of immunological factors are lower in mature HM [6,12,40,41]. Although our study did not involve HM collection in the same individuals over multiple timepoints, the sample size was large enough to identify a strong relationship between time of sampling postpartum and growth factor levels. We observed a strong relationship between growth factor levels and time postpartum both within colostrum, and between colostrum and mature milk samples, which was independent of geographical location. Although the difference between colostrum and mature milk composition is well established in the literature [6,12,40,41], our finding of a rapid decline in growth factor levels (HGF, TGFβ1, TGFβ3) and evidence for reduced detectability of cytokines (IL2, IL5, IL10, IFNγ) in colostrum with time postpartum has not been consistently demonstrated by others. Soto-Ramirez et al.

found none of the immune markers to correlate with the time of milk collection in a study conducted in the USA [42]; this may be partially explained by a wide range in collection times (week one to eight) and absence of colostral samples. In a study done in China with a narrower range of collection times, levels of TGF-β1 and TGF-β2 decreased significantly over time [3]. Studies which do not adequately account for variations in sampling time may explain some of the inconsistency of HM composition and its determinants in the literature [29].

Dilution could be a potential explanation of the growth factor decline over time. During the first week of life the infant's volume requirements are low. Later levels of the immune active molecules decrease as the volume and nutritional requirements of the infant increase. Immune active constituents of colostrum and breast milk represent a minor component but one of the most biologically active parts of HM total protein. In this study, we attempted to adjust for dilutional effects by correcting growth factor colostrum levels for total protein level in the same sample. Correction for colostrum total protein failed to consistently remove the relationship between factor level and time postpartum, and highlighted significant variation between factors in the kinetics of decline. This implies active transport of these growth factors using varied mechanisms specific to each factor. If we assume biological relevance, then these results suggest that infants need relatively higher amounts of TGFβ1 and TGFβ2 for longer than that of TGFβ3 or HGF. TGFβ3 is significantly different from TGFβ1 and TGFβ2 in its detailed tertiary structure of the active domain despite homology in amino acid sequence [43]. There is some evidence [43] that TGFβ3 may also have distinct functions to other TGFβ isoforms. TGFβ3 is up-regulated by milk stasis, and induces apoptosis in mammary gland epithelium during involution, in contrast to TGFβ1 and TGFβ2 [44]. The biological relevance of HM TGFβ is illustrated by the observed direct correlation between the levels of TGFβ in human milk and infant serum IgA [45]. As the infant's immune response matures there is likely to be less need for an extrinsic supply of immune stimulants.

The main limitations of our study are first that we did not assess maternal diet using a food frequency questionnaire, did not collect detailed information on the strain of probiotics and/or fish oil supplements used, and did not evaluate maternal genotype as a potentially important determinant or modulator of HM composition. This means that while we were able to explore our primary focus of maternal and demographic factors influence on HM composition, we were not able to reliably identify reasons for the difference in HM composition identified between sites. Second, we sampled single colostrum and HM specimens from each subject. Our findings regarding the kinetics of growth factor decline in colostrum and HM need to be explored further in prospective studies with longitudinal sampling at multiple timepoints within the same participants. Third, we only made preliminary attempts to adjust for the effect of time or milk maturity on compositional analysis. Since time postpartum may be a surrogate for milk/breast maturity, we aimed to identify a 'correction factor' that might reflect milk maturity. We did not find evidence that any growth factor concentration was related to HM protein concentration, but further work is needed to identify markers of HM maturity in order to control for this in compositional analysis of colostrum. Maternal body mass index (BMI) data has not been assessed due to a difficulty in one of the participating countries. Finally, due to logistical, funding, and sample size constraints our analysis covers only a small number of growth factors and cytokines, so may not be generalisable to all immune factors in HM.

5. Conclusions

In this large international cohort study of HM composition, we have found an important influence of time after birth on colostrum composition, which must be adjusted for in any further research. Despite adjusting for this and other factors, we identified unexplained and significant variation in HM immune composition between geographically distant populations. Overall, our data suggest that levels of human milk mediators decline at different rates post-partum, and this may suggest that these factors are likely to have specific biological roles in early postnatal development. An important aim of future research should be to optimize the analysis of HM composition, accounting for maturity of milk, and aim to better understand the biological roles and consequences for the developing infant of variations in HM immune composition.

Acknowledgments: We are grateful to the staff of birth centres and postnatal units involved and all the women and their babies, participating in our study. Robert Boyle and John Warner are supported by a National Institute for Health Research Biomedical Research Centre (BRC). Both JW and RB have received research grant income from Danone in relation to studies of the value of prebiotics in allergy prevention and Airsonette to evaluate Temperature controlled laminar airflow for asthma. JW is on a Danone, UCB and Airsonette scientific advisory board and both JW and RB have given paid lectures for the companies. DM has received travel funding from Nutricia. DG receives an unrestricted research grant from Medela AG and has received travel funding and support for lectures.

Author Contributions: J.O.W., R.J.B. and D.M. conceived and designed the experiments; D.M., S.D., L.Y.C., P.A. and S.S. performed the experiments; D.M., L.Y.C. collected data in London; D.G.P. and A.L.B. collected data in Verona; M.T. and A.P. collected data in Moscow; S.C. analysed the data; D.M., D.T.G., R.J.B. and J.O.W. wrote the paper. For research articles with several authors, a short paragraph specifying their individual contributions must be provided. The following statements should be used "X.X. and Y.Y. conceived and designed the experiments; X.X. performed the experiments; X.X. and Y.Y. analysed the data; W.W. contributed reagents/materials/analysis tools; Y.Y. wrote the paper". Authorship must be limited to those who have contributed substantially to the work reported.

Appendix A

Table A1. Lower limit of detection values (pg/mL) for cytokines and growth factors analysis and overall locations median concentrations for all immune active molecules (values below LLOD for all cytokines have been transformed into 1/2 of LLOD).

Immune Active Molecule	Median Lower Limit of Detection	Median (IQR) Colostrum	Median (IQR) HM
IFN-γ	3.49	1.23 (0.51–3.49)	3.49 (1.54–7.8)
IL2	2.06	0.6 (0.29–1.47)	0.98 (0.23–2.06)
IL4	1.83	1.83 (0.24–1.83)	1.83 (0.50–1.83)
IL5	2.89	1.44 (0.57–2.85)	1.57 (0.33–2.89)
IL10	1.50	2.67 (1.01–9.04)	1.5 (0.74–2.66)
IL12	3.50	1.85 (0.34–3.5)	2.13 (0.32–3.5)
IL13	4.60	4.6 (1.85–4.69)	4.6 (3.52–6.76)
HGF	73.00	2055.31 (964–6239)	784.041 (508–1189)
TGFβ1	8.73	731.534 (505–1142)	493.514 (375–653)
TGFβ2	265.00	42,209.88 (23,847–98,597)	14,040.62 (10,080–27,262)
TGFβ3	8.37	1535.081 (847–3395)	279.41 (183–395)

Standard curve ranges: IFN-γ, IL2, IL4, IL5, IL10, IL12, IL13 0—2500 pg/mL; HGF, TGFβ1, TGFβ2 0—100.000; TGFβ3 0—50.000. All values presented in pg/mL.

Table A2. Absolute and relative decline of growth factors over time.

Growth Factor Concentration (pg/mL)/Time of Collection	Raw Concentration (pg/mL)	Growth Factor/Protein Ratio
HGF	$r = -0.39, p < 0.001$ ↓	$r = -0.19, p = 0.003$ ↓
TGFβ1	$r = -0.21, p < 0.001$ ↓	$r = 0.25, p < 0.001$ ↑
TGFβ2	$r = -0.16, p = 0.01$ ↓	$r = 0.20, p = 0.004$ ↑
TGFβ3	$r = -0.35, p < 0.001$ ↓	$r = -0.06, p = 0.34$ ↓

↑—Positive correlation with time of collection; ↓—Negative correlation with time of collection.

References

1. Matheson, M.C.; Allen, K.J.; Tang, M.L. Understanding the evidence for and against the role of breastfeeding in allergy prevention. *Clin. Exp. Allergy* **2012**, *42*, 827–851. [CrossRef] [PubMed]
2. Hoppu, U.; Isolauri, E.; Laakso, P.; Matomaki, J.; Laitinen, K. Probiotics and dietary counselling targeting maternal dietary fat intake modifies breast milk fatty acids and cytokines. *Eur. J. Nutr.* **2012**, *51*, 211–219. [CrossRef] [PubMed]

3. Urwin, H.J.; Miles, E.A.; Noakes, P.S.; Kremmyda, L.S.; Vlachava, M.; Diaper, N.D.; Perez-Cano, F.J.; Godfrey, K.M.; Calder, P.C.; Yaqoob, P. Salmon consumption during pregnancy alters fatty acid composition and secretory IgA concentration in human breast milk. *J. Nutr.* **2012**, *142*, 1603–1610. [CrossRef] [PubMed]
4. Amoudruz, P.; Holmlund, U.; Schollin, J.; Sverremark-Ekstrom, E.; Montgomery, S.M. Maternal country of birth and previous pregnancies are associated with breast milk characteristics. *Pediatr. Allergy Immunol.* **2009**, *20*, 19–29. [CrossRef] [PubMed]
5. Holmlund, U.; Amoudruz, P.; Johansson, M.A.; Haileselassie, Y.; Ongoiba, A.; Kayentao, K.; Traore, B.; Doumbo, S.; Schollin, J.; Doumbo, O.; et al. Maternal country of origin, breast milk characteristics and potential influences on immunity in offspring. *Clin. Exp. Immunol.* **2010**, *162*, 500–509. [CrossRef] [PubMed]
6. Peroni, D.G.; Pescollderungg, L.; Piacentini, G.L.; Rigotti, E.; Maselli, M.; Watschinger, K.; Piazza, M.; Pigozzi, R.; Boner, A.L. Immune regulatory cytokines in the milk of lactating women from farming and urban environments. *Pediatr. Allergy Immunol.* **2010**, *21*, 977–982. [CrossRef] [PubMed]
7. Tomicic, S.; Johansson, G.; Voor, T.; Bjorksten, B.; Bottcher, M.F.; Jenmalm, M.C. Breast milk cytokine and IgA composition differ in Estonian and Swedish mothers-relationship to microbial pressure and infant allergy. *Pediatr. Res.* **2010**, *68*, 330–334. [CrossRef] [PubMed]
8. Striker, G.A.; Casanova, L.D.; Nagao, A.T. Influence of type of delivery on A, G and M immunoglobulin concentration in maternal colostrum. *J. Pediatr.* **2004**, *80*, 123–128. [CrossRef]
9. Bottcher, M.F.; Jenmalm, M.C.; Garofalo, R.P.; Bjorksten, B. Cytokines in breast milk from allergic and nonallergic mothers. *Pediatr. Res.* **2000**, *47*, 157–162. [CrossRef] [PubMed]
10. Laiho, K.; Lampi, A.M.; Hamalainen, M.; Moilanen, E.; Piironen, V.; Arvola, T.; Syrjanen, S.; Isolauri, E. Breast milk fatty acids, eicosanoids, and cytokines in mothers with and without allergic disease. *Pediatr. Res.* **2003**, *53*, 642–647. [CrossRef] [PubMed]
11. Prokesova, L.; Lodinova-Zadnikova, R.; Zizka, J.; Kocourkova, I.; Novotna, O.; Petraskova, P.; Sterzl, I. Cytokine levels in healthy and allergic mothers and their children during the first year of life. *Pediatr. Allergy Immunol.* **2006**, *17*, 175–183. [CrossRef] [PubMed]
12. Rigotti, E.; Piacentini, G.L.; Ress, M.; Pigozzi, R.; Boner, A.L.; Peroni, D.G. Transforming growth factor-beta and interleukin-10 in breast milk and development of atopic diseases in infants. *Clin. Exp. Allergy* **2006**, *36*, 614–618. [CrossRef] [PubMed]
13. Marek, A.; Zagierski, M.; Liberek, A.; Aleksandrowicz, E.; Korzon, M.; Krzykowski, G.; Kaminska, B.; Szlagatys-Sidorkiewicz, A. TGF-beta(1), IL-10 and IL-4 in colostrum of allergic and nonallergic mothers. *Acta Biochim. Pol.* **2009**, *56*, 411–414. [PubMed]
14. Sidor, K.; Jarmolowska, B.; Kaczmarski, M.; Kostyra, E.; Iwan, M.; Kostyra, H. Content of beta-casomorphins in milk of women with a history of allergy. *Pediatr. Allergy Immunol.* **2008**, *19*, 587–591. [CrossRef] [PubMed]
15. Snijders, B.E.; Damoiseaux, J.G.; Penders, J.; Kummeling, I.; Stelma, F.F.; van Ree, R.; van den Brandt, P.A.; Thijs, C. Cytokines and soluble CD14 in breast milk in relation with atopic manifestations in mother and infant (KOALA study). *Clin. Exp. Allergy* **2006**, *36*, 1609–1615. [CrossRef] [PubMed]
16. Bottcher, M.F.; Abrahamsson, T.R.; Fredriksson, M.; Jakobsson, T.; Bjorksten, B. Low breast milk tgf-beta2 is induced by lactobacillus reuteri supplementation and associates with reduced risk of sensitization during infancy. *Pediatr. Allergy Immunol.* **2008**, *19*, 497–504. [CrossRef] [PubMed]
17. Boyle, R.J.; Ismail, I.H.; Kivivuori, S.; Licciardi, P.V.; Robins-Browne, R.M.; Mah, L.J.; Axelrad, C.; Moore, S.; Donath, S.; Carlin, J.B.; et al. Lactobacillus GG treatment during pregnancy for the prevention of eczema: A randomized controlled trial. *Allergy* **2011**, *66*, 509–516. [CrossRef] [PubMed]
18. Prescott, S.L.; Wickens, K.; Westcott, L.; Jung, W.; Currie, H.; Black, P.N.; Stanley, T.V.; Mitchell, E.A.; Fitzharris, P.; Siebers, R.; et al. Supplementation with *Lactobacillus Rhamnosus* or *Bifidobacterium Lactis* probiotics in pregnancy increases cord blood interferon-gamma and breast milk transforming growth factor-beta and immunoglobin a detection. *Clin. Exp. Allergy* **2008**, *38*, 1606–1614. [CrossRef] [PubMed]
19. Rautava, S.; Kalliomaki, M.; Isolauri, E. Probiotics during pregnancy and breast-feeding might confer immunomodulatory protection against atopic disease in the infant. *J. Allergy Clin. Immunol.* **2002**, *109*, 119–121. [CrossRef] [PubMed]
20. Kuitunen, M.; Kukkonen, A.K.; Savilahti, E. Impact of maternal allergy and use of probiotics during pregnancy on breast milk cytokines and food antibodies and development of allergy in children until 5 years. *Int. Arch. Allergy Immunol.* **2012**, *159*, 162–170. [CrossRef] [PubMed]

21. Zanardo, V.; Nicolussi, S.; Cavallin, S.; Trevisanuto, D.; Barbato, A.; Faggian, D.; Favaro, F.; Plebani, M. Effect of maternal smoking on breast milk interleukin-1alpha, beta-endorphin, and leptin concentrations and leptin concentrations. *Environ. Health Perspect.* **2005**, *113*, 1410–1413. [CrossRef] [PubMed]
22. Burch, J.; Karmaus, W.; Gangur, V.; Soto-Ramirez, N.; Yousefi, M.; Goetzl, L.M. Pre- and perinatal characteristics and breast milk immune markers. *Pediatr. Res.* **2013**, *74*, 615–621. [CrossRef] [PubMed]
23. Min, J.K.; Lee, Y.M.; Kim, J.H.; Kim, Y.M.; Kim, S.W.; Lee, S.Y.; Gho, Y.S.; Oh, G.T.; Kwon, Y.G. Hepatocyte growth factor suppresses vascular endothelial growth factor-induced expression of endothelial ICAM-1 and VCAM-1 by inhibiting the nuclear factor-kappaB pathway. *Circ. Res.* **2005**, *96*, 300–307. [CrossRef] [PubMed]
24. Kobata, R.; Tsukahara, H.; Ohshima, Y.; Ohta, N.; Tokuriki, S.; Tamura, S.; Mayumi, M. High levels of growth factors in human breast milk. *Early Hum. Dev.* **2008**, *84*, 67–69. [CrossRef] [PubMed]
25. Horibe, N.; Okamoto, T.; Itakura, A.; Nakanishi, T.; Suzuki, T.; Kazeto, S.; Tomoda, Y. Levels of hepatocyte growth factor in maternal serum and amniotic fluid. *Am. J. Obstet. Gynecol.* **1995**, *173*, 937–942. [CrossRef]
26. Yamada, Y.; Saito, S.; Morikawa, H. Hepatocyte growth factor in human breast milk. *Am. J. Reprod. Immunol.* **1998**, *40*, 112–120. [CrossRef] [PubMed]
27. Strachan, D.P. Family size, infection and atopy: The first decade of the "hygiene hypothesis". *Thorax* **2000**, *55* (Suppl. 1), S2–S10. [CrossRef] [PubMed]
28. Strachan, D.P. Hay fever, hygiene, and household size. *BMJ* **1989**, *299*, 1259–1260. [CrossRef] [PubMed]
29. Munblit, D.; Boyle, R.J.; Warner, J.O. Factors affecting breast milk composition and potential consequences for development of the allergic phenotype. *Clin. Exp. Allergy* **2015**, *45*, 583–601. [CrossRef] [PubMed]
30. Ramirez-Santana, C.; Perez-Cano, F.J.; Audi, C.; Castell, M.; Moretones, M.G.; Lopez-Sabater, M.C.; Castellote, C.; Franch, A. Effects of cooling and freezing storage on the stability of bioactive factors in human colostrum. *J. Dairy Sci.* **2012**, *95*, 2319–2325. [CrossRef] [PubMed]
31. Jones, C.A.; Holloway, J.A.; Popplewell, E.J.; Diaper, N.D.; Holloway, J.W.; Vance, G.H.; Warner, J.A.; Warner, J.O. Reduced soluble CD14 levels in amniotic fluid and breast milk are associated with the subsequent development of atopy, eczema, or both. *J. Allergy Clin. Immunol.* **2002**, *109*, 858–866. [CrossRef] [PubMed]
32. Orivuori, L.; Loss, G.; Roduit, C.; Dalphin, J.C.; Depner, M.; Genuneit, J.; Lauener, R.; Pekkanen, J.; Pfefferle, P.; Riedler, J.; et al. Soluble immunoglobulin A in breast milk is inversely associated with atopic dermatitis at early age: The PASTURE cohort study. *Clin. Exp. Allergy* **2014**, *44*, 102–112. [CrossRef] [PubMed]
33. Savilahti, E.; Siltanen, M.; Kajosaari, M.; Vaarala, O.; Saarinen, K.M. IgA antibodies, TGF-beta1 and -beta2, and soluble CD14 in the colostrum and development of atopy by age 4. *Pediatr. Res.* **2005**, *58*, 1300–1305. [CrossRef] [PubMed]
34. Kondo, N.; Suda, Y.; Nakao, A.; Oh-Oka, K.; Suzuki, K.; Ishimaru, K.; Sato, M.; Tanaka, T.; Nagai, A.; Yamagata, Z. Maternal psychosocial factors determining the concentrations of transforming growth factor-beta in breast milk. *Pediatr. Allergy Immunol.* **2011**, *22*, 853–861. [CrossRef] [PubMed]
35. Ismail, I.H.; Licciardi, P.V.; Oppedisano, F.; Boyle, R.J.; Tang, M.L. Relationship between breast milk sCD14, Tgf-beta1 and total IgA in the first month and development of eczema during infancy. *Pediatr. Allergy Immunol.* **2013**, *24*, 352–360. [CrossRef] [PubMed]
36. Groer, M.W.; Shelton, M.M. Exercise is associated with elevated proinflammatory cytokines in human milk. *J. Obstet. Gynecol. Neonatal Nurs.* **2009**, *38*, 35–41. [CrossRef] [PubMed]
37. Walter, J.; Kuhn, L.; Ghosh, M.K.; Kankasa, C.; Semrau, K.; Sinkala, M.; Mwiya, M.; Thea, D.M.; Aldrovandi, G.M. Low and undetectable breast milk interleukin-7 concentrations are associated with reduced risk of postnatal HIV transmission. *J. Acquir. Immune Defic. Syndr.* **2007**, *46*, 200–207. [CrossRef] [PubMed]
38. Hawkes, J.S.; Bryan, D.L.; Neumann, M.A.; Makrides, M.; Gibson, R.A. Transforming growth factor beta in human milk does not change in response to modest intakes of docosahexaenoic acid. *Lipids* **2001**, *36*, 1179–1181. [CrossRef] [PubMed]
39. Lee, S.Y.; Kang, M.J.; Kwon, J.W.; Park, K.S.; Hong, S.J. Breastfeeding might have protective effects on atopy in children with the CD14C-159T CT/CC genotype. *Allergy Asthma Immunol. Res.* **2013**, *5*, 239–241. [CrossRef] [PubMed]
40. Takahata, Y.; Takada, H.; Nomura, A.; Ohshima, K.; Nakayama, H.; Tsuda, T.; Nakano, H.; Hara, T. Interleukin-18 in human milk. *Pediatr. Res.* **2001**, *50*, 268–272. [CrossRef] [PubMed]

41. Ustundag, B.; Yilmaz, E.; Dogan, Y.; Akarsu, S.; Canatan, H.; Halifeoglu, I.; Cikim, G.; Aygun, A.D. Levels of cytokines (IL-1beta, IL-2, IL-6, IL-8, TNF-alpha) and trace elements (Zn, Cu) in breast milk from mothers of preterm and term infants. *Mediat. Inflamm.* **2005**, *2005*, 331–336. [CrossRef] [PubMed]
42. Soto-Ramirez, N.; Karmaus, W.; Yousefi, M.; Zhang, H.; Liu, J.; Gangur, V. Maternal immune markers in serum during gestation and in breast milk and the risk of asthma-like symptoms at ages 6 and 12 months: A longitudinal study. *Allergy Asthma Clin. Immunol.* **2012**, *8*, 11. [CrossRef] [PubMed]
43. Laverty, H.G.; Wakefield, L.M.; Occleston, N.L.; O'Kane, S.; Ferguson, M.W. TGF-β3 and cancer: A review. *Cytokine Growth Factor Rev.* **2009**, *20*, 305–317. [CrossRef] [PubMed]
44. Nguyen, A.V.; Pollard, J.W. Transforming growth factor beta3 induces cell death during the first stage of mammary gland involution. *Development* **2000**, *127*, 3107–3118. [PubMed]
45. Ogawa, J.; Sasahara, A.; Yoshida, T.; Sira, M.M.; Futatani, T.; Kanegane, H.; Miyawaki, T. Role of transforming growth factor-beta in breast milk for initiation of IgA production in newborn infants. *Early Hum. Dev.* **2004**, *77*, 67–75. [CrossRef] [PubMed]

5

Effect of Human Milk Appetite Hormones, Macronutrients, and Infant Characteristics on Gastric Emptying and Breastfeeding Patterns of Term Fully Breastfed Infants

Zoya Gridneva [1,*], Sambavi Kugananthan [1,2], Anna R. Hepworth [1], Wan J. Tie [1], Ching T. Lai [1], Leigh C. Ward [3], Peter E. Hartmann [1] and Donna T. Geddes [1]

1 School of Chemistry and Biochemistry, The University of Western Australia, Crawley, Perth, Western Australia 6009, Australia; 21141062@student.uwa.edu.au (S.K.); anna.hepworth@uwa.edu.au (A.R.H.); ash.tie@uwa.edu.au (W.J.T.); ching-tat.lai@uwa.edu.au (C.T.L.); peter.hartmann@uwa.edu.au (P.E.H.); donna.geddes@uwa.edu.au (D.T.G.)

2 School of Anatomy, Physiology and Human Biology, The University of Western Australia, Crawley, Perth, Western Australia 6009, Australia

3 School of Chemistry and Molecular Biosciences, The University of Queensland, St. Lucia, Brisbane, Queensland 4072, Australia; l.ward@uq.edu.au

* Correspondence: zgridneva@gmail.com

Abstract: Human milk (HM) components influence infant feeding patterns and nutrient intake, yet it is unclear how they influence gastric emptying (GE), a key component of appetite regulation. This study analyzed GE of a single breastfeed, HM appetite hormones/macronutrients and demographics/anthropometrics/body composition of term fully breastfed infants (n = 41, 2 and/or 5 mo). Stomach volumes (SV) were calculated from pre-/post-feed ultrasound scans, then repeatedly until the next feed. Feed volume (FV) was measured by the test-weigh method. HM samples were analyzed for adiponectin, leptin, fat, lactose, total carbohydrate, lysozyme, and total/whey/casein protein. Linear regression/mixed effect models were used to determine associations between GE/feed variables and HM components/infant anthropometrics/adiposity. Higher FVs were associated with faster (−0.07 [−0.10, −0.03], $p < 0.001$) GE rate, higher post-feed SVs (0.82 [0.53, 1.12], $p < 0.001$), and longer GE times (0.24 [0.03, 0.46], $p = 0.033$). Higher whey protein concentration was associated with higher post-feed SVs (4.99 [0.84, 9.13], $p = 0.023$). Longer GE time was associated with higher adiponectin concentration (2.29 [0.92, 3.66], $p = 0.002$) and dose (0.02 [0.01, 0.03], $p = 0.005$), and lower casein:whey ratio (−65.89 [−107.13, −2.66], $p = 0.003$). FV and HM composition influence GE and breastfeeding patterns in term breastfed infants.

Keywords: human milk; term breastfed infants; gastric emptying; feeding frequency; ultrasound; stomach volumes; appetite hormones; macronutrients; feed volume; anthropometrics; body composition

---

1. Introduction

Breastfeeding and its longer duration are associated with reduced risks of developing obesity and other chronic non-communicable diseases later in life [1,2]. This unique protection could be the result of many mechanisms associated with both nutritive and non-nutritive components of human milk (HM) [3] as well as breastfeeding patterns and behaviour [4,5]. It has been shown that HM has the pleiotropic role, providing immune and anti-inflammatory protection [6,7] and endocrine, developmental, neural, and psychological benefits [2]. Non-nutritive HM components such as hormones, growth factors, neuropeptides, and anti-inflammatory and immune-modulating agents influence the growth, development, and function of the gastrointestinal (GI) tract during early infancy [8], while some micronutrients act as nutritional antioxidants, improving GI functions [9]; however, there is much to be learned about the spectrum of HM programming agents, how their patterns change throughout lactation period, and their short-term effect on the gastric emptying (GE) rate of the breastfed infants.

GE is a process by which ingested food is mechanically and chemically partially broken down and delivered to the duodenum at a controlled rate for further digestion and absorption [10,11]. While well studied in the preterm population [12–14], in healthy term fully breastfed infants the GE rate and its relationship with breastfeeding patterns are not fully understood.

GE rate and patterns are known to depend on the nature and macronutrient composition of the ingested meal. HM or formula in the infant stomach separates into two phases, a liquid phase consisting of water, whey proteins, lactose, etc., and a semi-solid phase consisting of curd formed by casein and lipids. The semi-solid phase typically empties more slowly than the liquid phase. Different proportions of these phases in part explain the difference between GE patterns of formula-fed and breastfed infants—linear and curvilinear, respectively [12,15].

HM has a unique composition, including nutrients, growth factors, immune factors, and hormones. Despite numerous investigations into the different effects of HM and formula, few components, including major macronutrients, have been studied in connection with the GE of breasted term infants.

Fatty acids profiles are not associated with GE rate in preterm infants [16], while in term infants more rapid GE has been attributed to the fat and protein components of feeds with similar lactose concentration and osmolality [17].

Both osmolality and carbohydrate content are known to influence the rate of GE in adults [18], but in infants results are dependent on the type of carbohydrate [19,20].

Proteins from different HM fractions such as whey and casein are resistant to proteolysis in the infant stomach [21] and the protein content of a food has also been shown to influence appetite and its regulation [22]. Infant formula generally empties more slowly than HM in term infants; further, formulas with different casein:whey protein ratio exhibit different GE rates, with casein-predominant formulas emptying slower than whey-predominant formulas [23]. Thus the casein:whey ratio of HM could play an important role in controlling GE in the breastfed infant.

HM lysozyme, also present in whey in a relatively high concentration, catalyzes the hydrolysis of specific bonds in Gram-negative bacteria cell walls and plays multiple roles in digestive strategy, such as controlling the microbiome in the stomach and speeding up the digestion of microbial protein, which may affect gastric motility and GE rate [24,25].

The satiety hormone leptin and the appetite-stimulating hormone adiponectin are also present in HM. Although not transferred to the infant circulation in direct manner, levels of HM leptin and adiponectin from HM have been found to correlate with levels of these hormones in infant serum [26,27] and are known to affect both appetite control and infant body composition (BC) [28,29], but are yet to be investigated in relation to GE in the term infant. In animal models (rat, mouse), injection of leptin into the fourth ventricle has been shown to delay GE [30] and oral administration reduced food intake [31]. Leptin in HM is by far the most studied appetite hormone, but predominantly in skim milk [32]. Leptin measured in skim HM was not associated with time between feeds [33,34] or GE [34] in term breastfed infants, emphasizing the need for studies including whole milk leptin, where the levels of leptin are shown to be higher [32]. Adiponectin has the highest concentration of any appetite hormone in HM. It is present in a biologically active form that is resistant to digestion [35]. In the animal model adiponectin inhibits tension-sensitive gastric vagal afferent mechanosensitivity, modulating satiety signals in both lean and obese animals, while simultaneously increasing the mechanosensitivity of mucosal gastric vagal afferent in the obesity-induced model [36]. In humans, elevated serum levels of adiponectin are associated with more rapid GE in diabetic patients [37]. It is not known whether adiponectin levels impact GE in the infant and this warrants further investigation.

The volume of milk taken at a single feed varies greatly both within and between infants [38]. This may be affected by HM composition, with greater breastfeeding frequency associated with lower total 24-h protein intakes and higher lactose concentrations [39]. This suggests that the variations in HM components between mothers may potentially influence GE rate and time, and therefore feeding patterns.

This study investigated the effects of HM appetite hormones (whole milk adiponectin and leptin, skim milk leptin) and macronutrients (fat, total carbohydrates, lactose, oligosaccharides, total protein, casein and whey protein, lysozyme) on feeding frequency and GE. Further exploration of infant demographics, anthropometrics, and BC was carried out to determine relationships with infant feeding and GE.

2. Materials and Methods

2.1. Participants

Lactating mothers and their infants (n = 27) were recruited predominantly through the Australian Breastfeeding Association. Inclusion criteria were: healthy singletons, gestational age $\geq$ 37 weeks, fully breastfed on demand at the point of measurement. Exclusion criteria were: infant health issues requiring medication that could potentially influence GE rate (e.g., reflux), indications of low maternal milk production or infant growth issues. All mothers provided written informed consent to participate in the study, which was approved by the University of Western Australia, Human Research Ethics Committee (RA/1/4253) and registered with the Australian New Zealand Clinical Trials Registry (ACTRN12616000368437).

2.2. Study Design

Participants arrived at our laboratory at King Edward Memorial Hospital for Women (Subiaco, Perth, WA, Australia) in the morning (09:30–11:30 a.m.) to avoid circadian influence on the outcomes, and stayed for two consecutive breastfeeding sessions. Before the first feed (F1) infants were weighed and had ultrasound stomach volumes recorded (pre-feed residual, R1). Mothers expressed a pre-feed sample (fore-milk) of milk from the feeding breast/breasts and then breastfed their infants as usual. Immediately after F1, infant stomach volumes images and infant weights were taken, and mothers expressed a post-feed (hind-milk) milk sample. Subsequent scans of the stomach were scheduled at 15–20 min intervals (although attending infants' needs caused some variation) until the infant cued for the next feed (F2), when a final stomach volume immediately before F2 was measured (pre-feed residual, R2).

To assess infant BC bioimpedance spectroscopy measurements were taken pre-feed, unless impractical—then they were taken post-feed [40]. Ultrasound skinfold, length, and head circumference measurements were taken post-feed. This combination of two methods for measuring infant BC was used to ensure safe, non-invasive and accurate assessment and to avoid the inherent limitations of a singular technique [41]. Clothing was removed for the measurements except for a dry diaper and a singlet.

2.3. Feeding Frequency

Mothers were asked how frequently their infant feeds, and the self-reported typical time between the feeds (e.g., every three hours) during the week prior to the study session was taken as a proxy measure of feeding frequency.

2.4. Feed Volume Measurement

The volume of milk transferred from a breast/breasts by the infant was determined by weighing the infant immediately before and after the breastfeed using electronic scales ($\pm$2.0 g, Medela Electronic Baby Weigh Scales, Medela Inc., McHenry, IL, USA). Milk intake (g) was calculated by deducting the initial weight from the final weight of the infant [42] and was converted to mL (feed volume; FV) using HM density of 1.03 g/mL [43].

2.5. *Stomach Measurements with Ultrasound*

The infant's stomach was scanned using the Aplio XG (Toshiba, Tokyo, Japan) machine, with a high-resolution PVT-674BT (6MHz) transducer and Parker ultrasonic gel (Fairfield, NJ, USA). Three to nine (median [IQR]: 5 [5; 6]) serial measurements of infant stomachs were taken 3 to 62 min apart (16 $\pm$ 10). Scans were performed with the infant in the semi-supine position according to the method validated in preterm infants [44]. Briefly, the sagittal and transverse planes of the stomach were used to measure the longitudinal (L), anterior-posterior (AP) and transverse (T) diameters directly from images on the ultrasound screen using electronic calipers (Figure 1). One experienced sonographer with good intra- and interrater reliability [44] performed all of the measurements. Gastric volume (mL) was calculated from the above measured diameters using following equation for an ellipsoidal body:

$$\textit{Stomach volume}\ (\text{mL}) = \text{L (mm)} \times \text{AP (mm)} \times \text{T (mm)} \times 0.52. \quad (1)$$

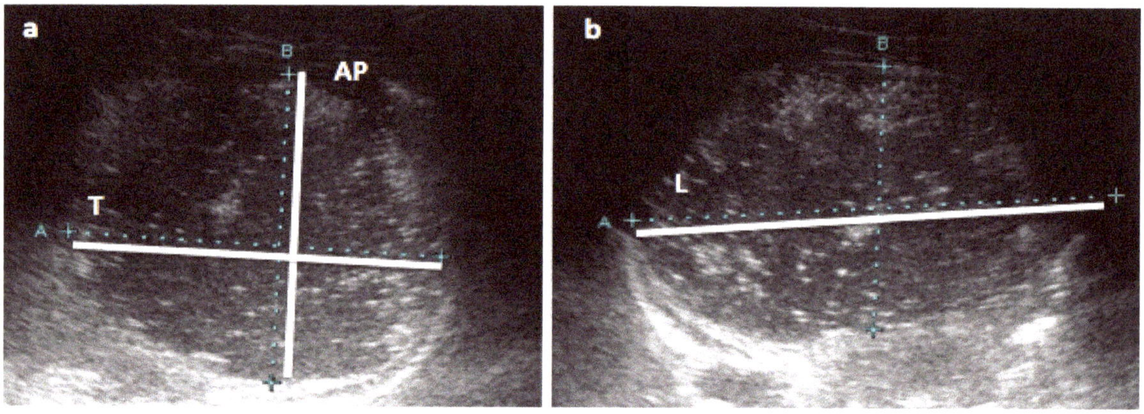

Figure 1. Measurements of infant's stomach with ultrasound. Ultrasound images of infant's stomach: (**a**) transverse view with anterior-posterior (AP) and transverse (T) diameter measurements; (**b**) longitudinal view with longitudinal (L) diameter (maximum length) measurement. Stomach volume (mL) = longitudinal diameter (mm) × anterior-posterior diameter (mm) × transverse diameter (mm) × 0.52.

2.6. *Milk Sample Collection*

Mothers hand-expressed or pumped small (1–2 mL) pre- and post-feed milk samples into separate 5-mL polypropylene plastic vials (Disposable Products, Adelaide, SA, Australia). Fat concentration was measured (below) and samples were frozen at −20 °C for further biochemical analysis.

2.7. *Biochemical Analysis*

2.7.1. Fat Content

Percentage fat was measured in pre- and post-feed samples immediately after sample collection with the creamatocrit method [45] using the Creamatocrit Plus device (Medela Inc., McHenry, IL, USA). Fat concentration of the pre- and post-feed milk samples (g/L) was calculated from the cream content of the milk samples, based on the equation [46]:

$$\textit{Fat}\ (\text{g/L}) = 3.56 + (5.917 \times \text{cream percentage}). \quad (2)$$

Fat concentration in the volume consumed by the infant was further calculated [47]:

$$Fat\ (g/L) = 0.53 \times \text{Fat}_{\text{pre-feed}} + 0.47 \times \text{Fat}_{\text{post-feed}}. \quad (3)$$

2.7.2. Sample Preparation

Prior to further analysis, all samples were thawed for two hours at room temperature (RT) and aliquoted into 1.5-mL tubes (Sarstedt, Numbrecht, Germany). Components' concentrations were determined in both pre- and post-feed samples in case of adiponectin, skim and whole milk leptin, fat, and lactose, and in pooled samples in case of total protein, casein, whey protein, total carbohydrates, and lysozyme. Concentrations of pre- and post-feed samples were averaged to arrive at the concentration used for statistical analyses. Whole milk was used for measuring whole milk adiponectin and leptin concentration. Milk samples were defatted (by centrifugation at RT in a Beckman Microfuge 11 (Aberdon Enterprise Inc., Elk Grove Village, IL, USA) at 10,000× *g* for 10 min and removing the fat layer by clipping it off with the top of the tube [48]) for analysis of skim milk leptin, total protein, lysozyme, lactose, and total carbohydrates concentrations. The standard assays were adapted for and carried out using a JANUS workstation (PerkinElmer, Inc., Waltham, MA, USA) and measured on EnSpire (PerkinElmer, Inc., Waltham, MA, USA).

2.7.3. Leptin

Leptin concentration in HM was measured using the R & D Systems Human Leptin enzyme linked immunosorbent assay (ELISA) DuoSet kit (Minneapolis, MN, USA) optimized to measure leptin in sonicated skim HM, as previously described by Cannon et al. [33] and further modified to measure leptin in skim and whole HM milk as described by Kugananthan et al. [32]. Recovery of leptin was 97.7% ± 9.7% (n = 10) with a detection limit of 0.05 ng/mL and an inter-assay CV of <7.2%.

2.7.4. Adiponectin

Adiponectin concentration in whole milk was measured using the Biovendor Human Adiponectin Sandwich ELISA kit (Life Technologies, Asheville, NC, USA). Adiponectin recovery was 96.2% ± 3.2% (n = 10) with a detection limit of 1 ng/mL and an inter-assay CV of <2.5%.

2.7.5. Protein

Casein and whey proteins were separated by the method fully described by Kunz and Lonnerdal [49], and Khan et al. [50]. Protein concentrations (total protein of skim HM, casein and whey proteins) were measured using the Bradford Protein Assay adapted from Mitoulas et al. [51]. Recovery of protein was 100.6% ± 5.2% (n = 5) with a detection limit of 0.031 g/L and an inter-assay CV of 7.8% (n = 18). Casein:whey ratio was calculated as follows:

$$\textit{Casein:whey ratio} = \text{casein concentration/whey protein concentration}. \quad (4)$$

2.7.6. Lysozyme

Lysozyme concentration was determined using a modified turbidimetric assay [52]. Hen egg white lysozyme (EC 3.2.1.17, Sigma, St. Louis, MA, USA) standards (range 0.00075–0.0125 g/L) and skim milk samples were diluted 10-fold with 0.1 M of Na_2HPO_4/1.1 mM of citric acid (pH 5.8) buffer. Twenty-five microliters of standards or diluted skim milk samples were placed into the wells of a plate (Greiner Bio-One, Frickenhausen, Germany), 175 μL of *Micrococcus lysodeiltikus* suspension (0.075% *w/v*, ATCC No. 4698, Sigma, St. Louis, MA, USA) was added into each well and plate was incubated at RT for 1 h. The absorbance was measured at 450 nm. Recovery of lysozyme was 97.0% ± 5.0% (n = 8) with a detection limit of 0.007 g/L and an inter-assay CV of 13.0% (n = 8).

2.7.7. Carbohydrates

Defatted milk was deproteinized with trichloroacetic acid [53] before dehydration by sulphuric acid [54]. This technique reliably estimates concentrations and carbon content for monosaccharides, disaccharides, and polysaccharides. Total carbohydrates were analyzed by UV-spectrophotometry. Recovery of total carbohydrates was 101.4% ± 2.1% (n = 7) with a detection limit of 0.007 g/L and an inter-assay CV of 3.3% (n = 7).

Lactose concentration was measured using the enzymatic spectrophotometric method of Kuhn and Lowenstein [55], adapted from Mitoulas et al. [51], with recovery of 98.2% ± 4.1% (n = 10), detection limit of 30 mM and inter-assay CV of 3.5%.

The human milk oligosaccharides (HMO) concentration (g) was calculated by deducting concentration of lactose (g) from concentration of total carbohydrates (g). The glucose and galactose were not measured or accounted for as their concentrations in HM are small and comparable or less than the assays errors [56].

2.8. Hormone and Macronutrient Dose

Doses were defined as the amount of hormone/macronutrient ingested during a breastfeed and calculated as average of the pre- and post-feed HM component concentration, multiplied by the corresponding FV. When an infant fed from both breasts at the breastfeeding session, hormone/macronutrient doses from these individual breastfeeds were calculated separately and added together.

2.9. Infants' Anthropometrics and Body Composition

2.9.1. Anthropometric Measurements

Infants' weight was determined by weighing before breastfeeding using Medela Electronic Baby Weigh Scales (±2.0 g; Medela Inc., McHenry, IL, USA). Clothing was removed except for a dry diaper and a singlet. Infant crown-heel length was measured once to the nearest 0.1 cm using non-stretch tape and headpiece and footpiece, both applied perpendicular to the hard surface. Infant head circumference was measured with non-stretch tape. Infant BMI was calculated according to the following formula:

$$BMI = \text{Body weight (kg)}/(\text{Height (m)})^2. \quad (5)$$

2.9.2. Body Composition with Bioelectrical Impedance Spectroscopy

Infants' whole body bioimpedance were measured using the Impedimed SFB7 bioelectrical impedance analyzer (ImpediMed, Brisbane, Queensland, Australia) applying an adult protocol (wrist to ankle) according to the manufacturer's instructions and analyzed with settings customized for each infant according to Lingwood et al. [57] and Gridneva et al. [41]. Values of resistance (ohm) at frequency of 50 kHz (R_{50}) were determined from the curve of best fit, averaged for analysis purposes and used in the Lingwood et al. age matched (3 and 4.5 mo infants) equations for fat-free mass (FFM) of 2 and 5 mo infants respectively [57]:

$$FFM\ 3\ \text{mo} = 1.458 + 0.498 \times W - 0.197 \times S + 0.067 \times L^2/R_{50} \quad (6)$$

$$FM\ 4.5\ \text{mo} = 2.203 + 0.334 \times W - 0.361 \times S + 0.185 \times L^2/R_{50}, \quad (7)$$

where L is body length (cm), R_{50} is resistance (Ω), S is sex (male = 1, female = 2) and W is infant weight (kg).

%FM was calculated as follows:

$$\%FM = 100(\text{Weight (kg)} - \text{FFM (kg)})/\text{Weight (kg)}. \quad (8)$$

2.9.3. Body Composition with Ultrasound Skinfold Measurements

Infant ultrasound skinfold measurements were carried out using the Aplio XG (Toshiba, Tokyo, Japan) ultrasound machine, PLT-1204BX 14-8 MHz transducer and sterile water-based Parker ultrasonic gel (Fairfield, NJ, USA). Single ultrasound scans of four anatomical sites (biceps, subscapular, suprailiac, and triceps) were performed on the left side of the body with minimal compression. Skinfold thickness (skin thickness and the skin–fat interface to fat–muscle interface distance) was measured directly from images on the screen using electronic calipers. One experienced sonographer (DG) with good intra- and interrater reliability [44] performed all of the measurements.

The doubled ultrasound skinfold thickness was used in Brook body density (d) age-matched (3–18 mo) equations [58] developed for skinfolds measured with calipers:

$$\text{Male } d = 1.1690 - 0.0788 \times \log\left(\sum \text{SFT}\right) \quad (9)$$

$$\text{Female } d = 1.2063 - 0.0999 \times \log\left(\sum \text{SFT}\right), \quad (10)$$

where d is infant body density (kg/L) and $\sum$SFT is a sum of four skinfolds (mm).

Predicted body density was converted to %FM using the Lohman equation [59]:

$$\%FM = 100 \times (5.28/d - 4.89), \quad (11)$$

where d is the infant body density (kg/L).

2.10. Statistical Analysis

Statistical analysis was performed in R 2.9.0 [60] for Mac OSX using additional packages nlme [61]; lattice [62], lattice extra [63], and car [64]; MASS [65], sfsmisc [66] and multcomp [67] for mixed effects modeling, data representation, robust regression, and multiple comparisons of means, respectively. Descriptive statistics are reported as mean ± standard deviation (SD) (range) or median (IQR) unless otherwise stated; model parameters are presented as estimate ± standard error (SE), and, where appropriate, an approximate 95% confidence interval (95% CI).

Measurements missing due to insufficient sample volume: skim milk leptin, whole milk leptin, adiponectin, total protein, whey and casein protein, lactose and total carbohydrate (n = 3); lysozyme (n = 5). Measurements of fat (n = 14) were missing as a result of either insufficient sample volumes or absence of separate feed volumes from breasts where both breast were offered during one feed. Also missing were feeding frequency as reported by mothers (n = 6), measurements of length, head circumference, infant BMI, %FM measured with bioelectrical spectroscopy (n = 4) and %FM measured with ultrasound skinfolds (n = 5).

GE time was determined as the time from the start of F1 to the start of F2 and included the time between two feeds and feed duration. Feed duration was included as up to 80% of HM consumed by term healthy breastfed infants in the first 4–5 min [68]. GE during breastfeeding was defined as the volume of milk to have left the stomach, calculated as the difference between the immediate post-feed stomach volumes and the sum of R1 and FV.

Due to the lack of term infant gastric-emptying studies focusing on stomach volume, no power calculation/sample size determination could be performed for this study. A goal of 20 infants at each two and five months was selected with the expectation that this would be sufficient to show overall patterns. When available, infants were included in both subsets to allow for investigation of longitudinal patterns. Linear mixed effects models allow us to treat the individual feeds as separate, without having to assume independence, when there may be correlations between feeds within infants.

Influences on GE rate were analyzed by first fitting a time curve to the sequential post-feed stomach volumes using linear mixed effects models; as curves differed significantly within and between infants ($p < 0.001$), random time curves were fitted to feeds within infants. Time terms (linear, square root) were selected as per the fractional polynomial method of [69]; this model also considered possible confounding effects of FV (median-centred) and feed duration (median-centred). Interaction terms involving the time curve indicated changes in the GE rate; main effects indicated overall effects on post-feed stomach volumes but not the GE rate. The addition of one term to this base model was used to investigate associations with (a) concentrations/doses of hormones/macronutrients; (b) infant characteristics/anthropometrics/BC; (c) R1. Whether the overall effect of HM component concentrations differs by feed volume was investigated by including interactions between FV and concentration measures. Models using the selected technique did not converge for fat concentration, lysozyme concentration, or lysozyme dose. Omitting the random effect of feed within infant provided converging models, but no evidence of an association with fat or lysozyme was seen. Given the complexity of linear mixed effects models used to analyze GE rate, no further adjustments were performed and $p < 0.05$ was considered to be statistically significant.

Associations between pre-feed residual stomach volumes, FV, immediate post-feed stomach volumes, feed duration, feeding frequency and both hormone and macronutrient concentrations and doses, and infant anthropometrics/BC parameters were tested using robust linear regression. Mixed effects models were considered, but were not significantly better ($p > 0.1$) Robust linear regression (rlm) was chosen so as to address heteroscedasticity in the data and points with high leverage in the majority of the predictors; MM-estimation (M-estimation with Tukey's biweight, initialized by a specific S-estimator) accounting for appropriate covariates was used [65]. Approximate p-values were determined using the Wald test. Multivariate models accounting for FV were used for testing the relationship with FV-dependent predictor (fat dose and concentration).

Possible age differences in HM components, infant characteristics, and GE/breastfeeding parameters were analyzed with either linear mixed effects models or robust linear regression models; model type was determined using likelihood ratio tests. Linear mixed effects models were used to analyze relationships of GE during feed time with HM components and infant characteristics. R1, FV and feed duration were not associated with stomach volume reduction during the feed time, therefore univariate models were run. Multivariate linear mixed effects models accounting for R1, FV and feed duration were used in analysis of relationships of immediate post-feed stomach volumes with HM components and infant characteristics.

Owing to the large number of comparisons, a false discovery rate adjustment [70] was performed on associated subgroupings of results with one or more p-values < 0.05. p-values were considered to be significant at <0.011 for GE time, <0.031 for feeding frequency, <0.038 for R2, and <0.008 for associations between HM components' concentrations.

3. Results

3.1. Participants

Characteristics of the 27 participants (2 months (n = 20; longitudinal: 7 females, 7 males; cross-sectional: 2 females, 4 males); 5 months (n = 21; longitudinal: 7 females, 7 males; cross-sectional: 6 females); overall n = 41 feeds) are described in Table 1. At the study session, infants fed from one (n = 23) or both (n = 18) breasts.

3.2. Influence of Infant Age

Infant anthropometrics and %FM measured with bioimpedance spectroscopy significantly differed by infant age ($p < 0.001$), while breastfeeding and GE parameters did not change significantly ($p > 0.067$) (Table 1).

Lower whey protein concentration (5.51 ± 0.96 g/L 5 mo vs. 6.41 ± 1.39 g/L 2 mo, $p = 0.034$) and subsequently a higher casein:whey ratio (0.32 ± 0.14 5 mo vs. 0.22 ± 0.07 2 mo, $p = 0.035$) were observed at 5 months. All other measured appetite hormones and macronutrient concentrations did not differ significantly by infant age ($p > 0.053$).

3.3. Analyzed Human Milk Components

Appetite hormones and macronutrient concentrations and doses per feed are presented in Table 2. Higher skim milk leptin concentrations were associated with lower whole milk leptin concentrations (−0.25 [−0.34, −0.16], $p < 0.001$) and higher protein concentrations were associated with higher whey protein concentrations (0.68 [0.41, 0.95], $p < 0.001$). Higher HMO concentrations were associated with higher total carbohydrates concentrations ($p < 0.001$) and lower lactose concentrations ($p < 0.001$).

Table 1. Participant characteristics expressed as mean ± SD and range.

Characteristics	2 mo [a]		5 mo [b]		Total [c]	
	Mean ± SD	Range	Mean ± SD	Range	Mean ± SD	Range
Infant characteristics						
Infant age (weeks)	9 ± 1	6–10	22 ± 1	18–23	16 ± 7	6–23
Infant length (cm)	57 ± 2	53–61	65 ± 2 ***	62–69	61 ± 4	53–69
Infant weight (kg)	5.3 ± 0.8	4.2–6.3	7.2 ± 1.0 ***	5.8–9.5	6.3 ± 1.3	4.2–9.5
Infant BMI	15.9 ± 1.3	13.9–18.1	17.6 ± 1.7 ***	14.9–20.4	16.7 ± 1.7	13.9–20.4
HC (cm)	39 ± 1	37–42	43 ± 2 ***	40–46	41 ± 2	37–46
Fat Mass with BIS (%)	21.4 ± 3.6	11.1–27.1	28.9 ± 3.2 ***	21.7–35.8	25.3 ± 5.0	11.1–35.8
Fat Mass with US (%)	24.2 ± 3.6	17.5–30.5	26.6 ± 3.6	20.8–35.9	25.5 ± 3.8	17.5–35.9
BF/GE characteristics						
Feed volume (mL)	86 ± 34	35–140	85 ± 33	36–180	86 ± 33	35–180
SV after feed 1 (mL)	87 ± 36	32–141	93 ± 41	22–189	90 ± 38	22–189
Feed duration (min)	28 ± 14	11–72	20 ± 8	6–37	24 ± 12	6–72
SV reduction (mL) [d]	5 ± 21	(−42)–33	4 ± 26	(−57)–56	4 ± 24	(−57)–56
GE time (min) [e]	94 ± 29	44–153	88 ± 18	50–140	91 ± 24	44–140
Residual 1 (mL)	6 ± 12	0–50	11 ± 19	0–62	9 ± 16	0–62
Residual 2 (mL)	20 ± 20	0–81	15 ± 15	0–55	18 ± 18	0–81
Feeding frequency (h) [f]	2.3 ± 0.7	1.0–4.0	2.7 ± 0.8	1.5–4.0	2.5 ± 0.7	1.0–4.0

Data are mean ± SD and ranges. [a] $n = 20$; [b] $n = 21$. [c] $n = 41$ feeds. [d] Stomach volume reduction during feed time is calculated as the difference between the sum of residual 1 and feed volume and the immediate stomach volume after Feed 1 . [e] GE time is the time from the start of Feed 1 to the start of Feed 2 (time between feeds plus feed duration). [f] Feeding frequency self-reported by mothers as to how often infant feeds (e.g., every three hours). *** Indicates significant differences ($p < 0.001$) between two- and five-month-old infants. Abbreviations: BF—breastfeeding; BIS—bioimpedance spectroscopy; GE—gastric emptying; HC—head circumference; SV—stomach volume; US—ultrasound.

Table 2. Concentrations and doses of measured HM hormones and macronutrients.

Components	Concentration		Dose Per Feed	
	Mean ± SD	Range	Mean ± SD	Range
Adiponectin (ng/mL, ng)	10.02 ± 4.08	6.18–22.58	868.62 ± 491.32	238.60–2536.91
WM leptin (ng/mL, ng)	0.51 ± 0.18	0.23–1.10	44.80 ± 24.30	10.15–115.03
SM leptin (ng/mL, ng)	0.28 ± 0.12	0.20–0.84	24.8 ± 15.0	6.91–73.00
Total protein (g/L, g)	11.29 ± 2.56	7.60–24.16	0.99 ± 0.39	0.35–2.29
Casein (g/L, g)	1.54 ± 0.53	0.69–3.45	0.14 ± 0.07	0.04–0.29
Whey protein (g/L, g)	5.97 ± 1.26	3.82–9.08	0.52 ± 0.19	0.17–0.95
Casein:whey ratio	0.27 ± 0.11	0.10–0.73	n/a [a]	n/a [a]
Lysozyme (g/L, g)	0.14 ± 0.12	0.05–0.48	0.01 ± 0.01	0.003–0.030
TCH (g/L, g)	82.72 ± 7.89	67.08–97.49	7.28 ± 2.62	3.28–15.18
Lactose (g/L, g)	65.84 ± 5.14	53.49–77.94	5.86 ± 2.22	2.19–12.06
HMO (g/L, g)	16.88 ± 9.89	(−10.86) [b]–35.77	1.42 ± 0.94	(−1.09) [b]–3.78
Fat (g/L, g)	42.74 ± 12.10	17.42–66.79	3.57 ± 1.45	0.64–6.40

Data are mean ± SD and ranges, $n = 41$ feeds. [a] Casein:whey ratios for doses are the same as for concentrations. [b] Negative values are seen for human milk oligosaccharides (HMO) when lactose measurements are higher than total carbohydrates. Abbreviations: SM—skim milk; TCH—total carbohydrates; WM—whole milk.

3.4. Gastric Emptying Rate

The overall decreasing curvilinear pattern of GE (linear: 0.04 [−0.17, 0.24], $p = 0.72$; square root: −10.5 [−12.7, −8.2], $p < 0.001$) is shown in Figure 2. Higher FVs were associated with faster

(−0.07 [−0.10, −0.03], $p < 0.001$) GE rate (Figure 3) and higher overall post-feed stomach volumes (0.82 [0.53, 1.12], $p < 0.001$). No association was seen between feed duration and post-feed stomach volume (−0.25 [−0.68, 0.18], $p = 0.23$).

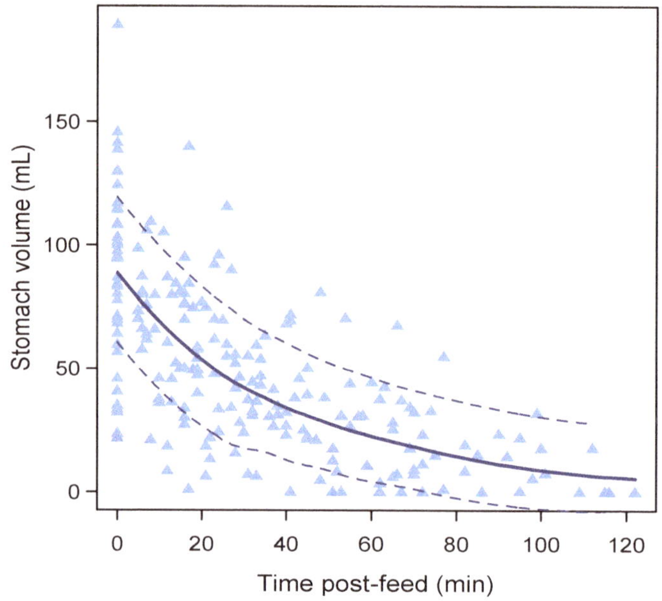

Figure 2. Overall curvilinear pattern of gastric emptying (n = 41 feeds). The lines represent the overall pattern of changes in stomach volume as measured by ultrasound imaging. Bold line represents local regression smoother (LOESS, span = 0.9). Dotted lines represent confidence interval.

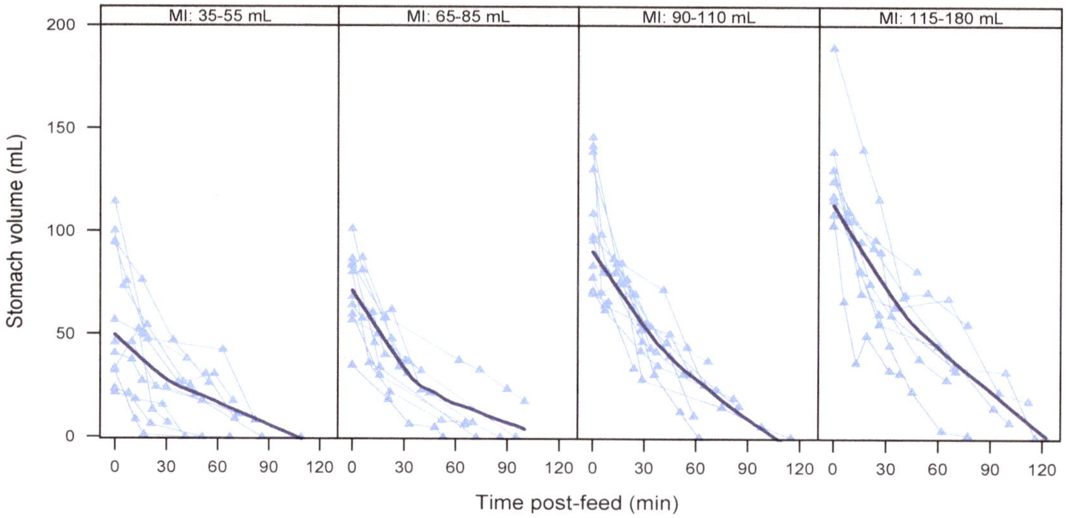

Figure 3. Gastric emptying of individual feeds in term breastfed infants (n = 41 feeds). Feeds are grouped by milk intake (MI) to illustrate the effect of the feed volumes; approximately equal numbers are included in each panel. Data points represent stomach volumes calculated from ultrasound images; connecting lines link measurements from the same feed. Bold line represents local regression smoother (LOESS, span = 0.9).

Immediate post-feed stomach volumes were not associated with R1 ($p = 0.91$).

After accounting for time post-feed, FV, and feed duration, as per the above model, larger R1 volumes (0.55 [0.24, 0.86], $p = 0.003$) and higher whey protein concentrations (4.99 [0.84, 9.13], $p = 0.023$) were associated with larger post-feed stomach volumes, while the casein:whey ratio (2.2 ± 0.88, $p = 0.030$) and lactose concentration (−0.04 ± 0.02, $p = 0.037$) modified the GE curve depending on

FV. Higher casein:whey ratios at lower FVs were associated with faster GE, and at higher FVs with slower GE, while higher lactose concentrations at lower FVs were associated with slower GE, and at higher FVs with faster GE. No other associations with post-feed stomach volumes or changes to the GE curves were found (Table 3).

Table 3. HM components and infant characteristics and their associations with feed variables and gastric emptying.

Predictors	Feed Volume [a]		Gastric Emptying Time [a]		Post-Feed Stomach Volumes [b]	
	Estimate ± SE (95% CI)	*p*-Value	Estimate ± SE (95% CI)	*p*-Value	Estimate ± SE (95% CI)	*p*-Value
Concentrations						
Adiponectin (ng/mL)	1 ± 1.3 (−36.6, 134.5)	0.44	2.3 ± 0.7 (0.9, 3.7)	**0.002** [c]	1.3 ± 0.7 (−0.2, 2.7)	0.081
Whole milk leptin (ng/mL)	9.9 ± 29.9 (−36.6, 134.5)	0.74	6.8 ± 15.8 (−24.2, 37.8)	0.67	−9.5 ± 13.3 (−35.8, 16.9)	0.48
Skim milk leptin (ng/mL)	49 ± 43.6 (−36.6, 134.5)	0.26	6.7 ± 24.3 (−41, 54.4)	0.78	39.8 ± 18.4 (−0.8, 80.3)	0.054
Total protein (g/L)	−2.1 ± 2.1 (−6.2, 1.9)	0.30	−0.9 ± 1.1 (−3.1, 1.3)	0.41	1.1 ± 1 (−1.2, 3.4)	0.30
Whey protein (g/L)	−5.5 ± 4.2 (−13.8, 2.7)	0.19	5.8 ± 2.2 (1.6, 10.1)	0.011	5 ± 1.9 (0.8, 9.1)	**0.023**
Casein (g/L)	2.6 ± 10.2 (−17.4, 22.5)	0.80	−12.4 ± 4.7 (−21.5, −3.2)	0.013	−2 ± 4.4 (−11.6, 7.6)	0.66
Casein:whey ratio	24.5 ± 46.1 (−65.9, 114.9)	0.59	−65.9 ± 21 (−107.1, −24.7)	**0.003**	−17.3 ± 20.1 (−61.4, 26.9)	0.41
Lysozyme (g/L)	−81.4 ± 46.2 (−172, 9.1)	0.079	−19.5 ± 28.3 (−75, 36)	0.49	23.3 ± 15.4 (−7.2, 53.8)	0.13
Total carbohydrates (g/L)	−1.1 ± 0.7 (−2.3, 0.2)	0.12	−0.6 ± 0.4 (−1.3, 0.1)	0.10	−0.5 ± 0.3 (−1.2, 0.1)	0.089
Lactose (g/L)	0.7 ± 1.1 (−1.4, 2.7)	0.51	0.2 ± 0.6 (−0.9, 1.3)	0.76	0.03 ± 0.49 (−1, 1.1)	0.96
HMO (g/L)	−0.8 ± 0.5 (−1.9, 0.2)	0.13	−0.4 ± 0.3 (−1, 0.2)	0.16	−0.4 ± 0.2 (−0.9, 0.1)	0.13
Fat (g/L)	−0.69 ± 0.6 (−1.8, 0.5)	0.26	−0.1 ± 0.3 (−0.6, 0.5)	0.79	−0.1 ± 0.3 (−0.9, 0.6)	0.71
Doses						
Adiponectin (ng)	n/a [d]	n/a [d]	0.02 ± 0.01 (0.01, 0.03)	**0.005**	0.01 ± 0.01 (−0.003, 0.03)	0.094
Whole milk leptin (ng)	n/a	n/a	−0.1 ± 0.2 (−0.4, 0.2)	0.44	−0.2 ± 0.2 (−0.5, 0.2)	0.28
Skim milk leptin (ng)	n/a	n/a	−0.2 ± 0.2 (−0.7, 0.3)	0.38	0.4 ± 0.2 (−0.1, 0.8)	0.086
Total protein (g)	n/a	n/a	−25.9 ± 12.4 (−50.2, −1.7)	0.040	15 ± 13.1 (−13.7, 43.7)	0.27
Whey protein (g)	n/a	n/a	47.6 ± 18.7 (10.8, 84.3)	0.015	50.6 ± 24.3 (−2.8, 104)	0.061
Casein (g)	n/a	n/a	−119 ± 53.3 (−223.4, −14.6)	0.030	0.4 ± 47.6 (−104.2, 105.1)	0.99
Lysozyme (g)	n/a	n/a	−276.2 ± 370.7 (−1002.9, 450.4)	0.46	395.5 ± 258.3 (−114.7, 905.6)	0.13
Total carbohydrates (g)	n/a	n/a	−4.1 ± 1.8 (−7.6, −0.5)	0.030	−4.6 ± 3 (−11.2, 2.1)	0.16
Lactose (g)	n/a	n/a	−5.8 ± 2.7 (−11.1, −0.6)	0.037	−3.1 ± 5.4 (−15.1, 8.9)	0.58
HMO (g)	n/a	n/a	−3.1 ± 3.1 (−9.2, 3)	0.32	−3.2 ± 2.7 (−9.1, 2.8)	0.27
Fat (g)	n/a	n/a	−2.8 ± 2.7 (−8.1, 2.4)	0.30	−4.9 ± 2.8 (−12.7, 2.8)	0.15

Table 3. *Cont.*

Predictors	Feed Volume [a]		Gastric Emptying Time [a]		Post-Feed Stomach Volumes [b]	
	Estimate ± SE (95% CI)	*p*-Value	Estimate ± SE (95% CI)	*p*-Value	Estimate ± SE (95% CI)	*p*-Value
Demographics						
Infant sex (Male)	−2.2 ± 10.7 (−23.1, 18.8)	0.84	−1.5 ± 7.5 (−16.3, 13.2)	0.84	−8.4 ± 4.6 (−17.8, 1.1)	0.081
Infant age (months)	−0.9 ± 3.6 (−7.9, 6)	0.80	−1.8 ± 2.5 (−6.6, 3)	0.47	−1.5 ± 1.4 (−4.5, 1.6)	0.32
Anthropometrics						
Infant length (cm)	−0.03 ± 1.3 (−2.6, 2.6)	0.98	−1.3 ± 0.9 (−3, 0.4)	0.15	−0.5 ± 0.6 (−1.8, 0.8)	0.44
Infant weight (kg)	0.7 ± 4.1 (−7.4, 8.8)	0.87	−2.3 ± 2.9 (−7.9, 3.4)	0.43	−2.3 ± 1.8 (−6.3, 1.7)	0.23
Head circumference (cm)	−2.5 ± 2.6 (−7.5, 2.5)	0.34	−1.4 ± 1.8 (−4.9, 2.1)	0.42	−1.8 ± 1.2 (−4.5, 0.8)	0.15
Infant BMI	−0.2 ± 3.2 (−6.5, 6)	0.94	−1.5 ± 2.2 (−5.8, 2.8)	0.48	−3.2 ± 1.5 (−6.6, 0.2)	0.062
Body composition						
Fat mass with US (%)	0.6 ± 1.4 (−2.2, 3.4)	0.67	−0.3 ± 0.9 (−2.2, 1.5)	0.71	−0.6 ± 0.7 (−2.1, 1.0)	0.42
Fat mass with BIS (%)	0.4 ± 1.1 (−1.8, 2.5)	0.74	−0.4 ± 0.7 (−1.9, 1)	0.56	−0.5 ± 0.5 (−1.5, 0.5)	0.35

Data are parameter estimate ± SE and 95% CI, n = 41 feeds. [a] Effects of predictors taken from univariate regression models; [b] Effects of predictors taken from linear mixed effects models that accounted for postprandial time, feed volume and feed duration. [c] After the false discovery rate adjustment the *p*-values were considered to be significant at <0.011 for GE time (bold font); [d] n/a—dosage is dependent on feed volume. Abbreviations: BIS—bioimpedance spectroscopy; HMO—human milk oligosaccharides; US—ultrasound skinfolds.

3.5. Feed Volume, Feed Duration, and Gastric Emptying during Breastfeeding

Higher FVs were associated with higher stomach volumes measured immediately post-feed (0.79 [0.51, 1.07], $p < 0.001$) and longer GE times (0.24 [0.03, 0.46], $p = 0.033$). FV was not associated with either concentrations of measured HM components or infant's characteristics/anthropometrics/BC (Table 3).

Feed duration was not associated with FV (0.06 [−0.03, 0.15], $p = 0.20$) or R1 volume (0.01 [−0.17, 0.19], $p = 0.91$).

After accounting for R1 (1.07 [0.47, 1.7], $p = 0.002$), FV (1.00 [0.71, 1.3], $p < 0.001$) and feed duration (−0.30 [−0.96, 0.36], $p = 0.34$), immediate post-feed stomach volumes were not associated with either measured HM components ($p > 0.068$) or infant's demographics/anthropometrics/BC ($p > 0.46$). Stomach volume reduction during breastfeeding was not associated with either measured HM components ($p > 0.11$); infant's demographics/anthropometrics/BC ($p > 0.48$); R1, FV or feed duration ($p > 0.34$).

3.6. Gastric Emptying Time

The GE time was not associated with feed duration (0.35 [−0.29, 0.98], $p = 0.28$), but was negatively associated with R2 (−0.63 [−1.05, −0.21], $p = 0.005$) after accounting for FV ($p < 0.001$). Longer GE times were associated with higher adiponectin concentration (2.3 [0.9, 3.7], $p = 0.002$) and dose (0.02 [0.01, 0.03], $p = 0.005$), and lower casein:whey ratio (−65.9 [−107.1, −24.7], $p = 0.003$). No associations with infant characteristics were seen (Table 3).

3.7. Pre-Feed Residuals

Infants cued for F1 and F2 with different residual volumes (R1 and R2) present in their stomachs (Table 1). Larger FVs were associated with smaller R1 volumes ($p = 0.002$), with each

−0.92 [−1.47, −0.37] mL of R1 volume resulting in extra mL of FV. Larger R2 volumes were associated with larger FVs ($p = 0.006$), each additional mL of FV resulting in 0.21 [0.07, 0.35] mL greater R2.

There was no association between R2 and R1 in univariate model (0.11 [−0.19, 0.42], $p = 0.46$). After accounting for FV and GE time ($p < 0.001$ for both) larger R2 volumes were associated with larger R1 volumes (0.36 [0.11, 0.60], $p = 0.005$).

After accounting for FV, R2 was not associated with any concentration of HM components ($p \geq 0.038$ after adjusting for multiple comparisons).

3.8. Feeding Frequency

A longer time between the feeds was seen when infants were longer, heavier, and had higher %FM measured with BIS (Table 4) in univariate models. The associations for length and weight were not significant after accounting for the other ($p > 0.38$); the association for %FM measured with BIS was not significant after accounting for infant length ($p = 0.095$).

Table 4. Associations between infant feeding frequency and HM components and infant characteristics.

Predictors	Feeding Frequency (h) [a]	
	Estimate ± SE (95% CI) [b]	*p*-Value
Concentrations		
Adiponectin (ng/mL)	−0.001 ± 0.03 (−0.06, 0.06)	0.96
Whole milk leptin (ng/mL)	−1.1 ± 0.7 (−2.5, 0.3)	0.13
Skim milk leptin (ng/mL)	0.8 ± 1.6 (−2.3, 4)	0.60
Total protein (g/L)	−0.05 ± 0.05 (−0.15, 0.04)	0.28
Whey protein (g/L)	−0.1 ± 0.1 (−0.3, 0.1)	0.42
Casein (g/L)	0.04 ± 0.2 (−0.4, 0.5)	0.86
Casein:whey protein ratio	0.4 ± 1.1 (−1.7, 2.5)	0.68
Lysozyme (g/L)	−0.4 ± 1.1 (−2.5, 1.7)	0.71
Total carbohydrates (g/L)	0.01 ± 0.02 (−0.03, 0.04)	0.73
Lactose (g/L)	−0.05 ± 0.02 (−0.1, −0.01)	0.031
HMO (g/L)	0.01 ± 0.02 (−0.03, 0.04)	0.73
Fat (g/L)	−0.02 ± 0.01 (−0.04, 0.01)	0.19
Doses		
Adiponectin (ng/mL)	0.0002 ± 0.0003 (−0.0004, 0.0008)	0.50
Whole milk leptin (ng/mL)	−0.002 ± 0.01 (−0.01, 0.01)	0.80
Skim milk leptin (ng/mL)	0.01 ± 0.01 (−0.01, 0.03)	0.59
Total protein (g/L)	0.1 ± 0.3 (−0.5, 0.8)	0.67
Whey protein (g/L)	0.1 ± 0.7 (−1.3, 1.5)	0.89
Casein (g/L)	2.1 ± 2 (−1.7, 5.9)	0.27
Lysozyme (g/L)	−5.7 ± 17.2 (−39.4, 27.9)	0.73
Total carbohydrates (g/L)	0.1 ± 0.1 (0, 0.2)	0.22
Lactose (g/L)	0.04 ± 0.06 (−0.08, 0.17)	0.49
HMO (g/L)	0.3 ± 0.1 (0, 0.5)	0.051
Fat (g/L)	−0.2 ± 0.1 (−0.5, 0)	0.085
Demographics		
Infant sex (Male)	−0.2 ± 0.3 (−0.7, 0.4)	0.53
Infant age (months)	0.2 ± 0.1 (0, 0.3)	0.078
Anthropometrics		
Infant length (cm)	0.1 ± 0.03 (0.04, 0.15)	**0.004** [c]
Infant weight (kg)	0.2 ± 0.1 (0.1, 0.4)	**0.010**
Head circumference (cm)	0.1 ± 0.1 (0, 0.2)	0.23
Infant BMI	0.13 ± 0.1 (0, 0.3)	0.10
Body composition		
% fat mass with US	0.07 ± 0.03 (0, 0.13)	0.040
% fat mass with BIS	0.08 ± 0.02 (0.03, 0.12)	**0.002**

Data are parameter estimate ± SE and 95% CI, $n = 41$ feeds. [a] Feeding frequency self-reported by mothers as to how often infant feeds (e.g., every three hours). [b] Effects of predictors are results of univariate regression model. [c] After the false discovery rate adjustment the p-values were considered to be significant at <0.031 (highlighted). Abbreviations: BIS—bioimpedance spectroscopy; HMO—human milk oligosaccharides; US—ultrasound skinfolds.

4. Discussion

Our research shows that HM components, such as adiponectin, whey protein, casein: whey ratios, lactose, total carbohydrates, and oligosaccharides are associated with gastric emptying and breastfeeding patterns of breastfed infants. GE is a mechanism involved in satiety, therefore milk components influencing GE have the potential to affect infant milk intake and therefore growth and development in early life and subsequently health later in life.

Given the assumption that HM composition potentially influences GE [14,71], in term infants we expected the appetite hormones to be associated with infant GE rate such that high concentrations and/or doses of leptin would result in slower GE [30], whereas adiponectin might induce faster GE [37] consistent with both animal and human models. However, neither the concentrations nor doses of these hormones were related to GE rate. Previously skim milk leptin was not found to be associated with either GE rate or GE time [33,34], which we have confirmed with this larger study cohort. It was speculated that whole milk leptin, which is known to be of higher concentration, might be the reason for the negative finding [32]. While our measures of whole milk leptin were typically higher, there is an opinion that values of this magnitude are unlikely to contribute considerably to infant serum levels [72] so only the local pathways would be engaged in GE regulation. As such we were unable to find a relationship between whole milk leptin and GE. This is in contrast to animal studies showing reduced GE [30] or food intake [31] after injection or oral administration of leptin, respectively. However, it is possible that the long-term energy expenditure regulatory effect of leptin [73] may mask its short-term satiety effect on GE. Alternatively, if levels of leptin are contributing significantly to serum levels, there is a possibility that the number of receptors in the stomach of the young infant is low. Further, short-term satiety signaling through hypothalamic neurons is not fully mature, both of which would allow the infant to maintain a high physiological drive to feed to ensure adequate growth [28,73]. Gender differences in infant serum leptin levels associated with adiposity [74] have also been speculated to play a role in gastric response to HM leptin, although we did not find any relationships between infant sex/adiposity and both GE rate and GE time.

In contrast to leptin, we found that increased levels and doses of adiponectin were associated with longer GE times. This finding may partially explain the growth-regulating effect of adiponectin in infants in the first six months of life [29], when high HM adiponectin concentration is associated with lower infant weight and adiposity. Further adiponectin is 20-fold higher in concentration compared to leptin and is therefore likely to have greater biological significance [75]. The lack of association between adiponectin and GE rate is in agreement with studies of rats that showed that gastric epithelium and glands are populated with adiponectin receptors, which downregulate gastric motility [36,76]. Conversely, the findings are in contrast to studies of type 2 diabetic adults, in which elevated levels of adiponectin were associated with faster GE [37]. Further, other HM hormones such as ghrelin, cholecystokinin, and insulin may counteract or interact synergistically with leptin [77,78] and/or adiponectin.

Our study examined an extensive array of macronutrients beyond fat, total protein and lactose. Consistent with the findings of Cannon et al. [34] there were no associations with fat and total protein and either GE rate or GE time. Studies in dogs indicate that all three major macronutrients activate the ileal brake, resulting in reduction of GE; limited human studies support the findings for fat and carbohydrates while associations with protein are not so straightforward [79,80]. We were unable to find associations between the HM fat content and GE consistent with findings of Khan et al. [39] and Kent et al. [38] regarding the feeding frequency. This may be because lipids initiate the ileal brake when they reach the ileum via hydrolysis of triacylglycerol into fatty acids, thereby producing a delay in GE in humans [79]. Further analysis of HM fatty acids may shed more light on GE in breastfed infants.

However, we have found that higher whey protein concentrations are associated with larger post-feed stomach volumes, although we did not see any interaction with time, so no effect on GE rate was detected. This contradicts the results of studies of GE conducted on breastfed and formula-fed infants or studies of formula with different casein:whey ratio [15,81] in which a fast or slow GE rate was explained by concentrations of whey protein or casein, respectively. Previous studies, however, could not adequately analyze the effect of the whey protein concentration in conjunction with volume, as they only reported gastric half-emptying time, restricted monitoring time, and/or controlled infants' volume intakes. The whey fraction of HM is highly soluble in the gastric juices and rapidly empties from the stomach compared to other proteins such as casein. Whey isolate, however, was associated with a lower gastric inhibitory polypeptide (GIP) response in adults, consistent with decreased rate of GE [82]. It may very well be that whey protein speeds up the initial stage of GE (probably during the breastfeeding time), but once it activates jejunal or ileal brakes the overall GE is reduced.

While lactose is related to GE rate, it is affected by FV; at the middle range FVs (71–108 mL) lactose has no relationship with GE, whereas at lower FVs higher lactose concentrations are associated with slower GE, and at higher FVs with faster GE. These results are consistent with Khan et al. [39], who reported an association of higher lactose concentration with increased feeding frequency. These findings could be an important addition to the evaluation of the digestive and metabolic effect of lower breastfeeding frequency and larger FVs, common in Western countries, contrary to the lactation practices in traditional societies [83].

In terms of casein:whey ratios the effect is opposite to that of lactose where at lower FVs higher casein:whey ratios are associated with faster GE, and at higher FVs with slower GE, which may explain the contradictory findings for casein associations with GE rate in previous studies [14,23]. Cows' milk casein was found to activate the ileal brake in adults, resulting in reduced food intake, although its effect on GE was not significant [84]. The finding of smaller volumes resulting in more rapid GE rate might be explained by the time casein spends in the acidic environment of the stomach. While soluble whey proteins rapidly enter the small intestine mostly intact, casein transit is delayed due to the curd formation. When it exits the stomach it is mainly in the form of degraded peptides [85]. If the FVs are small some casein may exit intact, thereby speeding up GE, while if the FVs are large, casein curdles and degrades to the opioid peptides that slow down GE [86]. However, this mechanism does not explain why higher casein:whey ratios of HM were associated with shorter GE time, which could be due to the smaller amounts of whey protein reaching the small intestine and having less effect on jejunal or ileal brakes [80]. Our finding that higher whey protein concentrations are associated with larger post-feed stomach volumes further supports this possible explanation.

Further, *k*-casein has been shown to inhibit the binding of *Helicobacter pylori* to human mucosa in vitro [87]. *Helicobacter pylori* are Gram-negative bacteria present in the stomach, and are known to downregulate levels of ghrelin and leptin in the stomach [88], which may significantly affect GE. The protective action of HM *k*-casein is reinforced by lysozyme, one of the major whey proteins. While we have not seen any significant associations between lysozyme and GE, lysozyme contributes to the control of the GI bacterial population [89], and could be upregulated to control the bacterial population in the GI tract [90] and increase digestion of microbial protein [24], all of which could potentially influence GE. In a clinical study of preterm infants, lysozyme added to donor HM or formula was associated with increased body weight, normalization of the stool, and improved feed tolerance [91]. While all of this suggests that lysozyme could potentially have an effect on GE in certain circumstances, given that we have studied a healthy population the magnitude of the effect could be insignificant.

GE during feed administration has been previously documented in preterm infants. In this study, an average of 20% of feed volume is emptied from the stomach during breastfeeding compared with 10% in preterm [92]. This is probably due to a more mature GI tract in term infants and the effect of both larger FVs and present pre-feed residuals, which were associated with faster GE rate, but not to the longer feed duration time in term infants or milk composition as no associations were found.

While we speculated that milk composition might regulate the milk intake of the infant and/or the residual volume in the stomach prior to cueing for the next feed, we were unable to show this. Rather, FV is more strongly associated with GE rate than variations in milk composition.

Gastric mechanosensation is an important factor in the regulation of satiation during food intake. Indeed, gastric distention is an important determinant of GE [93], and volume-related suppression of GE rate has been reported in animal models [94]. The observed volume-related acceleration of GE with larger FVs emptying more quickly in term breastfed infants is consistent with our previous findings [34]. The biggest effect of volume was seen after the feed and as the post-prandial period progressed the magnitude of this effect decreased (Figure 2). This may also explain the variability in the time between each feed for an infant over a 24-h period [33,38]. Feeding frequency decreases between one and three months of lactation, while milk intake during each breastfeeding session increases, with both parameters remaining constant up to six months [95]. This is attributed to the fact that as infants mature they become able to consume larger FVs [38], resulting in a longer time between feeds. Also, larger FVs are generally consumed at night or in the early morning when the frequency of feeding declines [33,38]. This decline in feeding frequency also coincides with higher nocturnal concentrations of leptin and fat, and lower concentrations of lactose in HM [33], although relationships between both feeding frequency and FV and these components' concentrations are yet to be evaluated.

The recommendations for breastfeeding are to feed on demand. Interestingly, we found that the majority of infants cued for a feed when milk was still present in the stomach, albeit in variable volumes (Table 1). This suggests that the reduction of gastric distension, which regulates hunger sensations, plays a greater role in signaling time to feed [96]. Further, it may be beneficial to the developing infant to have the gastric mucosa exposed to HM anti-inflammatory components such as lysozyme or immunomodulatory agents and growth factors, all of which contribute to the maturation of the GI tract [8]. Thus it may be detrimental to prescribe decreasing the frequency of feeding in breastfed infants or expect the infant stomach to be empty in order to feed again [97].

Furthermore, interesting associations were observed between infant milk intake and volumes remaining in the stomach prior to the first and second feed. Smaller residual volumes prior to the first feed were associated with greater milk intakes, and greater milk intakes were associated with larger volumes in the stomach prior to feeding again. This suggests that breastfed infants may appear to be consuming HM volumes in a variable pattern, but due to varying residuals may actually be feeding to a predetermined stomach volume, which is also supported by the positive relationship between both pre-feed residuals (R1, R2). In fasting adults ghrelin was found to increase and spontaneously decrease at the time points of the customary meals [98], supporting the involvement of the brain in GI tract regulation. Further studies monitoring two or more consecutive feeds or even 24-h GE measurements and analyses of ghrelin in HM would clarify this finding.

In healthy adults post-lag GE and colonic transfer is reported to be faster in men than in women [99]. In this study infant sex, age, anthropometrics, and BC were not associated with GE and breastfeeding parameters, with the exception of feeding frequency. Feeding frequency decreases in the first three months of lactation and then remains stable until six months [95,100]. The absence of a significant association between feeding frequency and age, together with associations with anthropometric and body composition parameters, illustrates that feeding frequency is dictated by the growth and development of an infant rather than the infant age. These findings further underline the need for breastfeeding on demand, with the frequency linked to individual infant growth rates rather than scheduled feeding, which could exert a detrimental effect on infant growth.

While the monitoring of a single feed limits the analysis possibilities, examination of multiple feeds requires the study to be carried out in the mother's home for long periods of time. The sample size is not a limitation of the study, as although no associations between milk composition and GE rate were detected, we were able to clearly show a relationship between FV and GE rate as well as associations between milk composition and other GE parameters.

5. Conclusions

Human milk appetite hormones and macronutrients and feed volume affect gastric emptying and feeding patterns in term breastfed infants. Adiponectin, whey protein, and casein:whey ratio are associated with GE, while the effects of casein:whey ratios and lactose concentrations on GE vary with feed volume. Larger feed volumes result in a faster GE rate. Thus, milk composition and feed volume play an important role in appetite regulation via gastric function.

Acknowledgments: All authors read and approved the final manuscript. The authors are grateful to all participants for their time and effort. The authors would like to thank Anna M. Cannon for establishing the methodology of appetite hormones assays (leptin) in human milk. This study was supported by an Australian Postgraduate Award from the University of Western Australia (Australia) and an unrestricted research grant from Medela AG (Switzerland).

Author Contributions: Zoya Gridneva conceived and designed of the study, collected the data, performed biochemical analysis, performed the statistical analyses, and wrote the manuscript; Sambavi Kugananthan adapted the methods for measuring adiponectin and leptin in whole milk, performed the hormone analysis, and critically reviewed the manuscript; Anna R. Hepworth was involved in research design, data analysis, and interpretation, and critically reviewed the manuscript; Wan J. Tie performed biochemical analysis and critically reviewed the manuscript; Ching T. Lai performed biochemical analysis, provided technical support, and critically reviewed the manuscript; Leigh C. Ward provided technical and educational support, contributed to the design of the study, and critically reviewed the manuscript; Peter E. Hartmann substantially contributed to the conception and design of the study, contributed reagents/materials/analysis tools for research, and critically reviewed the manuscript; Donna T. Geddes conceived and designed of the study, carried out the ultrasonography component of the study, provided the ultrasound images, and critically reviewed the manuscript. All authors have read and approved the final manuscript as submitted and agree to be accountable for all aspects of the work.

1. Geddes, D.; Prescott, S. Developmental origins of health and disease: The role of human milk in preventing disease in the 21(st) century. *J. Hum. Lact.* **2013**, *29*, 123–127. [CrossRef] [PubMed]
2. Marseglia, L.; Manti, S.; D'Angelo, G.; Cuppari, C.; Salpietro, V.; Filippelli, M.; Trovato, A.; Gitto, E.; Salpietro, C.; Arrigo, T. Obesity and breastfeeding: The strength of association. *Women Birth* **2015**, *28*, 81–86. [CrossRef] [PubMed]
3. Savino, F.; Liguori, S.; Fissore, M.; Oggero, R. Breast milk hormones and their protective effect on obesity. *Int. J. Pediatr. Endocrinol.* **2009**. [CrossRef]
4. Bartok, C. Babies fed breastmilk by breast versus by bottle: A pilot study evaluating early growth patterns. *Breastfeed. Med.* **2011**, *6*, 117–124. [CrossRef] [PubMed]
5. Sievers, E.; Oldigs, H.D.; Santer, R.; Schaub, J. Feeding patterns in breast-fed and formula-fed infants. *Ann. Nutr. Metab.* **2001**, *46*, 243–248. [CrossRef]
6. Le Huërou-Luron, I.; Bouzerzour, K.; Ferret-Bernard, S.; Ménard, O.; Le Normand, L.; Perrier, C.; Le Bourgot, C.; Jardin, J.; Bourlieu, C.; Carton, T.; et al. A mixture of milk and vegetable lipids in infant formula changes gut digestion, mucosal immunity and microbiota composition in neonatal piglets. *Eur. J. Nutr.* **2016**, 1–14. [CrossRef] [PubMed]
7. Manti, S.; Lougaris, V.; Cuppari, C.; Tardino, L.; Dipasquale, V.; Arrigo, T.; Salpietro, C.; Leonardi, S. Breastfeeding and il-10 levels in children affected by cow's milk protein allergy: A restrospective study. *Immunobiology* **2016**. [CrossRef] [PubMed]
8. Goldman, A.S. Modulation of the gastrointestinal tract of infants by human milk. Interfaces and interactions. An evolutionary perspective. *J. Nutr.* **2000**, *130*, S426–S431.
9. Hanson, C.; Lyden, E.; Furtado, J.; Van Ormer, M.; Anderson-Berry, A. A comparison of nutritional antioxidant content in breast milk, donor milk, and infant formulas. *Nutrients* **2016**, *8*, 681. [CrossRef] [PubMed]
10. Hunt, J. A possible relation between the regulation of gastric emptying and food intake. *Am. J. Physiol.* **1980**, *239*, G1–G4. [PubMed]

11. Hellstrom, P.; Gryback, P.; Jacobsson, H. The physiology of gastric emptying. *Best Pract. Res. Clin. Anaesthesiol.* **2006**, *20*, 397–407. [CrossRef] [PubMed]
12. Gomez, H.; Hornoy, P.; Liehn, J. Ultrasonography and gastric emptying in children: Validation of a sonographic method and determination of physiological and pathological patterns. *Pediatr. Radiol.* **2003**, *33*, 522–529. [CrossRef] [PubMed]
13. Carlos, M.; Babyn, P.; Marcon, M.; Moore, A. Changes in gastric emptying in early postnatal life. *J. Pediatr.* **1997**, *130*, 931–937. [CrossRef]
14. Perrella, S.; Hepworth, A.; Simmer, K.; Geddes, D. Influences of breast milk composition on gastric emptying in preterm infants. *J. Paediatr. Gastroenterol. Nutr.* **2015**, *60*, 264–271. [CrossRef] [PubMed]
15. Cavell, B. Gastric emtying in preterm infants. *Acta Paediatr. Scand.* **1979**, *68*, 725–730. [CrossRef] [PubMed]
16. Armand, M.; Hamosh, M.; Mehta, N.; Angelus, P.; Rhilpott, J.; Henderson, T.; Dwyer, N.; Lairon, D.; Hamosh, P. Effect of human milk or formula on gastric function and fat digestion in the premature infant. *Pediatr. Res.* **1996**, *40*, 429–437. [CrossRef] [PubMed]
17. Cavell, B. Gastric emptying in infants fed human milk or infant formula. *Acta Paediatr. Scand.* **1981**, *70*, 639–641. [CrossRef] [PubMed]
18. Vist, G.; Maughan, R. The effect of osmolality and carbohydrate content on the rate of gastric emptying of liquids in man. *J. Physiol.* **1995**, *486*, 523–531. [CrossRef] [PubMed]
19. Hunt, L.; Antonson, D.; Paxson, C.J.; Vanderhoff, J. Osmolality of carbohydrate solutions and gastric emptying in the newborn. *Am. J. Dis. Child.* **1982**, *136*, 448–451. [CrossRef] [PubMed]
20. Husband, J.; Husband, P.; Mallinson, C. Gastric emptying of starch meals in the newborn. *Lancet* **1970**, 290–292. [CrossRef]
21. Lonnerdal, B. Bioactive proteins in human milk: Mechanisms of action. *J. Pediatr.* **2010**, *156*, S26–S30. [CrossRef] [PubMed]
22. Michaelsen, K.; Larnkjaer, A.; Molgaard, C. Amount and quality of dietary proteins during the first two years of life in relation to NCD risk in adulthood. *Nutr. Metab. Cardiovasc. Dis.* **2012**, *22*, 781–786. [CrossRef] [PubMed]
23. Billeaud, C.; Guillet, J.; Sandler, B. Gastric emptying in infants with or without gastro-oesophageal reflux according to type of milk. *Eur. J. Clin. Nutr.* **1990**, *44*, 577–583. [PubMed]
24. Wang, G.; Lo, L.; Forsberg, L.; Maier, R. Helicobacter pylori peptidoglycan modifications confer lysozyme resistance and contribute to survival in the host. *mBio* **2012**, *3*, e00409-12. [CrossRef] [PubMed]
25. Artym, J.; Zimecki, M. Milk-derived proteins and peptides in clinical trials. *Postepy Hig. Med. Dosw.* **2013**, *67*, 800–816. [CrossRef]
26. Savino, F.; Sardo, A.; Rossi, L.; Benetti, S.; Savino, A.; Silvestro, L. Mother and infant body mass index, breast milk leptin and their serum leptin values. *Nutrients* **2016**, *8*, 383. [CrossRef] [PubMed]
27. Wang, Y.Y.; Zhang, Z.J.; Yao, W.; Morrow, A.; Peng, Y.M. Variation of maternal milk adiponectin and its correlation with infant growth. *Zhonghua Er Ke Za Zhi* **2011**, *49*, 338–343. [PubMed]
28. Miralles, O.; Sanchez, J.; Palou, A.; Pico, C. A physiological role of breast milk leptin in body weight control in developing infants. *Obesity* **2006**, *14*, 1371–1377. [CrossRef] [PubMed]
29. Woo, J.; Guerrero, M.; Altaye, M.; Ruiz-Palacios, G.; Martin, L.; Dubert-Ferrandon, A.; Newburg, D.; Morrow, A. Human milk adiponectin is associated with growth in two independent cohorts. *Breastfeed. Med.* **2009**, *4*, 101–109. [CrossRef] [PubMed]
30. Smedh, U.; Hakansson, M.L.; Meister, B.; Uvnas-Moberg, K. Leptin injected into the fourth ventricle inhibits gastric emptying. *Neuroreport* **1998**, *9*, 297–301. [CrossRef] [PubMed]
31. Sanchez, J.; Oliver, P.; Miralles, O.; Ceresi, E.; Pico, C.; Palou, A. Leptin orally supplied to neonate rats is directly uptaken by the immature stomach and may regulate short-term feeding. *Endocrinology* **2005**, *146*, 2575–2582. [CrossRef] [PubMed]
32. Kugananthan, S.; Lai, C.T.; Gridneva, Z.; Mark, P.J.; Geddes, D.T.; Kakulas, F. Leptin levels are higher in whole compared to skim human milk, supporting a cellular contribution. *Nutrients* **2016**, *8*, 711. [CrossRef] [PubMed]
33. Cannon, A.; Kakulas, F.; Hepworth, A.; Lai, C.; Hartmann, P.; Geddes, D. The effects of leptin on breastfeeding behaviour. *Int. J. Environ. Res. Public Helath* **2015**, *12*, 12340–12355. [CrossRef] [PubMed]

34. Cannon, A.M.; Gridneva, Z.; Hepworth, A.; Lai, C.T.; Tie, W.J.; Khan, S.; Hartmann, P.E.; Geddes, D.T. The relationship of human milk leptin and macronutrients with gastric emptying in term breastfed infants. *Pediatr. Res.* **2016**, under review.
35. Newburg, D.; Woo, J.; Morrow, A. Characteristics and potential functions of human milk adiponectin. *J. Pediatr.* **2010**, *156*, S41–S46. [CrossRef] [PubMed]
36. Kentish, S.J.; Ratcliff, K.; Li, H.; Wittert, G.A.; Page, A.J. High fat diet induced changes in gastric vagal afferent response to adiponectin. *Physiol. Behav.* **2015**, *152*, 354–362. [CrossRef] [PubMed]
37. Iwase, M.; Iino, K.; Oku, M.; Nohara, S.; Asano, T.; Doi, Y.; Iida, M. Serum high-molecular weight adiponectin is related to early postprandial glycemic increases and gastric emptying in patients with type 2 diabetes mellitus. *Diabetes Metab. Res. Rev.* **2009**, *25*, 344–350. [CrossRef] [PubMed]
38. Kent, J.C.; Mitoulas, L.R.; Cregan, M.D.; Ramsay, D.T.; Doherty, D.A.; Hartmann, P.E. Volume and frequency of breastfeedings and fat content of breast milk throughout the day. *Pediatrics* **2006**, *117*, e387–e395. [CrossRef] [PubMed]
39. Khan, S.; Hepworth, A.R.; Prime, D.K.; Lai, C.T.; Trengove, N.J.; Hartmann, P.E. Variation in fat, lactose, and protein composition in breast milk over 24 h: Associations with infant feeding patterns. *J. Hum. Lact.* **2013**, *29*, 81–89. [CrossRef] [PubMed]
40. Gridneva, Z.; Hepworth, A.; Ward, L.; Lai, C.T.; Hartmann, P.; Geddes, D.T. Bioimpedance spectroscopy in the infant: Effect of milk intake and extracellular fluid reservoirs on resistance measurements in term breastfed infants. *Eur. J. Clin. Nutr.* **2016**, *70*, 843–851. [CrossRef] [PubMed]
41. Gridneva, Z.; Hepworth, A.R.; Ward, L.C.; Lai, C.T.; Hartmann, P.E.; Geddes, D.T. Determinants of body composition in breastfed infants using bioimpedance spectroscopy and ultrasound skinfolds—Methods comparison. *Pediatr. Res.* **2016**, in press. [CrossRef] [PubMed]
42. Arthur, P.; Hartmann, P.; Smith, M. Measurement of the milk intake of breast-fed infants. *J. Paediatr. Gastroenterol. Nutr.* **1987**, *6*, 758–763. [CrossRef]
43. Neville, M.C.; Keller, R.; Seacat, J.; Lutes, V.; Neifert, M.; Casey, C.; Allen, J.; Archer, P. Studies in human lactation: Milk volumes in lactating women during the onset of lactation and full lactation. *Am. J. Clin. Nutr.* **1988**, *48*, 1375–1386. [PubMed]
44. Perrella, S.; Hepworth, A.; Simmer, K.; Geddes, D. Validation of ultrasound methods to monitor gastric volume changes in preterm infants. *J. Paediatr. Gastroenterol. Nutr.* **2013**, *57*, 741–749. [CrossRef] [PubMed]
45. Fleet, I.; Linzell, J. A rapid method of estimating fat in very small quantities of milk. *J. Physiol.* **1964**, *175*, 15–17.
46. Meier, P.; Engstrom, J.; Zuleger, J.; Motykowski, J.; Vasan, U.; Meier, W.; Hartmann, P.E.; Williams, T.M. Accuracy of a user-friendly centrifuge for measuring creamatocrits on mothers' milk in the clinical setting. *Breastfeed. Med.* **2006**, *1*, 79–87. [CrossRef] [PubMed]
47. Mitoulas, L.R. Short- and Long-Term Variation in the Production, Content and Composition of Human Milk Fat. Ph.D. Thesis, The University of Western Australia, Crawley, WA, Australia, 2000.
48. Keller, R.; Neville, M. Determination of total protein in human milk: Comparison of methods. *Clin. Chem.* **1986**, *32*, 120–123. [PubMed]
49. Kunz, C.; Lonnerdal, B. Human milk proteins: Separation of whey proteins and their analysis by polyacrylamide gel electrophoresis, fast protein liquid chromatography (FPLC) gel filtration, and anion-exchange chromatography. *Am. J. Clin. Nutr.* **1989**, *49*, 464–470. [PubMed]
50. Khan, S.; Casadio, Y.; Lai, C.; Prime, D.; Hepworth, A.; Trengove, N.; Hartmann, P. Investigation of short-term variations in casein and whey proteins in breast milk of term mothers. *Hepatol. Nutr.* **2012**, *55*, 136–141. [CrossRef] [PubMed]
51. Mitoulas, L.R.; Kent, J.C.; Cox, D.B.; Owens, R.A.; Sherriff, J.L.; Hartmann, P.E. Variation in fat, lactose and protein in human milk over 24 h and throughout the first year of lactation. *Br. J. Nutr.* **2002**, *88*, 29–37. [CrossRef] [PubMed]
52. Selsted, M.; Martinez, R. A simple and ultrasensitive enzymatic assay for the quantitative determination of lysozyme in the picogram range. *Anal. Biochem.* **1980**, *109*, 67–70. [CrossRef]
53. Euber, J.; Brunner, J. Determination of lactose in milk products by high-performance liquid chromatography. *J. Dairy Sci.* **1979**, *62*, 685–690. [CrossRef]
54. Albalasmeh, A.; Berhe, A.; Ghezzehei, T. A new method for rapid determination of carbohydrate and total carbon concentrations using UV spectrophotometry. *Carbohydr. Polym.* **2013**, *97*, 253–261. [CrossRef] [PubMed]

55. Kuhn, N.; Lowenstein, J. Lactogenesis in the rat. Changes in metabolic parameters at parturition. *Biochem. J.* **1967**, *105*, 995–1002. [CrossRef] [PubMed]
56. Newburg, D.; Neubauer, S. Carbohydrates in milks: Analysis, quantities, and significance. In *Handbook of Milk Composition*; Jensen, R., Ed.; Academic Press, Inc.: San Diego, CA, USA, 1995; pp. 273–349.
57. Lingwood, B.; Van Leeuwen, A.; Carberry, A.; Fitzgerald, E.; Callaway, L.; Colditz, P.; Ward, L. Prediction of fat-free mass and percentage of body fat in neonates using biolelectrical impedance analysis and anthropometric measures: Validation against pea pod. *Br. J. Nutr.* **2012**, *107*, 1545–1552. [CrossRef] [PubMed]
58. Brook, C. Determination of body composition of children from skinfold measurements. *Arch. Dis. Child.* **1971**, *46*, 182–184. [CrossRef] [PubMed]
59. Lohman, T. Body composition in children and youth. In *Advances in Pediatric Sport Sciences*; Boileau, R.A., Ed.; Human Kinetics Publishers: Champaign, IL, USA, 1984; pp. 29–57.
60. R Core Team. *R: A Language and Environment for Statistical Computing*; R Foundation for Statistical Computing: Vienna, Austria, 2009.
61. Pinheiro, J.; Bates, D.; DebRoy, S.; Sarkar, D.; Team, T.R.C. nlme: Linear and Nonlinear Mixed Effects Models. R Package Version 3.1-128. 2016. Available online: http://CRAN.R-project.org/package=nlme (accessed on 20 May 2016).
62. Sarkar, D. *Lattice: Multivariate Data Visualization with R*; Springer: New York, NY, USA, 2008.
63. Sarkar, D.; Andrews, F. *LatticeExtra: Extra Graphical Utilities Based on Lattice*, R Package Version 0.6-28, 2016. Available online: http://CRAN.R-project.org/package=latticeExtra (accessed on 20 May 2016).
64. Fox, J.; Weisberg, S. *An R Companion to Applied Regression*; Sage: Thousand Oaks, CA, USA, 2011.
65. Venables, W.N.; Ripley, B.D. *Modern Applied Statistics with S*, 4th ed.; Springer: New York, NY, USA, 2002.
66. Maechler, M. Sfsmisc: Utilities from Seminar Fuer Statistik Eth Zurich. R Package Version 1.1-0. 2016. Available online: http://cran.r-project.org/package=sfsmisc (accessed on 20 May 2016).
67. Hothorn, T.; Bretz, F.; Westfall, P. Simultaneous inference in general parametric models. *Biom. J.* **2008**, *50*, 346–363. [CrossRef] [PubMed]
68. Cannon, A.M.; Sakalidis, V.S.; Lai, C.T.; Perrella, S.L.; Geddes, D.T. Vacuum characteristics of the sucking cycle and relationships with milk removal from the breast in term infants. *Early Hum. Dev.* **2016**, *96*, 1–6. [CrossRef] [PubMed]
69. Royston, P.; Altman, D.G. Regression using fractional polynomials of continuous covariates: Parsimonious parametric modelling. *J. R. Stat. Soc. Ser. C Appl. Stat.* **1994**, *43*, 429–467. [CrossRef]
70. Curran-Everett, D. Multiple comparisons: Philosophies and illustrations. *Am. J. Physiol. Regul. Integr. Comp. Physiol.* **2000**, *279*, R1–R8. [PubMed]
71. Meyer, R.; Foong, R.; Thapar, N.; Kritas, S.; Shah, N. Systematic review of the impact of feed protein type and degree of hydrolysis on gastric emptying in children. *BMC Gastroenterol.* **2015**, *15*, 137. [CrossRef] [PubMed]
72. Lonnerdal, B.; Havel, P.J. Serum leptin concentrations in infants: Effects of diet, sex, and adiposity. *Am. J. Clin. Nutr.* **2000**, *72*, 484–489. [PubMed]
73. Bouret, S.G.; Draper, S.J.; Simerly, R.B. Trophic action of leptin on hypothalamic neurons that regulate feeding. *Science* **2004**, *304*, 108–110. [CrossRef] [PubMed]
74. Petridou, E.; Mantzoros, C.S.; Belechri, M.; Skalkidou, A.; Dessypris, N.; Papathoma, E.; Salvanos, H.; Lee, J.H.; Kedikoglou, S.; Chrousos, G.; et al. Neonatal leptin levels are strongly associated with female gender, birth length, IGF-I levels and formula feeding. *Clin. Endocrinol.* **2005**, *62*, 366–371. [CrossRef] [PubMed]
75. Savino, F.; Benetti, S.; Liguori, S.; Sorrenti, M.; Cordero Di Montezemolo, L. Advances of human milk hormones and protection against obesity. *Cell. Mol. Biol.* **2013**, *59*, 89–98. [PubMed]
76. Gonzalez, C.R.; Caminos, J.E.; Gallego, R.; Tovar, S.; Vazquez, M.J.; Garces, M.F.; Lopez, M.; Garcia-Caballero, T.; Tena-Sempere, M.; Nogueiras, R.; et al. Adiponectin receptor 2 is regulated by nutritional status, leptin and pregnancy in a tissue-specific manner. *Physiol. Behav.* **2010**, *99*, 91–99. [CrossRef] [PubMed]
77. Perry, B.; Wang, Y. Appetite regulation and weight control: The role of gut hormones. *Nutr. Diabetes* **2012**, *2*, e26. [CrossRef] [PubMed]
78. Chaudhri, O.; Small, C.; Bloom, S. Gastrointestinal hormones regulating appetite. *Philos. Trans. R. Soc. Lond. B Biol. Sci.* **2006**, *361*, 1187–1209. [CrossRef] [PubMed]
79. Maljaars, P.W.J.; Peters, H.P.F.; Mela, D.J.; NMasclee, A.A.M. Ileal brake: A sensible food target for appetite control. A review. *Physiol. Behav.* **2008**, *95*, 271–281. [CrossRef] [PubMed]

80. Van Citters, G.W.; Lin, H.C. Ileal brake: Neuropeptidergic control of intestinal transit. *Curr. Gastroenterol. Rep.* **2006**, *8*, 367–373. [CrossRef] [PubMed]
81. Khoshoo, V.; Brown, S. Gastric emptying of two whey-based formulas of different energy density and its clinical implication in children with volume intolerance. *Eur. J. Clin. Nutr.* **2002**, *56*, 656–658. [CrossRef] [PubMed]
82. Stanstrup, J.; Schou, S.S.; Holmer-Jensen, J.; Hermansen, K.; Dragsted, L.O. Whey protein delays gastric emptying and suppresses plasma fatty acids and their metabolites compared to casein, gluten, and fish protein. *J. Proteome Res.* **2014**, *13*, 2396–2408. [CrossRef] [PubMed]
83. Hale, T.W.; Hartmann, P.E. *Hale and Hartmann's Textbook of Human Lactation*, 1st ed.; Hale Publishing, L.P.: Amarillo, TX, USA, 2007.
84. Van Avesaat, M.; Troost, F.J.; Ripken, D.; Hendriks, H.F.; Masclee, A.A.M. Ileal brake activation: Macronutrient-specific effects on eating behavior? *Int. J. Obes.* **2015**, *39*, 235–243. [CrossRef] [PubMed]
85. Boirie, Y.; Dangin, M.; Gachon, P.; Vasson, M.P.; Maubois, J.L.; Beaufrere, B. Slow and fast dietary proteins differently modulate postprandial protein accretion. *Proc. Natl. Acad. Sci. USA* **1997**, *94*, 14930–14935. [CrossRef] [PubMed]
86. Daniel, H.; Vohwinkel, M.; Rehner, G. Effect of casein and beta-casomorphins on gastrointestinal motility in rats. *J. Nutr.* **1990**, *120*, 252–257. [PubMed]
87. Stromqvist, M.; Falk, F.; Bergstrom, S.; Hansson, L.; Lonnerdal, B.; Normark, S.; Hernell, O. Human milk kappa-casein and inhibition of helicobacter pylori adhesion to human gastric mucosa. *J. Pediatr. Gastroenterol. Nutr.* **1995**, *21*, 288–296. [CrossRef] [PubMed]
88. Francois, F.; Roper, J.; Joseph, N.; Pei, Z.; Chhada, A.; Shal, J.R.; Olivares De Perez, A.Z.; Perez-Perez, G.I.; Blaser, M.J. The effect of *H. pylori* eradication on meal-associated changes in plasma ghrelin and leptin. *BMC Gastroenterol.* **2011**, *11*, 37. [CrossRef] [PubMed]
89. Montagne, P.; Cuilliere, M.L.; Mole, C.; Bene, M.C.; Faure, G. Changes in lactoferrin and lysozyme levels in human milk during the first twelve weeks of lactation. *Adv. Exp. Med. Biol.* **2001**, *501*, 241–247. [PubMed]
90. Rubio, C.A. The natural antimicrobial enzyme lysozyme is up-regulated in gastrointestinal inflammatory conditions. *Pathogens* **2014**, *3*, 73–92. [CrossRef] [PubMed]
91. Bol'shakova, A.M.; Shcherbakova, E.G.; Ivanova, S.D.; Medvedeva, M.M.; Zhuravleva, T.P. Lysozyme in the feeding of premature infants with mixed pathology. *Antibiotiki* **1984**, *29*, 784–790. [PubMed]
92. Perrella, S.L.; Hepworth, A.R.; Simmer, K.N.; Hartmann, P.E.; Geddes, D.T. Repeatability of gastric volume measurements and intragastric content using ultrasound in preterm infants. *J. Pediatr. Gastroenterol. Nutr.* **2014**, *59*, 254–263. [CrossRef] [PubMed]
93. Hellstrom, P.; Naslund, E. Interactions between gastric emptying and satiety, with special reference to glucagon-like peptide-1. *Physiol. Behav.* **2001**, *74*, 735–741. [CrossRef]
94. Lorenz, D.N. Gastric emptying of milk in rat pups. *Am. J. Physiol.* **1985**, *248*, R732–R738. [PubMed]
95. Kent, J.; Hepworth, A.; Sherriff, J.; Cox, D.; Mitoulas, L.; Hartmann, P. Longitudinal changes in breastfeeding patterns from 1 to 6 months of lactation. *Breastfeed. Med.* **2013**, *8*, 401–407. [CrossRef] [PubMed]
96. Sepple, C.P.; Read, N.W. Gastrointestinal correlates of the development of hunger in man. *Appetite* **1989**, *13*, 183–191. [CrossRef]
97. Lawrence, R.A.; Lawrence, R.M. Practical management of the mother-infant nursing couple. In *Breastfeeding: A Guide for Medical Profession*, 7th ed.; Lawrence, R.A., Lawrence, R.M., Eds.; Mosby/Elsevier: Maryland Heights, MO, USA, 2011; pp. 232–283.
98. Natalucci, G.; Riedl, S.; Zidel, T.; Frisch, H. Spontaneous 24-h ghrelin secretion pattern in fasting subjects: Maintenance of a meal-related pattern. *Eur. J. Endocrinol.* **2005**, *152*, 845–850. [CrossRef] [PubMed]
99. Degen, L.P.; Phillips, S.F. Variability of gastrointestinal transit in healthy women and men. *Gut* **1996**, *39*, 299–305. [CrossRef] [PubMed]
100. Butte, N.; Garza, C.; Smith, E.; Nichols, B. Human milk intake and growth in exclusively breast-fed infants. *J. Pediatr.* **1984**, *104*, 187–195. [CrossRef]

6

Compliance with WHO IYCF Indicators and Dietary Intake Adequacy in a Sample of Malaysian Infants Aged 6–23 Months

Geok Lin Khor [1,*], Sue Yee Tan [1], Kok Leong Tan [1], Pauline S. Chan [2] and Maria Sofia V. Amarra [2]

1 Department of Nutrition and Dietetics, International Medical University, Kuala Lumpur 57000, Malaysia; sueyee_tan@imu.edu.my (S.Y.T.); kokleong_tan@imu.edu.my (K.L.T.)

2 International Life Sciences Institute South East Asia Region, Singapore 238959, Singapore; paulinechan@ilsisea.org.sg (P.S.C.); sofiaamarra@ilsisea.org.sg (M.S.V.A.)

* Correspondence: khor.geoklin@gmail.com

Abstract: Background: The 2010 World Health Organisation (WHO) Infant and Young Child Feeding (IYCF) indicators are useful for monitoring feeding practices. Methods: A total sample of 300 subjects aged 6 to 23 months was recruited from urban suburbs of Kuala Lumpur and Putrajaya. Compliance with each IYCF indicator was computed according to WHO recommendations. Dietary intake based on two-day weighed food records was obtained from a sub-group (N = 119) of the total sample. The mean adequacy ratio (MAR) value was computed as an overall measure of dietary intake adequacy. Contributions of core IYCF indicators to MAR were determined by multinomial logistic regression. Results: Generally, the subjects showed high compliance for (i) timely introduction of complementary foods at 6 to 8 months (97.9%); (ii) minimum meal frequency among non-breastfed children aged 6 to 23 months (95.2%); (iii) consumption of iron-rich foods at 6 to 23 months (92.3%); and minimum dietary diversity (78.0%). While relatively high proportions achieved the recommended intake levels for protein (87.4%) and iron (71.4%), lower proportions attained the recommendations for calcium (56.3%) and energy (56.3%). The intake of micronutrients was generally poor. The minimum dietary diversity had the greatest contribution to MAR (95% CI: 3.09, 39.87) (p = 0.000) among the core IYCF indicators. Conclusion: Malaysian urban infants and toddlers showed moderate to high compliance with WHO IYCF indicators. The robustness of the analytical approach in this study in quantifying contributions of IYCF indicators to MAR should be further investigated.

Keywords: infant and young child feeding; dietary adequacy; core complementary feeding indicators; micronutrients; dietary diversity

---

1. Introduction

Culture- and age-appropriate infant and young child feeding (IYCF) practices are well recognized as imperative for child health and survival. In 2008, the World Health Organization (WHO) recommended a set of population-level breastfeeding practices and food-related aspects of child feeding practices appropriate for children aged 6 to 23 months [1]. The questionnaire comprises eight core indicators and seven optional indicators of feeding practices, and offers the advantage of inter-country comparisons of IYCF practices.

In examining indicators of infant and young child feeding practices using data from Demographic and Health Surveys (DHS) of 46 countries between 2002 and 2008, Lutter et al. [2] reported that: (i) few infants and young children benefited from optimal complementary feeding practices; and (ii) less than one-third and only 21% of children aged 6 to 23 months met the minimum criteria for dietary diversity and received a minimum acceptable diet, respectively. Based on India's National Family Health Survey

(2005–2006), involving over 18,000 children aged zero to 23.9 months, Menon et al. [3] reported overall poor status of IYCF practices, especially indicators for complementary feeding, with 16% and 9% complying with minimum dietary diversity and minimum acceptable diet, respectively. A similar finding was reported by Marriot et al. [4], in assessing the WHO IYCF indicators of 14 low-income countries in Africa and Asia. The mean minimum dietary diversity adherence was found low, ranging from 11.3% for ages 6 to 11 months to 25.1% among those aged 18–23 months. The low prevalence of dietary diversity was reflected in poor compliance with minimum acceptable diet which was only 7.7% for infants 6 to 11 months of age and 16.3% for those aged 18–23 months. These recent reviews indicate room for improvement in young child feeding practices in low- to middle-income countries.

The International Life Sciences Institute of Southeast Asia region (ILSI SEA) Expert Panel on Infant and Young Child Nutrition, at its meeting in 2012, highlighted the importance for the region to undertake country-specific assessment of the IYCF indicators in association with measured dietary intakes and nutritional status of infants and young children [5]. In this respect, Cambodia, Indonesia, Philippines and Vietnam have periodic updates on IYCF practices, as reported by Demographic and Health Surveys (DHS) and/or Multiple Indicator Cluster Surveys (MICS) for these countries.

Malaysia is not covered by either the DHS or MICs, and relies instead on its National Health and Morbidity Surveys (NHMS) for IYCF data, such as the Third NHMS undertaken in 2006 [6] and the just-completed 2016 NHMS. There are concerns for inadequate feeding practices in Malaysia in view of recent findings of rather high prevalence of stunting and underweight among young children. Stunting among urban children nationwide was reported at 23.9% in ages 0.5–0.9 years [7], and underweight was reported at 19.6% among children aged 0–4 years [8]. Over-reliance on milk, leading to a lack of dietary diversity, was reported among Malaysian urban children aged one to three years [9]. Hence, this study was undertaken to assess the quality of young child feeding practices and dietary intake adequacy in a sample of infants and toddlers.

2. Methodology

This cross-sectional study was undertaken with the following objectives:

2.1. Objectives

1. To estimate the prevalence of compliance with the WHO IYCF indicators in a total sample of 300 infants and toddlers aged 6.0–23.9 months;
2. To determine dietary intake using a two-day weighed food records of a sub-group of infants and toddlers ($N = 119$), matched for age and sex with the total sample, with dietary intake adequacy computed as the mean adequacy ratio (MAR);
3. To determine the contributions of the WHO core complementary feeding indicators to the MAR values of the sub-group of subjects.

2.2. Subjects

The inclusion criteria for the selection of the study subjects were:

- Infants and children aged 6.0 to 23.9 months
- Malay ethnicity
- Families residing in the urban suburbs of Kuala Lumpur and Putrajaya
- Subjects attending licensed child care centers (registered with the Social Welfare Department of the Ministry of Women, Family and Community Development (Licensed child care centers are obliged to adhere to government regulations including caregiver to child ratio, standards of hygiene and menu guidelines.))
- Consent of the child care center management and parents/caregivers

The exclusion criteria were:

- Mentally or physically disabled infants and children
- Ill at the time of data collection
- Having dietary restrictions

The rationale for including only Malay infants and children of families from urban areas is to minimize the influence of cultural and socio-economic factors on feeding practices of infants and toddlers. Malay is the predominant ethnicity of the Malaysian population.

2.3. Total Sample Size for Determining Compliance with IYCF Indicators

The total sample size was estimated according to the guidelines of the WHO "Indicators for assessing infant and young child feeding practices [1] (Part 2 Measurements). Based on assuming an indicator estimate of 50% and a 95% confidence interval, a minimum number of 225 infants and young children aged 6.0–23.9 months was recommended. It was decided to have a total sample size of 300 subjects in case of dropouts and incomplete questionnaires. Data collection was carried out in 2013–2014.

A list of the licensed child care centers was compiled from various sources including the Association of Registered Care Providers of Selangor and the Ministry of Health Nutrition Division. The child care centers were contacted through emails and phone calls. Out of approximately 100 centers, about one-fifth gave permission for the conduct of this study. Using the snow-ball approach in going from one center to the next, approximately 100 infants and children who met the inclusion criteria were recruited for each of these age groups: 6.0–11.9 months, 12.0–17.9 months and 18.0–23.9 months, with almost an equal proportion of males and females in each age group. As the participants were recruited by convenience sampling, they are not deemed as representative of urban Malay toddlers.

The WHO IYCF indicators questionnaire was translated to the Malay language and pretested before use on five Malay mothers. This is to improve the language, technical contents and length of time used for the interview. Calculation for compliance with each IYCF indicator was in accordance with the formula recommended by WHO [1] (Part 2 Measurements).

2.4. Sub-Group of Toddlers for Two-Day Weighed Food Records and Compliance with Core Complementary Feeding

Only a sub-group of subjects was included for the two-day weighed food records part of the study, given that weighing of food intake was time-consuming. The sub-group of subjects was matched for age and sex to the total sample. In this way, the sub-sample comprised approximately 40 subjects in each of the three age groups of 6.0–11.9 months, 12.0–17.9 months and 18.0–23.9 months, making a total of 120 subjects. This age disaggregation is in accordance with the recommendation for studying the core complementary feeding indicators [1]. Each of the age groups consisted of approximately an equal proportion of male and female subjects. At the end, 119 subjects were included as one questionnaire was found to be incomplete.

Trained research assistants with at least a bachelor-level qualification in nutrition or dietetics carried out the weighing of food intake for two days when the child was in the center from about 7 a.m. until 5 p.m., Monday to Friday. All foods consumed were weighed for two consecutive weekdays but not on a weekend, as the day care centers are closed during the weekends.

For solid or semi-solid foods, the research assistants prepared a duplicate plate of the food items that were given to the child. The individual items were weighed using a kitchen scale that has a weight capacity of 2 kg and a weight graduation of 1 gm (TANITA-KD160WH). The amounts not consumed by the child were deducted from the total amounts weighed. The research assistants checked for ingredients used in preparing the food items by asking the center manager or person who prepared the foods or beverages.

For recording food and beverages consumed by children who were fed individually by the center helpers, the research assistants first identified the ingredients used in preparing the food or beverage, and then estimated the amounts of the food/beverage consumed by the child, based on the serving spoon or cup. As the entire procedure of observation, weighing and calculation for each child was time-consuming, a research assistant could complete the procedure for only three to four subjects a day, on average.

Parents/caregivers were instructed to record foods and beverages, in terms of description and quantity, taken by their child from the time he/she was picked up from the child care center until the following morning when the child was brought back to the center. The research assistants checked the forms and sought clarifications from parents/care givers, particularly for the quantities and types of constituents in the food or beverage consumed at home or outside.

3. Statistical Analyses

Compliance with the IYCF indicators was reported in percentage. Dietary intake was computed in terms of percentage of meeting the Malaysian dietary recommendations (Recommended Nutrient Intakes (RNIs) [10]. The mean adequacy ratio (MAR) was used as an overall measure of dietary adequacy. Several studies have reported MAR values to be positively associated with other indexes of dietary quality [4,11]. In order to compute MAR, one has to calculate first the nutrient adequacy ratio (NAR), which is defined as the ratio of a subject's nutrient intake to the recommended nutrient intake (RNI) of the assessed nutrient, appropriate for the age and sex of the subject.

$$\text{NAR} = \text{Actual nutrient intake (per day)/Recommended nutrient intake (RNI)} \tag{1}$$

The value for MAR is calculated as the total of all the NARs divided by the total expressed as a percentage. MAR has a range from 0% to 100% with 100% as the ideal [12].

$$\text{MAR} = \sum \text{NARs/Total number of nutrients} \tag{2}$$

For computing MAR, each of the NARs was truncated as 1, so that a high intake of one nutrient could not compensate for the low intake of another nutrient, as originally conceived by Malden et al. [13] and cited by Vieux et al. [14].

Multinomial logistic regression was used to assess the odds of compliance with the core complementary feeding indicators as the nominal independent variable, and MAR values as the dependent variable. All analyses were performed with SPSS version 22.0 (SPSS Inc., Chicago, IL, USA). A level of <0.05 was set for statistical significance.

Ethics Approval and Consent

The study proposal was approved by the Joint Committee on Research and Ethics of the International Medical University, Kuala Lumpur, Malaysia on 23 September 2013. (Project ID No. IMU R 123/2013). The Study Information Sheet and Written Consent Form in the Malay and English language were also approved by the IMU ethics committee. The Study Information Sheet comprised the following information: What is the purpose of this research? Why you are invited to this research? What is involved in this research? Is there any danger? How does this research help me? Contact persons for further information. After we had explained the information to the parents, one of them signed the Written Consent Form allowing their child to participate in the study.

4. Results

4.1. Total Sample Compliance with IYCF Indicators (N = 300)

The total sample size of 300 children consisted of 105 subjects aged 6.0–11.9 months, 87 aged 12.0–17.9 months, and 98 aged 18.0–23.9 months, with about an equal proportion of male and female subjects in each age group. These children were from young families with mothers having an average age of 30.9 ± 0.3 years, and with 1.4 ± 0.1 of children aged three years or less per family, on average.

Out of the WHO set of 15 IYCF indicators, data was collected for 12 indicators only, as the other three indicators referred to feeding practices for infants aged from zero to under 6 months, whereas these study subjects were aged 6.0–23.9 months. The subjects showed high compliance for several of the assessed indicators, namely (i) Children ever breastfed (99.3%); (ii) Timely introduction of complementary foods at 6–8 months (97.9%); (iii) Minimum meal frequency among non-breastfed children aged 6–23 months (95.2%); and (iv) Consumption of iron-rich foods at 6–23 months (92.3%) (Table 1). In contrast, the other indicators were achieved by relatively lower proportions of the subjects, and these include indicators related to breastfeeding beyond 6 months of age: (i) Continued breastfeeding at 2 years (38.3%); (ii) Continued breastfeeding at 1 year (57.1%); and (iii) Age-appropriate breastfeeding among children aged 6–23 months receiving breast milk as well as solids in the previous day (55.9%).

The minimum acceptable diet indicator was also found to have relatively low compliance among the non-breastfed children (39.5%) and breastfed children (50.6%). The minimum acceptable diet indicator combines compliance with the minimum dietary diversity and minimum meal frequency indicators. Actually, the subjects showed quite high compliance with meeting the latter two indicators separately, which is 78% for minimum dietary diversity, and 95.2% and 69.3% for minimum meal frequency among non-breastfed and breastfed children, respectively. However, in computing the minimum acceptable diet indicator for non-breastfed subjects, the formula includes the criteria of receiving two milk feeds, in addition to meeting the criteria for dietary diversity and meal frequency; moreover, the dairy group is excluded when calculating dietary diversity to avoid "double counting" [1] (WHO Part 2 Measurements). Consequently, the acceptable diet formula becomes more stringent to attain, resulting in a relatively lower prevalence of compliance among the non-breastfed.

Table 1. Compliance (%) with WHO IYCF indicators [1] (WHO, 2010) by total sample (N = 300).

Core Indicators	**% (*N*) ***
1. Early initiation of breastfeeding	
Proportion of children born in the last 24 months who were put to the breast within one hour of birth	76.3 (300)
2. Exclusive breastfeeding under 6 months	-
3. Continued breastfeeding at 1 year	
Proportion of children aged 12–15 months who are fed breast milk during the previous day	57.1 (56)
4. Timely introduction of solid, semi-solid or soft foods	
Proportion of infants aged 6–8 months who receive solid, semi-solid or soft foods during the previous day	97.9 (47)
5. Minimum dietary diversity	
Proportion of children aged 6–23 months who received foods from 4 or more food groups during the previous day	78.0 (300)
6. Minimum meal frequency	
Breastfed children: Proportion of breastfed children aged 6–23 months who received solid, semi-solid, or soft foods the minimum number of times or more during the previous day	69.3 (163)
Non-breastfed children: Proportion of children aged 6–23 months who received solid, semi-solid or soft foods or milk feeds the minimum number of times or more during the previous day	95.2 (125)
Total:	80.6 (288)

Table 1. *Cont.*

7. Minimum acceptable diet	
Breastfed children: Proportion of children aged 6–23 months who had at least a minimum dietary diversity and the minimum meal frequency during the previous day	50.6 (166)
Non-breastfed children: Proportion of children aged 6–23 months who received at least 2 milk feedings and had at least the minimum dietary diversity and the minimum meal frequency during the previous day	39.5 (129)
Total:	45.8 (295)
8. Consumption of iron-rich or iron-fortified foods	
Proportion of children aged 6–23 months who receive an iron-rich food or iron-fortified food that is specially designed for infants and young children, or that is fortified in the home during the previous day	92.3 (298)
Optional Indicators	
9. Children ever breastfed	
Proportion of children born in the last 24 months who were ever breastfed	99.3 (300)
10. Continued breastfeeding at 2 years	
Proportion of children aged 20–23 months who received breast milk during the previous day	38.3 (47)
11. Age-appropriate breastfeeding	-
Proportion of children aged 6–23 months who received breast milk, as well as solid, semi-solid or soft foods during the previous day	55.9 (161)
12. Predominant breastfeeding under 6 months (0–5.9 months)	-
13. Duration of breastfeeding (0–5.9 months)	-
14. Bottle feeding	
Proportion of children aged 0–23 months who are fed with a bottle during the previous day	80.4 (296) **
15. Milk feeding frequency for non breastfed children	
Proportion of non-breastfed children 6–23 months of age who received at least 2 milk feedings during the previous day	91.3 (127)

* Number of eligible subjects; ** Age studied 6.0–23.9 months.

4.2. Compliance with Core Complementary Feeding Indicators by Sub-Group (N = 119)

Compliance with four of the five core indicators for complementary feeding was investigated among the sub-group of subjects, as only a small number ($N = 13$) of subjects (aged 6 to 8 months) was eligible for computing the indicator on "Timely introduction of solids", which was hence excluded. The sub-group showed generally high compliance with the core complementary feeding indicators (Table 2). There was high compliance with (i) Timely introduction of solid, semi-solid or soft foods (92.3%); (ii) Consumption of iron-rich foods (92.4%); (iii) Minimum meal frequency among both breastfed and non-breastfed children aged 6–23 months (91.7% and 85.5%, respectively); as well as (iv) Minimum dietary diversity (83.2%). A low prevalence for the minimum acceptable diet indicator for non-breastfed (34.6%) and breastfed (68.8%) infants was recorded for the sub-group.

Table 2. Compliance (%) with WHO core complementary feeding indicators by sub-group ($N = 119$).

* Core Complementary Feeding Indicators	Compliance% (N)
Minimum dietary diversity	83.2 (119)
Minimum meal frequency	
Breastfed	85.5 (62)
Non-breastfed	91.7 (48)
Minimum acceptable diet	
Breastfed	68.8 (64)
Non-breastfed	34.6 (52)
Consumption of iron-rich or iron-fortified foods	92.4 (119)

* Timely introduction of solid, semi-solid or soft foods indicator was excluded owing to the small number of subjects who were eligible ($N = 13$ aged 6 to 8 months).

4.3. Dietary Intake Adequacy of Sub-Group (N = 119)

Based on the two-day weighed food intake, dietary intake adequacy was computed and described as meeting the Malaysian recommendations for energy and nutrient intake (RNI) [10]. The nutrient adequacy ratio (NAR) value exceeded 1.0 for energy, protein, calcium and iron, indicating that their intakes achieved more than 100% of the recommended levels (RNIs) (Table 3). Mean iron and protein intake were double the RNI recommendation levels, while those for energy and calcium exceeded 100%. The likely dietary sources for these nutrients were animal food including milk, chicken meat, fish and eggs. As for the NAR values for the rest of the nutrients, they ranged from 0.50 for vitamin A to 0.84 for zinc, denoting intake of these nutrients met 50% to 84% of the RNIs, respectively. Relatively high proportions of the subjects achieved the RNI for protein (87.4%) and iron (71.4%), while just over half managed to do so for calcium (56.3%) and energy (56.3%). The proportions of the subjects meeting the rest of the micronutrients were low and these include vitamin A, thiamin, vitamin C niacin, riboflavin and zinc. This finding suggests that the subjects were not consuming sufficient vegetables, fruits, legumes and whole grains.

Table 3. Energy and nutrient intake adequacy ($N = 119$).

Dietary Intake †	Percentage of the Recommended Nutrient Intake (RNI) Achieved % ± SD	[a] Nutrient Adequacy Ratio (NAR) Value Mean ± SE
energy	110.7 ± 49.2	1.14 ± 0.05
protein	202.8 ± 101.9	2.07 ± 0.10
calcium	127.5 ± 92.6	1.32 ± 0.10
iron [b]	216.7 ± 181.2	2.44 ± 0.21
zinc	75.7 ± 70.2	0.84 ± 0.10
thiamin	47.6 ± 34.6	0.55 ± 0.06
riboflavin	76.0 ± 51.5	0.82 ± 0.06
niacin	66.5 ± 53.5	0.77 ± 0.07
vitamin C	41.5 ± 39.7	0.57 ± 0.07
vitamin A	42.2 ± 39.6	0.50 ± 0.06
[c] Mean adequacy ratio (MAR)		0.67 ± 0.02

† based on two-day weighed food record; [a] NAR for a given nutrient is the ratio of a subject's nutrient intake to the recommended nutrient intake of the assessed nutrient, appropriate for the age and sex of the subject; [b] based on 15% bioavailability; [c] Mean adequacy ratio (MAR) was calculated as the total of all the NARs ($\sum$ NAR for energy and nine nutrients) divided by the total, expressed as a percentage.

For this study, it was arbitrarily decided to compute NAR for energy and nutrients taken by the subjects that met at least 40% of the Malaysian RNIs. Hence, NAR was determined for energy and the following nine nutrients: protein, calcium, iron, zinc, vitamin A, vitamin C, thiamin, riboflavin and niacin. The value for MAR was then calculated as $\sum$ NARs divided by the total (10 in this case) expressed as a percentage.

Overall, the mean adequacy ratio (MAR) value computed was 0.67, indicating that the dietary intake of the subjects met, on average, 67% of the combined RNIs for energy and the nine nutrients under consideration in this study.

4.4. Contributions of Core Complementary Feeding Indicators to Dietary Intake Adequacy (N = 119)

Multinomial logistic regression was used to determine the contributions of the four WHO core complementary feeding indicators as the independent variables to dietary intake adequacy based on MAR values as the dependent variables. Since MAR = 0.67 was generated from the weighed dietary intake in this study, MAR > 0.6 was selected for comparison with MAR ≤ 0.5. Among the core complementary feeding indicators, minimum dietary diversity contributed highest to dietary intake adequacy (OR 11.10; 95% CI: 3.09, 39.87) (p = 0.000) (Table 4). The other core complementary feeding indicators showed lower odds of contributing to intake adequacy for the same MAR values. The minimum dietary diversity indicator also showed the highest odds of leading to dietary intake adequacy (OR 5.49; 95% CI: 1.35, 22.22) (p = 0.017) with MAR set at a lower level of (0.5 < MAR ≤ 0.6) that is, overall dietary adequacy between 50.1% and 60% (Table 4). Hence, these results suggest that, for this sample of Malaysian urban toddlers, compliance with minimum dietary diversity is of key importance towards attaining dietary intake adequacy.

Table 4. Contributions of WHO core complementary feeding indicators to dietary intake adequacy (N = 119) †.

Dietary Intake Adequacy Based on Mean Adequacy Ratio (MAR)	Minimum Dietary Diversity	Minimum Meal Frequency	Minimum Acceptable Diet	Consumption of Iron-Rich/Fortified Food
	Odds Ratio (95% CI)			
[b] MAR > 0.6 (more than 60.0%)	11.10 (3.09, 39.87), p = 0.000	6.70 (1.44, 31.16), p = 0.015	4.03 (1.17, 13.87), p = 0.027	2.73 (0.45, 16.48), p = 0.273
0.5 < [a] MAR ≤ 0.6 (50.1%–60.0%)	5.49 (1.35, 22.22), p = 0.017	1.60 (0.35, 7.30), p = 0.544	2.96 (0.75, 11.67), p = 0.121	1.33 (0.20, 9.00), p = 0.768

Above results generated using multinomial logistic regression whereby the reference category is MAR ≤ 0.5; † Dietary adequacy defined as meeting the combined RNIs for energy and nine nutrients (protein, calcium, iron, zinc, vitamin A, vitamin C, thiamin, riboflavin and niacin); NAR = 10 Nutrient adequacy ratio (NAR) for a given nutrient is the ratio of a subject's intake to the current recommended nutrient intake of the assessed nutrient, appropriate for the age and sex of the subject. Mean adequacy ratio (MAR) is the total of all the NARs ($\sum$ NAR for energy and nine nutrients) divided by the 10, expressed as a percentage; 0.5 < [a] MAR ≤ 0.6: meeting between 50.1% to 60.0% of the combined RNIs for the 10 NARs; [b] MAR > 0.6: meeting more than 60% of the combined RNIs for the 10 NARs.

5. Discussion

In a sample of urban Malaysian infants and toddlers aged 6 to 23 months, this study highlighted (i) moderate rates of continued breastfeeding beyond 6 months of age; (ii) high proportions of compliance with timely introduction of complementary foods and receiving iron-rich foods; and (iii) moderate to low proportions met the acceptable diet indicator (minimum dietary diversity and minimum meal frequency). Achieving the indicator on acceptable diet is important as it reflects compliance with both the qualitative and quantitative aspects of complementary feeding. Studies have well documented the significant relationships between attaining a minimum acceptable diet and child nutritional status. In assessing the WHO IYCF indicators of 14 low-income countries in Africa and Asia, Marriot et al. [4] found children consuming a minimum acceptable diet had a significantly lower overall probability of being underweight and stunted. Based on India's National Family Health Survey (2005–2006), involving over 18,000 children aged zero to 23.9 months, Menon et al. [3] showed the acceptable diet indicator as a strong predictor of stunting and underweight.

Dietary intake adequacy in terms of MARs was shown to be influenced most by the minimum dietary diversity indicator. This finding is in line with growing global evidence of the usefulness of dietary diversity in predicting dietary quality, including micronutrient intake adequacy among infants and young children [12,15–17]. In evaluating cross-country patterns based on DHS data, Jones et al. [18] reported that achieving minimum dietary diversity reduced the odds of stunting among children in India, Bangladesh and Zambia. Data from the 2007 Bangladesh Demographic and Health Survey of 1508 children aged 6 to 23 months also showed that those who achieved minimum dietary diversity had a significantly higher height for their age [19]. Nguyen et al. [20] reported a strong positive association between maternal and child dietary diversity in Bangladesh, Vietnam and Ethiopia, and hence advocated the measurement of both maternal and child dietary diversity. A low dietary diversity score was significantly associated with poor nutritional status of indigenous children in Malaysia [21]. A lack of dietary diversity is often reported in low-income populations as their diets are predominantly based on starchy staples, as animal food sources are costly and may not be readily available.

Countries are encouraged to conduct periodic surveys using the WHO IYCF indicators to enable comparing trends of breastfeeding and complementary feeding practices within countries and among countries, as well as for identifying populations at risk and evaluating the impacts of interventions [18]. Countries in Southeast Asia generally showed higher compliance with timely introduction of complementary foods than that for dietary diversity, meal frequency and acceptable diet (Table 5). These findings suggest that complementary foods are provided in a timely manner, but the diets tend to lack variety and frequency as recommended. Hence, owing to low achievements of dietary diversity and meal frequency, compliance with a minimum acceptable diet is generally low in the region.

Table 5. Comparison of WHO IYCF practices among countries in Southeast Asia *.

Core Complementary Feeding Indicators	Cambodia 2014 DHS	Indonesia 2012 DHS	Philippines 2008 DHS	Vietnam 2013–2014 MICS5	** Malaysia 2013–2014 Present Study
Timely introduction of complementary foods	82	91.0	89	90.7	97.9
Minimum dietary diversity	48.0	58.2	78.7	76.9	78.0
Minimum meal frequency					
breastfed					
Non-breastfed	74.0	61.4	80.7		69.3
Total	68.0	78.7	48.2	90.5	95.2
Minimum acceptable diet					
breastfed	32.0	34.2	68.2	62.4	50.6
Non-breastfed	26.0	43.0	40.5	54.5	39.5
Consumption of iron-rich/iron-fortified foods	75.8	67.5	78.3		92.3

* Cambodia, Indonesia, Philippines and Vietnam covered by Demographic and Health Surveys (DHS) or Multiple Indicators Cluster Surveys (MICS) [22–25]; ** $N = 300$.

Limitations of Study

The relatively small sample size and the homogeneous subjects preclude generalizing the results to other socio-economic and ethnic population groups of Malaysia. As a cross-section study, interpretation of causality of the data is restricted. The accuracy of the results is also limited by the methods of data collection, particularly relying on weighing of foods and food intake recording by parents/caregivers. There may be bias in the selection of subjects using the convenient snow-ball approach. The dietary results obtained should not be extended to children who do not attend licensed day care centers where the menus are based on the recommendations of the Ministry of Health.

6. Conclusions

Continued efforts remain essential for improving feeding practices to ensure adequate and quality complementary feeding in Malaysia and the region. This study provides an analytic approach at examining the contributions of core complementary feeding indicators to dietary intake adequacy. This approach should be validated with larger subject samples from different socio-economic statuses to verify its usefulness at different population levels.

Acknowledgments: The cooperation of the Nutrition Division, Ministry of Health Malaysia, is much appreciated. Grateful appreciation is also expressed to Chua Ee Yin for data entry and statistical analysis. The authors duly acknowledged the funding of the study by the International Life Sciences, Southeast Asia Region (ILSI SEA Region).

Author Contributions: Khor Geok Lin, Pauline Chan and Sofia Amarra conceptualized the initial proposal. Khor Geok Lin, Tan Sue Yee and Tan Kok Leong designed and supervised the study. Khor Geok Lin was responsible for data analysis, drafting and editing the manuscript. All authors read and approved the final manuscript.

1. World Health Organization, Department of Child and Adolescent Health and Development. *Indicators for Assessing Infant and Young Child Feeding Practices. Part II: Measurement*; World Health Organization: Geneva, Switzerland, 2010.
2. Lutter, C.K.; Daelmans, B.M.E.G.; de Onis, M.; Kothari, M.T.; Ruel, M.T.; Arimond, M.; Deitchler, M.; Dewey, K.G.; Blossner, M.; Borghi, E. Undernutrition, poor feeding practices, and low coverage of key nutrition interventions. *Pediatrics* **2011**, *128*, e1418–e1427. [CrossRef] [PubMed]
3. Menon, P.; Bamezai, A.; Subandoro, A.; Ayoya, M.A.; Aguayo, V. Age-appropriate infant and young child feeding practices are associated with child nutrition in India: Insights from nationally representative data. *Matern. Child Nutr.* **2015**, *11*, 73–87. [CrossRef] [PubMed]
4. Marriot, B.P.; White, A.J.; Hadden, L.; Davies, J.C.; Wallingford, J.C. World Health Organization (WHO) infant and young child feeding indicators: Associations with growth measures in 14 low-income countries. *Matern. Child Nutr.* **2012**, *8*, 354–370. [CrossRef] [PubMed]
5. Amarra, M.S.V.; Chan, P.M.S. Proceedings of the 3rd Expert Consultation and Planning Meeting on Infant and Young Child Nutrition-(Part 2). *Malays. J. Nutr.* **2013**, *19*, 139–142. [PubMed]
6. Ministry of Health Malaysia, Institute for Public Health (IPH). *The Third National Health and Morbidity Survey (NHMS III) 2006: Nutritional Status of Adults Aged 18 Years and Above*; Ministry of Health Malaysia: Kuala Lumpur, Malaysia, 2008.
7. Poh, B.K.; Ng, B.K.; Haslinda, M.D.S.; Shanita, S.N.; Wong, J.E.; Budin, S.B.; Ruzita, A.B.; Lai, O.N.; Khouw, I.; Norimah, A.K. Nutritional status and dietary intakes of children aged 6 months to 12 years: Findings of the Nutrition Survey of Malaysian Children (SEANUTS Malaysia). *Br. J. Nutr.* **2013**, *110*, S21–S35. [CrossRef] [PubMed]
8. Ministry of Health Malaysia, Institute for Public Health (IPH). *National Health and Morbidity Survey 2011. Non-Communicable Diseases*; Ministry of Health Malaysia: Kuala Lumpur, Malaysia, 2011.
9. Khor, G.L.; Zalilah, M.S.; Sariman, S.; Huang, S.L.M.; Mohamad, M.; Chan, Y.M.; Chin, Y.S.; Barakatun, N.M.Y. Milk drinking patterns among Malaysian urban children of different household income status. *J. Nutr. Health Sci.* **2015**. [CrossRef]
10. Ministry of Health Malaysia, National Coordinating Committee for Food and Nutrition (NCCFN). *Recommended Nutrient Intakes for Malaysia*; Ministry of Health: Putrajaya, Malaysia, 2005.
11. Torheim, L.E.; Ouattara, F.; Diarra, M.M.; Thiam, F.D.; Barikmo, I.; HatlØy, A.; Oshaug, A. Nutrient adequacy and dietary diversity in rural Mali: Association and determinants. *Eur. J. Clin. Nutr.* **2004**, *58*, 594–604. [CrossRef] [PubMed]
12. Steyn, N.P.; Nel, J.; Labadarios, D.; Maunder, E.M.W.; Salome, H.; Kruger, H.S. Which dietary diversity indicator is best to assess micronutrient adequacy in children 1 to 9 years? *Nutrition* **2014**, *30*, 55–60. [CrossRef] [PubMed]
13. Madden, J.P.; Goodman, S.J.; Guthrie, H.A. Validity of the 24-hr. recall. Analysis of data obtained from elderly subjects. *J. Am. Diet. Assoc.* **1976**, *68*, 143–147. [PubMed]
14. Vieux, F.; Soler, L.G.; Touazi, D.; Darmon, N. High nutritional quality is not associated with low greenhouse gas emissions in self-selected diets of French adults. *Am. J. Clin. Nutr.* **2013**, *97*, 569–583. [CrossRef] [PubMed]
15. Arimond, M.; Ruel, M.T. Dietary diversity is associated with child nutritional status: Evidence from 11 demographic and health surveys. *J. Nutr.* **2004**, *134*, 2579–2585. [PubMed]

16. Kennedy, G.L.; Pedro, M.R.; Seghieri, C.; Nantel, G.; Brouwer, I. Dietary diversity score is a useful indicator of micronutrient intake in non-breastfeeding Filipino children. *J. Nutr.* **2007**, *137*, 472–477. [PubMed]
17. Moursi, M.M.; Arimond, M.; Dewey, K.G.; Tre'che, S.; Ruel, M.T.; Delpeuch, F. Dietary diversity is a good predictor of the micronutrient density of the diet of 6- to 23-month-old children in Madagascar. *J. Nutr.* **2008**, *138*, 2448–2453. [CrossRef] [PubMed]
18. Jones, A.D.; Ickes, S.B.; Smith, L.E.; Mbuya, M.N.N.; Chasekwa, B.; Heidkamp, R.A.; Menon, P.; Zongrone, A.A.; Stoltzfus, R.J. World Health Organization infant and young child feeding indicators and their associations with child anthropometry: A synthesis of recent findings. *Matern. Child Nutr.* **2014**, *10*, 1–17. [CrossRef] [PubMed]
19. Zongrone, A.; Winskell, K.; Menon, P. Infant and young child feeding practices and child undernutrition in Bangladesh: Insights from nationally representative data. *Public Health Nutr.* **2010**, *15*, 1697–1704. [CrossRef] [PubMed]
20. Nguyen, P.H.; Avula, R.; Ruel, M.T.; Saha, K.K.; Ali, D.; Tran, L.M.; Frongillo, E.A.; Menon, P.; Rawat, R. Maternal and child dietary diversity are associated in Bangladesh, Vietnam, and Ethiopia. *J. Nutr.* **2013**, *143*, 1176–1183. [CrossRef] [PubMed]
21. Chua, E.Y.; Zalilah, M.S.; Chin, Y.S.; Norhasmah, S. Dietary Diversity is associated with nutritional status of Orang Asli children in Pahang. *Malays. J. Nutr.* **2012**, *18*, 1–13.
22. National Institute of Statistics, Directorate General for Health, ICF International. *Cambodia Demographic and Health Survey, 2014*; National Institute of Public Health, National Institute of Statistics, Directorate General for Health, ORC Macro: Phnom Penh, Cambodia; ICF International: Rockville, MD, USA, 2015.
23. Statistics Indonesia, National Population and Family Planning Board, Ministry of Health, ICF International. *Indonesia Demographic and Health Survey 2012*; Statistics Indonesia, National Population and Family Planning Board, Ministry of Health: Jakarta, Indonesia; ICF International: Calverton, MD, USA, 2013.
24. Philippine Statistics Authority, ICF International. *Philippines National Demographic and Health Survey 2008*; National Statistics Office (NSO): Quezon City, Philippines; ICF Macro: Calverton, MD, USA, 2009.
25. General Statistics Office, The United Nations Children's Fund. *Viet Nam Multiple Indicator Cluster Survey 2014, Final Report*; General Statistics Office: Hanoi, Vietnam; The United Nations Children's Fund: New York, NY, USA, 2015.

7

Breastmilk Production in the First 4 Weeks after Birth of Term Infants

Jacqueline C. Kent *, Hazel Gardner and Donna T. Geddes

School of Chemistry and Biochemistry, The University of Western Australia, Crawley 6009, Australia; Hazel.Gardner@uwa.edu.au (H.G.); Donna.Geddes@uwa.edu.au (D.T.G.)

* Correspondence: Jacqueline.Kent@uwa.edu.au

Abstract: Breastmilk provides the ideal nutrition for the infant, and exclusive breastfeeding is recommended for the first 6 months. Adequate milk production by the mother is therefore critical, and early milk production has been shown to significantly affect milk production during established lactation. Previous studies indicate that milk production should reach the lower limit of normal for established lactation (440 mL per day) by day 11 after birth. We have used test-weighing of term infants before and after each breastfeed over 24 h to measure milk production in the first 4 weeks of lactation in mothers with and without perceived breastfeeding problems to provide information on how often milk production is inadequate. Between days 11 and 13, two-thirds of the mothers had a milk production of less than 440 mL per day, and between days 14 and 28, nearly one-third of the mothers had a milk production of less than 440 mL per day. The high frequency of inadequate milk production in early lactation and the consequence of suboptimal milk production in later lactation if left untreated suggest that objective measurement of milk production can identify mothers and infants at risk and support early intervention by a lactation specialist.

Keywords: breastfeeding; milk production; insufficient milk

---

1. Introduction

There is a sound evidence base for the health advantages of breastfeeding for infants and their mothers, and a dose-response relationship has been demonstrated [1]. As such, any breastfeeding should be encouraged and full breastfeeding achieved if possible. Milk production and adequacy at 6 weeks after birth, for mothers of both healthy breastfeeding term infants and non-nursing preterm infants, have been shown to have a significant relationship with milk production 4–6 days after birth [2,3]. Hill et al. therefore suggest that interventions that promote an adequate milk supply by the first week postpartum are critical [2]. These include skin-to-skin contact and milk removal (breastfeeding or expressing) within an hour of birth and frequent milk removal during the first 24 h after birth. Early initiation of lactation, particularly breastfeeding or expressing within an hour of birth, has been shown to lead to a higher rate of breastfeeding beyond 6 weeks for term infants [4]. Skin-to-skin contact between mother and infant for the first hour after birth results in earlier effective breastfeeding [5] and an increased likelihood of breastfeeding 1–4 months after birth than when the infant was swaddled in blankets [6]. There is also a positive effect of the number of breastfeeds in the first 24 h on milk production on days 3 and 5 after birth [7]. It is important, therefore, to know if milk production is adequate during early lactation. The lower limit of normal daily milk production for established lactation has been calculated to be 440 g [8]. During the first week of lactation, on day 5, daily milk transfer during breastfeeding is 415 $\pm$ 123 g (combined data from a total of 305 breastfeeding mothers [7,9–14]). For mothers who were exclusively expressing breastmilk, one study of mothers of term infants measured a milk production of 973 $\pm$ 176 g per day on day 5 [15]. There is limited data on milk production during the second week after birth, but data from 10 mothers showed a daily milk transfer of 653 ± 154 g with a slightly higher milk yield of 668 ± 163 g due to some mothers occasionally pumping their breastmilk [11]. Hill et al. reported a lower milk production of 556 ± 187 g, but some of those mothers were supplementing [3]. Taken together, published data indicate that 92% of term mothers produce at least 440 g per day by 2 weeks of lactation.

It has been reported that 58% of term mothers experience problems with breastfeeding, including a perception of insufficient milk supply, in the first 2 weeks and this is associated with a lack of confidence in breastfeeding [16]. A perception of insufficient milk supply is given as a reason for the introduction of supplementary infant formula [17,18]. If breastmilk supply is actually inadequate supplementary feeds are necessary. If supplementary feeds are given instead of breastfeeds they could have a negative impact on milk supply. Measurement of milk production using in-home 24-h test-weighing is being used increasingly by lactation consultants and general practitioners as a clinical tool to either reassure mothers that their breastfeeding patterns and milk production are normal, or to guide advice to increase or decrease milk production or breastmilk transfer [19]. We aim to use 24-h milk profiles during the establishment of lactation to try to verify that full milk production is achieved by 2 weeks of lactation in mothers without perceived breastfeeding problems and, in a vulnerable population, how frequently milk supply is not adequate indicating that intervention would be appropriate.

2. Materials and Methods

A convenience sample of mothers within 4 weeks after the birth of a singleton, term infant (≥37 weeks gestational age at delivery, birth weight ≥2500 g) who were fully or partially breastfeeding [20] were invited to participate between June 2009 and April 2016. We recruited mothers under the care of general practitioners or lactation consultants for perceived breastfeeding problems, and volunteers for studies undertaken by the research group (e.g., Prime et al. [21]) who were without perceived breastfeeding problems. Demographics were recorded and the participants were loaned accurate digital scales (BabyWeigh™, Medela Inc., McHenry, IL, USA, resolution 2 g, accuracy ± 0.034%) to measure their milk profile. This involved the participants test-weighing their infants in their own homes [22] before and after each breastfeed or supplementary feed and recording amounts of breastmilk expressed. All measurements of breastfeed amounts and milk production are measured in grams but expressed in mL because the density of milk is 1.03 $g \cdot mL^{-1}$. Data were recorded either on paper or entered on a password-protected website accessed by invitation only. Breastfeeding parameters were calculated: the total amount of milk transferred from the mother to the infant while breastfeeding (total breastfeeding transfer), the amount of breastmilk expressed during the 24-h period (total breastmilk expressed), the total amount of milk produced by both breasts in the 24-h period (total breastmilk production = total breastfeeding transfer + total breastmilk expressed), and the total infant milk intake (total breastfeeding transfer plus expressed breastmilk and/or supplementary formula). The duration of each feed was taken from the time of weighing before to the time of weighing after the feeding.

Analysis used R version 3.2.1 GUI Snow Leopard (The R Foundation for Statistical Computing, Vienna, Austria) [23] with the base package and the library nlme [24] for linear mixed effects models. Summary statistics are presented as mean ± SD where the Shapiro-Wilk test indicated normality, or median (interquartile range) otherwise. Groups were compared on demographic and milk intake variables using two-tailed independent samples Student's *t*-test where the Shapiro-Wilk test indicated normality, and Kruskal-Wallis rank sum test otherwise. Linear mixed effects analyses of the relationship between demographic and milk intake variables and total milk production were carried out with random effects of different intercepts for each mother. Differences were considered to be significant where $p < 0.05$.

All participants supplied written, informed consent to participate in the studies, which were approved by the Human Research Ethics Committee at The University of Western Australia (RA/4/1/4103) and Women and Newborn Health Service (1746/ew).

3. Results

Sixty-two percent of participants who agreed to participate completed 24-h milk profiles between 6 and 28 days after birth. There were 13 participants without perceived breastfeeding problems (6 female infants, all Caucasian, 4 primiparous, 12 vaginal delivery) and 103 participants with perceived breastfeeding problems (50 female infants). Complete demographics were available for 48 participants (43 Caucasian, 32 primiparous, 28 vaginal delivery). Seventy-six of these provided information regarding their breastfeeding problems. The most common was a perception of insufficient milk supply (59 participants), but pain (11 participants) and positioning and attachment (10 participants) were also mentioned. Seventy-five of the participants with perceived breastfeeding problems were supplementing their infants with expressed breastmilk and/or infant formula, 45 using expressed breastmilk alone, 25 using infant formula and expressed breastmilk, and 5 participants used formula but no expressed breastmilk. The characteristics of the participants are presented in Table 1.

Table 1. Characteristics and breastfeeding parameters of participants without and with perceived breastfeeding problems.

	Perceived Breastfeeding Problems		p Value
	No	Yes	
n	13	103	
Birth weight (g)	3498 (293)	3450 (3206, 3739)	0.051
Gestational age at delivery (weeks^{+days})	39^{+2} (1^{+3})	39^{+6} (38^{+7}, 40^{+3})	0.025
Feed frequency (breasts)	12 (3)	12 (4)	0.50
Average feed duration (min)	17 (5)	15 (13, 21)	0.052
Average feed amount (mL)	63 (27)	30 (20, 45)	<0.001
Total breastfeeding transfer (mL·day^{-1})	693 (174)	399 (211)	<0.001
Total breastmilk expressed (mL·day^{-1})	160 (n = 1)	168 (78, 272) (n = 68)	
Supplementary infant formula (mL·day^{-1})	0	135 (80, 272) (n = 72)	
Total infant milk intake (mL·day^{-1})	699 (168)	567 (164)	0.007

Data are presented as mean (SD) or median (IQR). Comparisons between measures for participants with and without perceived breastfeeding problems were made using Student's t-test where the Shapiro-Wilk test indicated normality, and Kruskal-Wallis rank sum test otherwise.

There were no significant differences between the groups for birth weight, frequency of breastfeeds, duration of breastfeeds, or total breastmilk production, but there were significant differences between the two groups for gestational age at delivery, average feed amount, total breastfeeding transfer, and total infant milk intake. Those with perceived breastfeeding problems who were supplementing with infant formula had a significantly lower average feed amount and total breastfeeding transfer ($p < 0.001$).

There were no significant relationships between infant age, birth weight, gestational age at delivery or average feed duration on total breastfeeding transfer ($p > 0.13$), but there were significant relationships between average feed duration and average feed amount ($R^2 = 0.08$, $p = 0.003$), feed frequency and average feed amount ($R^2 = 0.10$, $p = 0.010$), feed frequency and total breastfeeding transfer ($R^2 = 0.05$, $p = 0.018$), and average feed amount and total breastfeeding transfer ($R^2 = 0.62$, $p < 0.001$).

All measurements of total milk production are shown in Figure 1. Twenty-nine measurements were made between 6 and 13 days of lactation. For those with perceived breastfeeding problems the total breastmilk production of 14 was ≥440 mL and 12 was <440 mL. Of the participants without perceived breastfeeding problems two had a total breastmilk production of 624 and 678 mL, and one who had a total breastmilk production of 338 mL at 1.4 weeks was an experienced breastfeeding mother (parity 4) who subsequently produced 722 mL at 5.1 weeks.

Eighty-seven measurements were made between 14 and 28 days of lactation. For the 77 of those with perceived breastfeeding problems, the total breastmilk production of 53 was ≥440 mL, and for 24 was <440 mL. All 10 participants without perceived breastfeeding problems had a total breastmilk production of ≥ 440 mL.

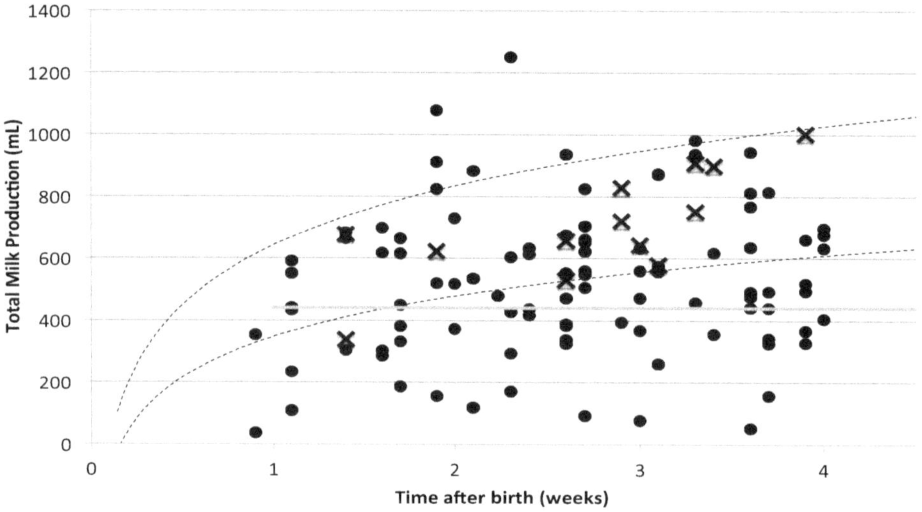

Figure 1. Total milk production of mothers with (circles) and without (crosses) perceived breastfeeding problems. The dotted lines indicate the mean ± SD of milk production derived from the literature [7,9–14,25]. The horizontal grey line indicates the lower limit of normal for established lactation [8].

4. Discussion

The current data from all but one of the participants who did not have any perceived breastfeeding problems support the findings of limited published data suggesting that full milk production is normally reached by the second week of lactation. Even for mothers with perceived breastfeeding problems, over half were producing more than 440 mL per day in the first 13 days after birth.

It is normal for infants to lose weight after birth, and a recent study has demonstrated that the time of the nadir of weight occurs 52.3 h after birth with a loss of 218 g and a weight ratio (weight divided by birth weight) of 0.933 [26]. Compared with infants who were breastfed less than 7 times a day in the first 24 h after birth, infants who were breastfed 7 or more times received significantly more breastmilk, had a maximum weight loss that was 1% lower (5.8% compared with 6.8%), started to regain weight 19 h earlier, and had more than regained their birth weight by 7 days after birth [9]. Although there was no statistically significant difference in the feed frequency between those with and without breastfeeding problems, we observed that 11 of the participants with perceived breastfeeding problems had a feed frequency of <7, a mean total breastfeeding transfer of 195 mL, and a mean total breastmilk production of 344 mL. It is possible that this low production is a result of early infrequent breastfeeding. We suggest that if fully breastfed infants have not regained their birth weight by 7 days after birth the mother's milk profile should be measured during the second week. If it is shown to be low (<440 mL) then early remedial action could be taken, which could include correction of positioning and attachment, increase in feeding frequency, and use of galactogogues. If an ample milk supply is demonstrated the infant should be assessed.

There were small effects of average feed duration and frequency on average feed amount, and a small effect of feed frequency on total breastfeeding transfer. However, the frequency and duration of breastfeeds for this population was very close to the average for mothers of exclusively breastfed infants between 4 and 26 weeks of lactation [17]. The most significant factor affecting total breastfeeding transfer was the average feed amount. This suggests that, while infants should be fed often and feed times should not be unnecessarily restricted, the major contributor to low total breastfeeding transfer is the amount of milk transferred during each breastfeed. About two-thirds of the mothers with perceived breastfeeding problems were already expressing breastmilk, suggesting that milk was possibly available but the infant was unable to remove sufficient milk during breastfeeding. The attention of the lactation specialist on good positioning and attachment and investigation of other possible reasons for poor milk transfer is reinforced by these data. The one participant who had a low measured milk production at 1.4 weeks gave only one extra breastfeed but doubled the amount transferred during each breastfeed and more than doubled her milk production by 5 weeks, illustrating that milk production can be increased during the early weeks as the infant becomes more effective at breastfeeding.

5. Study Limitations

Investigation of breastmilk production of mothers with and without breastfeeding problems in early lactation would benefit from a more detailed history of the initiation of lactation from the time of birth, including time of first breastfeed, skin-to-skin care, assessment of attachment, frequency of breastfeeds, and frequent measurements of the infants' weights in the first week after birth. Measurement of 24-h milk profiles at 7 and 14 days after birth would allow identification of the factors that are most important in optimizing breastfeeding milk transfer. Weighing an infant before and after every feeding for 24 h can be demanding, so while this technique is very useful, it is not appropriate for all lactating mothers.

6. Conclusions

The high frequency of inadequate milk production in early lactation and the consequence of suboptimal milk production in later lactation if left untreated underline the importance of early identification of mothers and infants at risk. Measurement of milk profile during the second week of lactation provides an objective measure of breastfeeding milk transfer and total breastmilk production. These measures, considered with the infant's weight changes, can provide an indication that early intervention by a lactation specialist to improve milk production is warranted.

Acknowledgments: The authors thank the mothers for their participation. Funding was provided by an unrestricted research grant from Medela AG, Baar, Switzerland.

Author Contributions: J.K. and D.G. conceived and designed the experiments; J.K. performed the experiments; J.K. analyzed the data; H.G. retrieved and analysed published data for comparison; J.K. wrote the paper, in consultation with H.G. and D.G.

References

1. Allen, J.; Hector, D. Benefits of breastfeeding. *N. S. W. Public Health Bull.* **2005**, *16*, 42–46. [PubMed]
2. Hill, P.D.; Aldag, J.C. Milk volume on day 4 and income predictive of lactation adequacy at 6 weeks of mothers of nonnursing preterm infants. *J. Perinat. Neonatal Nurs.* **2005**, *19*, 273–282. [CrossRef] [PubMed]
3. Hill, P.D.; Aldag, J.C.; Chatterton, R.T.; Zinaman, M. Comparison of milk output between mothers of preterm and term infants: The first 6 weeks after birth. *J. Hum. Lact.* **2005**, *21*, 22–30. [CrossRef] [PubMed]
4. DiGirolamo, A.M.; Grummer-Strawn, L.M.; Fein, S.B. Effect of maternity-care practices on breastfeeding. *Pediatrics* **2008**, *122*, S43–S49. [CrossRef] [PubMed]
5. Moore, E.R.; Anderson, G.C. Randomized controlled trial of very early mother-infant skin-to-skin contact and breastfeeding status. *J. Midwifery Womens Health* **2007**, *52*, 116–125. [CrossRef] [PubMed]

6. Moore, E.R.; Anderson, G.C.; Bergman, N. Early skin-to-skin contact for mothers and their healthy newborn infants. *Cochrane Database Syst. Rev.* **2012**. [CrossRef]
7. Yamauchi, Y.; Yamanouchi, I. Breast-feeding frequency during the first 24 h after birth in full-term neonates. *Pediatrics* **1990**, *86*, 171–175. [PubMed]
8. Kent, J.C.; Mitoulas, L.; Cox, D.B.; Owens, R.A.; Hartmann, P.E. Breast volume and milk production during extended lactation in women. *Exp. Physiol.* **1999**, *84*, 435–447. [CrossRef] [PubMed]
9. Casey, C.E.; Hambidge, K.M.; Neville, M.C. Studies in human lactation: Zinc, copper, manganese and chromium in human milk in the first month of lactation. *Am. J. Clin. Nutr.* **1985**, *41*, 1193–1200. [PubMed]
10. Casey, C.E.; Neifert, M.R.; Seacat, J.M.; Neville, M.C. Nutrient intake by breast-fed infants during the first five days after birth. *Am. J. Dis. Child.* **1986**, *140*, 933–936. [CrossRef] [PubMed]
11. Neville, M.C.; Keller, R.; Seacat, J.; Lutes, V.; Neifert, M.; Casey, C.; Allen, J.; Archer, P. Studies in human lactation: Milk volumes in lactating women during the onset of lactation and full lactation. *Am. J. Clin. Nutr.* **1988**, *48*, 1375–1386. [PubMed]
12. Saint, L.; Smith, M.; Hartmann, P.E. The yield and nutrient content of colostrum and milk of women from giving birth to 1 month post-partum. *Br. J. Nutr.* **1984**, *52*, 87–95. [CrossRef] [PubMed]
13. Evans, K.C.; Evans, R.G.; Royal, R.; Esterman, A.J.; James, S.L. Effect of caesarean section on breast milk transfer to the normal term newborn over the first week of life. *Arch. Dis. Child. Fetal Neonatal Ed.* **2003**, *88*, F380–F382. [CrossRef] [PubMed]
14. Arthur, P.G.; Smith, M.; Hartmann, P.E. Milk lactose, citrate, and glucose as markers of lactogenesis in normal and diabetic women. *J. Pediatr. Gastroenterol. Nutr.* **1989**, *9*, 488–496. [CrossRef] [PubMed]
15. Roderuck, C.; Williams, H.H.; Macy, I.G. Metabolism of women during the reproductive cycle; the utilization of thiamine during lactation. *J. Nutr.* **1946**, *32*, 249–265. [PubMed]
16. Ertem, I.O.; Votto, N.; Leventhal, J.M. The timing and predictors of the early termination of breastfeeding. *Pediatrics* **2001**, *107*, 543–548. [CrossRef] [PubMed]
17. Righard, L. Are breastfeeding problems related to incorrect breastfeeding technique and the use of pacifiers and bottles? *Birth* **1998**, *25*, 40–44. [CrossRef] [PubMed]
18. Segura-Millan, S.; Dewey, K.G.; Perez-Escamilla, R. Factors associated with perceived insufficient milk in a low-income urban population in Mexico. *J. Nutr.* **1994**, *124*, 202–212. [PubMed]
19. Kent, J.C.; Hepworth, A.R.; Langton, D.B.; Hartmann, P.E. Impact of measuring milk production by test weighing on breastfeeding confidence in mothers of term infants. *Breastfeed Med.* **2015**, *10*, 318–325. [CrossRef] [PubMed]
20. Labbok, M.; Krasovec, K. Toward consistency in breastfeeding definitions. *Stud. Fam. Plan.* **1990**, *21*, 226–230. [CrossRef]
21. Prime, D.K.; Garbin, C.P.; Hartmann, P.E.; Kent, J.C. Simultaneous breast expression in breastfeeding women is more efficacious than sequential breast expression. *Breastfeed Med.* **2012**, *7*, 442–447. [CrossRef] [PubMed]
22. Arthur, P.G.; Hartmann, P.E.; Smith, M. Measurement of the milk intake of breast-fed infants. *J. Pediatr. Gastroenterol. Nutr.* **1987**, *6*, 758–763. [CrossRef] [PubMed]
23. R Development Core Team. *R: A Language and Environment for Statistical Computing*; R Foundation for Statistical Computing: Vienna, Austria, 2011.
24. Pinheiro, J.; Bates, C.J.; DebRoy, S.; Sarkar, D.; R Development Core Team. *Nlme: Linear and Nonlinear Mixed Effects Models*, R package version 3.1-102; R Foundation for Statistical Computing: Vienna, Austria, 2011.
25. Dollberg, S.; Lahav, S.; Mimouni, F.B. A comparison of intakes of breast-fed and bottle-fed infants during the first two days of life. *J. Am. Coll. Nutr.* **2001**, *20*, 209–211. [CrossRef] [PubMed]
26. Fonseca, M.J.; Severo, M.; Santos, A.C. A new approach to estimating weight change and its reference intervals during the first 96 h of life. *Acta Paediatr.* **2015**, *104*, 1028–1034. [CrossRef] [PubMed]

8

Implementation of a Nutrition Program Reduced Post-Discharge Growth Restriction in Thai Very Low Birth Weight Preterm Infants

Suchada Japakasetr [1], Chutima Sirikulchayanonta [2,*], Umaporn Suthutvoravut [3], Busba Chindavijak [4], Masaharu Kagawa [5] and Somjai Nokdee [6]

1 Department of Nutrition, Faculty of Public Health, Mahidol University, Bangkok 10400, Thailand; scdj01@yahoo.com
2 College of Medicine, Rangsit University, Bangkok 10400, Thailand
3 Department of Pediatrics, Faculty of Medicine, Ramathibodi Hospital, Mahidol University, Bangkok 10400, Thailand; u_suthut@yahoo.com
4 Department of Pharmacy, Faculty of Pharmacy, Mahidol University, Bangkok 10400, Thailand; pybcd@mahidol.ac.th
5 Institute of Nutrition Sciences, Kagawa Nutrition University, Saitama Prefecture 350-0288, Japan; mskagawa@eiyo.ac.jp
6 Nursing Department, Buddhasothorn Hospital, Chachoengsao 24000, Thailand; somjainokdee@gmail.com
* Correspondence: chutimabk@yahoo.com

Abstract: Very low birth weight (VLBW) preterm infants are vulnerable to growth restriction after discharge due to cumulative protein and energy deficits during their hospital stay and early post-discharge period. The current study evaluated the effectiveness of the preterm infant, post-discharge nutrition (PIN) program to reduce post-discharge growth restriction in Thai VLBW preterm infants. A prospective, non-randomized interventional cohort study was undertaken to assess the growth of 22 VLBW preterm infants who received the PIN program and compared them with 22 VLBW preterm infants who received conventional nutrition services. Infant's growth was recorded monthly until the infants reached six months' corrected age (6-moCA). Intervention infants had significantly greater body weights ($p = 0.013$) and head circumferences ($p = 0.009$). Also, a greater proportion of the intervention group recovered their weight to the standard weight at 4-moCA ($p = 0.027$) and at 6-moCA ($p = 0.007$) and their head circumference to the standard head circumference at 6-moCA ($p = 0.004$) compared to their historical comparison counterparts. Enlistment in the PIN program thus resulted in significantly reduced post-discharge growth restriction in VLBW preterm infants. Further research on longer term effects of the program on infant's growth and development is warranted.

Keywords: very low birth weight preterm infant; growth restriction; post-discharge; nutrition program

---

1. Introduction

Very low birth weight (VLBW) preterm infants are those born before 37 weeks gestation weighing less than 1500 g, and they comprise between 4% and 8% of neonatal live-births [1,2]. Survival of these small infants has significantly improved mainly due to the advancement of medical intervention in neonatal intensive care units (NICU) [2,3]. However, the extra-uterine growth restriction (EUGR), defined as a decrease in z-score greater than two standard deviations (SD) between birth to discharge [4], is common in the preterm population [5]. A recent cohort study estimated that a prevalence of being small for gestational age (SGA) among VLBW infants (birth weight 750–1500 g) born between 2005 and 2012 to be 44.4%–58.8% at discharge [6]. This may be caused by several health problems such as need for respiratory support, unstable glucose levels, early sepsis, risk of necrotizing enterocolitis and feeding intolerance during NICU stay. These concerns impact highly on the prescribed feeding regimen and result in unrecovered early protein and energy deficits accumulated during hospital admission [7]. Moreover, post-discharge growth restriction also usually occurs in these infants at 28%–40% until 18–22 months corrected age (moCA) [8]. These poor postnatal growths are potentially associated with developmental delay [8], obesity and related complications, such as cardiovascular disease, type II diabetes mellitus and hypertension during adulthood [4,8,9].

In order to compensate for these nutritional deficits and improve the EUGR, the initiation of aggressive parenteral nutrition (PN) in the first week of life and fortified human milk (HM) to this population has been suggested during their hospital stay [10–12]. Furthermore, enriching HM or formula is widely recommended to decrease post-discharge growth restriction and accelerate catch-up growth [10,13]. However, the HM feeding rate in preterm infants usually declines after discharge [14]. Enriched-nutrient formula (EF) is therefore supplemented to provide adequate intakes of energy and nutrients to meet the infant's needs [15–17].

In 2012, a preliminary study was performed at Buddhasothorn Hospital, Chachoengsao, Thailand. It investigated the nutritional care services and growth outcomes in 85 VLBW preterm infants at pre- and post-discharge. The findings revealed that the HM feeding rate was decreased from 87% at discharge to 7% at 6-moCA. After discharge, these infants received unfortified HM and/or standard term formula (TF). Moreover, 85% of VLBW preterm infants were below the standard growth at discharge and 43% remained as below the standard growth at 6-moCA.

In order to reduce post-discharge growth restriction in this population, the preterm infant, post-discharge nutrition (PIN) program was developed and implemented at Buddhasothorn hospital in early 2014. Based on recent recommendations [10,15,18], it focuses on providing an EF in addition to fortified HM with regular monitoring after discharge to ensure infant nutritional intakes. The aim of the present study was to compare growth outcomes in VLBW preterm infants who enlist in the PIN program with those who received conventional nutrition services.

2. Materials and Methods

A prospective non-randomized interventional cohort study was conducted at Buddhasothorn Hospital, located in Chachoengsao province, Thailand. The present study was approved by the Institutional Review Boards of the Faculty of Public Health, Mahidol University (COA. No. MUPH 2014-002), Buddhasothorn Hospital (COA. No.EC-CA 007/2556) and Chachoengsao provincial health office (COA. No. PH_CCO_REC 003/56). The current study used the subgroup of the study that registered as a clinical trial with the Thai clinical trials registration number of TCTR20160211001.

2.1. Participants

A total of 22 VLBW preterm infants who were admitted and discharged from the NICU between March 2014 and February 2015 and given the PIN program were invited to participate in the current study. Detailed verbal and written explanations were given to parents of VLBW preterm infants and informed written consent was obtained from the parents of each participant. These infants were compared with records of 22 VLBW preterm infants who were born and discharged from the NICU between January 2012 and December 2013. The intervention group was enlisted in the PIN program after discharge to 6-moCA whereas; the comparison group received a conventional nutrition service at post-discharge for the same period of time.

A sample size of 22 preterm infants for each group was determined based on a previous study using a power of 80% and a significance level of 5% to detect a program effect of an increase of 5% on the body weight with favorable outcomes at 6-moCA [19]. Inclusion criteria of the study include: (1) birth at $\leq$34 weeks gestation; (2) birth weight ranged between 750 and 1499 g; (3) no use of any medical feeding tube at discharge; and (4) residence in Chachoengsao. On the other hand, infants were excluded if they had: (1) severe respiratory problems; (2) serious congenital anomalies; (3) more than or equal to grade III periventricular or intraventricular hemorrhage; (4) surgical necrotizing enterocolitis; (5) gastrointestinal perforation; (6) severe retinopathy of prematurity; (7) severe birth asphyxia [6,19]; and also if (8) the mothers cannot communicate with researchers.

2.2. Recruitment Process of the Participants

Figure 1 describes the recruitment process of 22 VLBW preterm infants for both intervention and comparison group. The infants born in the comparison period were randomly assigned to the historical comparison group, stratified for sex and birth weight.

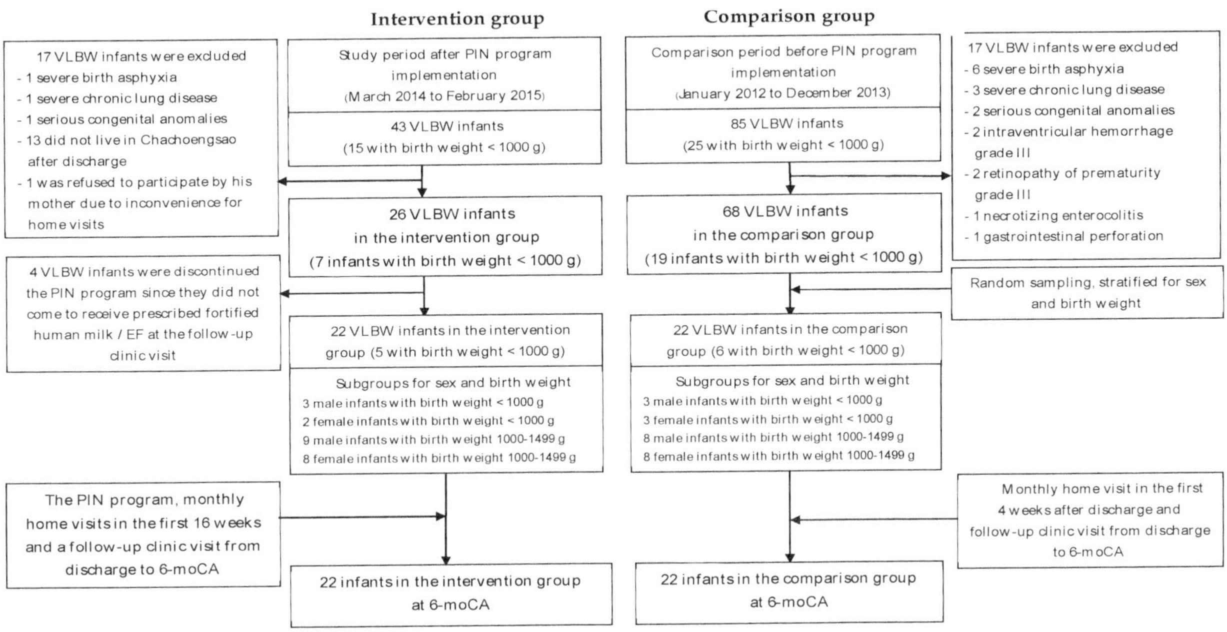

Figure 1. Recruitment process of participants. VLBW = very low birth weight, PIN = preterm infant post-discharge nutrition, EF = enriched-nutrient formula, g = gram, moCA = months corrected age.

2.3. Nutritional Strategies Conducted for Both Groups during Hospital Admission

Until their discharge from hospital, both groups received parenteral and enteral nutrition. Infants in both groups received individualized PN formulation in the first few weeks of life. When the infant's clinical status was improved, trophic oral feeding was introduced until the full feedings of at least 120–150 mL/kg/day were achieved [20]. All preterm infants mainly received their mother's own milk. Mothers were instructed by NICU nurses to assess volume intake of breast milk by test-weighing procedure [21] before discharge. In order to increase energy density from 20 to 24 or 27 kcal/oz during NICU stay as recommended by recent studies [22–24], infants were given fortified HM that was prepared by adding preterm formula (PF) into expressed HM (calculated by definite formula) once their volume of feeding reached 100 mL/kg/day [20,25].

2.4. The PIN Program Conducted for the Intervention Group

The PIN program is a post-discharge nutritional plan of feeding fortified HM and/or EF for VLBW preterm infants from discharge to 6-moCA. It is based on a commentary by the European Society for Pediatric Gastroenterology, Hepatology, and Nutrition (ESPGHAN) committee on nutrition [22] and a nutrition care practice guideline developed by the Oregon Pediatric Nutrition Practice Group (OPNPG) [15]. The program was developed based on outcomes from focused group discussions of a multi-disciplinary team in the hospital. Four experts—including two pediatricians, one neonatologist, and one nurse—reviewed and approved the program. It was implemented as a routine nutritional service at Buddhasothorn hospital since January 2014. The program also includes education on mothers prior to their discharge such as benefits of breastfeeding to preterm infants [26], essential knowledge for lactating mothers [27,28], preparation method of fortified HM, feeding practices [29,30], and personal hygiene for their infant care after hospital discharge [29,30]. The contents of the education program were based on previous studies that recommended the importance of these variables [31,32].

2.4.1. Enriched Milk Intake

The fortified HM suggested in the program was prepared by adding a given calibrated spoon (0.42 g, contains 2.1 kcal) of a powdered preterm formula (PF) (Pre-Nan Abott, Bangkok, Thailand) per oz (30 cc) of expressed HM to prepare milk with energy density of 22 kcal/oz. All intervention infants received fortified HM at discharge. If its volume was less than 50% of daily total volume intake, EF (Enfalac catch up care, Mead Johnson, Bangkok, Thailand) was supplemented to meet the infant needs with a goal of energy including 85–120 kcal/kg/day and 1.5–2.5 g/kg/day of protein according to their corrected age [10,15,22].

Specific written instructions on the fortification of HM and reconstitution of EF powder as well as containers for the preparation and storage of reconstituted milk were provided to each parent. In addition, the written instructions were repeated verbally and parental understanding was confirmed by research personnel. Dietary intake records were given to parents at discharge to assess actual milk and complementary food intake of infants. At the follow-up clinic, the mothers or caregivers were asked for more detailed information of their records. Volume of fortified expressed HM, EF, and other fluid intakes were determined by measuring in oz according to the label on the milk bottle.

2.4.2. Introduction of Semi-Solid Foods

The introduction of semi-solid foods was commenced if: (1) they reached 4–6 months after birth; (2) body weight was not less than 5 kg; (3) they had no extrusion reflex; (4) they had well controlled neck and chair sitting posture; (5) they developed an ability to receive spoon feeding; and (6) they developed an ability to show desire or refusal of food [33–36]. Type and formula of semi-solid foods recommended in the PIN program was based on guidelines of complementary foods for Thai infant and toddlers by Thai Ministry of Public Health [36]. In the PIN program, Thai foods such as a pulp of Thai rice, pumpkin, egg yolk, some kinds of Thai vegetable, such as Coccinia grandis (dtam-leung) were recommended to the infants from 6 to 9 months after birth. In addition, half a teaspoon of vegetable oil per 250 g of semisolid foods was added to prevent fat soluble vitamin deficiencies [36].

2.4.3. Biochemical Blood Tests and Nutrient Supplementation

Biochemical blood profiles were also assessed monthly as a high-risk follow-up clinic. One mL of blood sample was taken at blood drawing unit from all infants and hematocrit (Hct), calcium (Ca), phosphorus (P), alkaline phosphatase (ALP), and blood urea nitrogen (BUN) were examined in order to monitor iron deficiency anemia [37], bone health [38], and nutritional status, including sufficiency of protein. All analyses were conducted at the laboratory unit in the hospital. However, the historical group did not conduct a regular biochemical blood tests after discharge at the follow-up clinic visit. As a result, with an exception of Hct, a nutritional status of historical group was unable to be compared with the intervention group during 1- to 6-moCA and therefore did not include in the results of the current study. Moreover, monthly home visits were performed to monitor HM fortification procedure and infant feeding practices [19].

All infants received 2 mg/kg/day of iron at discharge. When abnormal levels of biochemical markers were identified, special nutrient supplementations were prescribed by a pediatrician at a follow-up clinic as these follows:

- Hct < 35%: Increase dose of ferrous sulfate/fumarate solution from 2 to 4–5 mg/kg/day [17,37].
- Total Ca < 8.0 mg/dL: Supplement calcium suspension 100–140 mg/kg/day [15,17]

- Phosphorus < 5.5 mg/day and/or ALP > 450 IU/L: Supplement phosphate solution 60–90 mg/kg/day [15,17]
- BUN > 20 mg/dL: Consider substitution with unfortified HM and/or standard term formula (TF) [10].

The infants also received 0.5 mL/day of multivitamin drop (MVD) (1 mL of MVD—composed of 2000 international unit (IU) of vitamin A, 400 IU of vitamin D and other water soluble vitamins)—until infants received total daily milk intake of >32 oz (1000 mL) [15]. However, non-fortified HM and/or TF was substituted when infants cannot tolerate with fortified HM and/or EF, or had an excessive rate of weight gain, and also showed Ca, P, and BUN above their normal levels [10].

Estimated volume of breastfeeding was derived by test weighing procedure [21]. Energy and selected nutrients intakes (protein, vitamin A and D, calcium, phosphorus, zinc, and iron), at 2-, 4-, and 6-moCA were estimated using HM composition values from literatures [39,40] manufacturer label claims for PF, EF and TF, drug label of MVD and ferrous fumarate drop, commercial complementary feeding formula and complementary foods composition recommended by the Thai Ministry of Public Health [36].

A nutritionist explained to the mothers/caregiver about the procedure of recording actual amount of all milk feeding, complementary food intake, and nutrient supplementation before infant discharge and also re-checked their practices monthly at the follow-up clinic visit. These records were kept by mothers/caregivers at home and by a nutritionist during home visit and at a follow-up clinic visit.

2.5. The Conventional Nutrition Services Conducted for the Comparison Group

Prior to their infant discharge, parents in the comparison group received general education such as latching technique and observations of feeding intolerance without specific nutritional education. After discharge, infants received unfortified HM and/or TF. They were provided with 2–5 mg/kg/day of ferrous fumarate solution and 0.5–1 mL/day of MVD according to a decision of the in-charge pediatrician at a follow-up clinic. Hematocrit was also tested for all infants at every clinic visits; while the other chemical blood tests, including Ca, P, ALP and BUN were performed at some visits according to pediatricians' decisions.

Enteral intake data of the comparison group was also obtained from dietary intake recorded by mothers/caregivers and nutritional records by a nutritionist at a follow-up clinic as performed in the intervention group. Differences of the nutritional activities between the groups are described in Table 1.

Table 1. Comparisons of activities in the preterm infant post-discharge nutrition (PIN) program and conventional nutrition services.

The PIN Program Activities	Conventional Nutrition Activities
I. Pre-discharge activities	
Giving formal nutritional education to parents/caregivers	No formal nutritional education for parents/caregivers
II. Post-discharge activities	
Giving enriched-nutrient HM and/or EF to the infants from discharge to 6-moCA	Giving unfortified HM and/or TF from discharge to infant weaning
Using revised biochemical blood tests and nutrition supplements protocol	Using biochemical blood tests according to decisions by in-charge pediatricians
Using revised criteria to start and recommended types of semi-solid foods to preterm infants	Suggestions mainly about time to start semi-solid foods at six months after birth without other specific criteria to start semi-solid foods
Monthly home visit until preterm infants reached 6-moCA	Home visit only one time after hospital discharge

moCA = months corrected age; HM = human milk; EF = enriched-nutrient formula; TF = term formula.

2.6. Differences in Milk Formula between the Groups

The energy and nutrients values of fortified HM and EF used in the intervention group and unfortified HM [39,40] and TF used in the comparison group are shown in Table 2. Brands of TF formula were derived from nutritional records at a follow-up clinic in the historical group. Composition of TF is obtained from the average amount of ingredients from four commercial brands of TF in Thailand (S-26, Dumex Hi-Q, Lactogen and Enfalac A^{+}) which contains equal energy density and protein per 100 mL, but are slightly different for the remaining nutrients.

The energy density of fortified HM and reconstituted formula of EF is 21.8 and 22.5 kcal/oz; while those of unfortified HM and TF is 19.7 and 20.1 kcal/oz, respectively. Fortified HM contains higher protein than unfortified HM and TF by 12.5% and 22.5%, respectively, but the remaining nutrients are equal to or less than TF. EF also contains higher protein, calcium, phosphorus, vitamin D and zinc by 42.9%, 79.2%, 70.6%, 33.8%, and 20.0%, respectively, and >100% of vitamin A and iron compared to those in TF.

Table 2. Composition of energy and selected nutrients in fortified human milk (HM) and enriched-nutrient formula (EF) in the intervention group versus unfortified HM and term formula (TF) in the comparison group.

Composition	Intervention Group		Comparison Group	
	Fortified HM	EF	Unfortified HM	TF
Energy (kcal)	72.60	75.00	65.60	67.00
Protein (g)	1.80	2.10	1.60	1.47
Vitamin A (IU)	122.40	343.30	72.00	160.83
Vitamin D (IU)	20.50	63.00	12.00	47.07
Calcium (mg)	38.03	82.00	29.00	45.77
Phosphorus (mg)	19.03	48.00	14.00	28.13
Zinc (mg)	0.63	0.72	0.53	0.60
Iron (mg)	0.25	1.37	0.13	0.63

HM = human milk, Fortified HM = expressed HM + preterm formula (PF: as a human milk fortifier), EF = enriched formula, TF = term formula, Milk composition is per 100 mL as provided by the literature and manufacturer, EF and TF were available cow milk protein-based formula.

The differences of feeding type and nutrient supplementation between the groups are summarized in Table 3.

Table 3. Comparisons of feeding type and nutrient supplementations for preterm infants after discharge between the intervention and comparison group.

	Intervention Group	Comparison Group
I. Feeding type		
1.1 Milk intake at discharge to 6-moCA	Fortified HM and/or EF with energy density of 22 kcal/oz	Unfortified HM and/or TF with energy density of 20 kcal/oz
1.2 Semi-solid foods	Recommended formula based on complementary food guideline for infants and toddlers by Thai MOPH	Commercial formula and/or any formula based on caregivers' decision
II. Nutrient supplementations		
2.1 At discharge		
Iron	2 mg/kg/day, increase to 4–5 mg/kg/day if Hct < 35%	2–5 mg/kg/day *
MVD	0.5 mL/day until infants had total daily milk intake of >32 oz	0.5–1 mL/kg/day *
Calcium suspension	100–140 mg/kg/day if total Ca < 8.0 mg/dL	90–120 mg/kg/day *
Phosphate solution	60–90 mg/kg/day if P < 5.5 mg/day and/or ALP > 450 IU/L	60–90 mg/kg/day *

* refers to dose of nutrient supplementation based on pediatricians' decisions, HM = human milk, EF = enriched formula, TF = term formula, moCA = months corrected age, MOPH = Ministry of Public Health, Hct = hematocrit, MVD = multivitamin drop, Ca = calcium, dL = deciliter, P = phosphorus, ALP = alkaline phosphatase.

2.7. Growth Assessments Conducted with Both Groups

Body weight, length and head circumference of infants in both groups were measured monthly, using revised anthropometric protocol for newborn by the same staff at the follow-up clinic. The hospital staff who perform growth measurement was trained and validated their measuring techniques every three months by the supervisor who is an expert in infant growth measurement. A digital balance (MS 2400; two decimals, maximum load 20 kg, maximum length measured 80 cm) was used for both weight and length measurements and a tape measure (Hochestmass 1.9 × 150 mm) was used for a head circumference measurement.

All data of the infants in the comparison group were recorded from patient charts during hospitalization and out-patient profiles at a follow-up clinic as secondary data until infants reached 6-moCA. Infant growth status was assessed by the Fenton [41] and WHO growth charts [42,43].

2.8. Statistical Analysis

Differences in energy and nutrient intakes between the groups were assessed by the Mann-Whitney *U* test. Comparisons of anthropometric variables between the two groups from 1- to 6-moCA were examined using multivariate of covariance (MANOVA) repeated measures. Mixed model analysis was used to adjust multiple measurements of each infant. The categorical data were compared using chi-squared test. Data analyses were conducted using PASW SPSS statistics (version 18.0, SPSS Inc., Chicago, IL, USA). All statistical analyses were examined with a significance level of 0.05.

3. Results

3.1. Baseline Characteristics of the Participants

Descriptive characteristics of infants were shown in Table 4. There were no statistically significant differences in baseline characteristics between the groups.

Table 4. Baseline characteristics of the intervention and comparison group.

Variables	Intervention Group (n = 22)	Comparison Group (n = 22)	p-Value
Sex, n (%)	Male, 13 (59.0)	Male, 11 (50.0)	0.763
GA at birth, week ± day	29 ± 12 day	30 ± 14 day	0.501
Twin, n (%)	3 (13.6)	6 (27.3)	0.457
Growth status at birth			
Birth weight, g	1192 ± 202	1151 ± 208	0.502
Length, cm	39.1 ± 2.6	38.4 ± 3.7	0.525
Head circumference, cm	26.1 ± 1.8	26.4 ± 1.9	0.626
SGA at birth			
Body weight, n (%)	1 (4.5)	2 (9.1)	1.000
Length, n (%)	1 (4.5)	1 (4.5)	1.000
Head circumference, n (%)	2 (9.1)	2 (9.1)	1.000
SGA at discharge			
Body weight, n (%)	19 (86.4)	20 (90.9)	1.000
Length, n (%)	10 (45.5)	14 (63.6)	0.364
Head circumference, n (%)	15 (68.2)	12 (54.5)	0.453
PMA at discharge, week ± day	37 ± 12 day	38 ± 20 day	0.199
LOS, days	52 ± 12	53 ± 17	0.895
Feeding type at discharge, n (%)			
Breast milk feeding	18 (81.8)	17 (77.3)	1.000
Mixed feeding	3 (13.6)	4 (18.2)	1.000
Standard formula	1 (4.5)	2 (9.1)	1.000
Growth status at term (40 weeks)			
Body weight, g	2631 ± 538	2426 ± 531	0.145
Length, cm	47.7 ± 2.7	46.9 ± 2.9	0.318
Head circumference, cm	33.1 ± 1.6	32.2 ± 2.3	0.470
Maternal age (years)	22.5 ± 4.8	25.3 ± 5.5	0.087

n = number of infant; GA = gestational Age; SGA = small of gestational age; PMA = postmenstrual age; LOS = length of hospital stay. Data are expressed as mean ± SD. The differences between the groups were determined by chi-squared test.

3.2. Human Milk Feeding and Introduction of Semi-Solid Foods

The volume of HM consumed (mL/kg/day) and proportion of HM volume per total volume of all milk feeds per day (%) among infants in the intervention group was greater than those of the comparison group ($p < 0.05$) at 6-moCA, but not 2-and 4-moCA. However, the total duration of HM feeding did not differ significantly between two groups. The length of time from birth to the introduction of semi-solids was also not significantly different (Table 5).

Table 5. Comparisons of exclusively human milk feeding, feeding duration and a timing of introducing semisolid foods between the groups.

	Intervention Group (n = 22) Median (Q1–Q3)	Comparison Group (n = 22) Median (Q1–Q3)	p-Value
Exclusively of HM feeding			
2-moCA			
HM intake, mL/kg/day	40.37 (5.51–111.14)	61.20 (3.05–139.55)	0.234
Proportion of HM volume per Total volume of milk feeds per day, %	35.50 (10.17–79.17)	48.50 (20.21–120.21)	0.381
4-moCA			
HM intake, mL/kg/day	24.67 (13.34–61.55)	27.45 (10.00–57.80)	0.761
Proportion of HM volume per Total volume of milk feeds per day, %	22.82 (15.09–61.09)	21.86 (16.33–56.33)	0.859
6-moCA			
HM intake, mL/kg/day	11.73 (3.16–13.51)	3.05 (1.12–11.43)	0.044 *
Proportion of HM volume per Total volume of milk feeds per day, %	11.82 (4.43–16.43)	2.27 (0.56–7.94)	0.041 *
Total HM feeding duration, weeks after birth	16.00 (10.00–26.00)	18.00 (12.00–24.00)	0.427
Time at introduction of semisolid foods, weeks after birth	20.00 (17.00–23.00)	21.00 (19.00–24.00)	0.625

n = number of infant, Q1 = the first quartile, Q3 = the third quartile, HM = human milk. moCA = months corrected age. Total HM feeding duration refers to duration of exclusively HM feeding and/or mixed feeding (HM feedings plus formula feedings). Differences between groups were assessed by Mann-Whitney U test. * refers to statistically significant differences.

3.3. Nutritional Intake

Table 6 shows differences in daily energy and nutrient intakes of both groups. The intervention group showed greater energy and nutrient intakes except in zinc and iron compared to the comparison group at 2-, 4- and 6-moCA. It was also found that a median iron intake in both groups were slightly greater than the daily recommendation for healthy term infants.

Table 6. Comparisons of daily energy and nutrient intakes of preterm infants between the groups.

Energy/Nutrient	Intervention Group (n = 22) Median (Q1–Q3)	Comparison Group (n = 22) Median (Q1–Q3)	p-Value	RDA
Energy, kcal/kg				
2-moCA	91.08 (89.27–93.46)	88.40 (85.85–91.74)	0.014	85–120
4-moCA	86.39 (82.15–88.22)	76.67 (72.65–78.16)	0.001	
6-moCA	82.07 (80.11–88.63)	69.22 (66.49–71.98)	<0.001	
Protein, g/kg				
2-moCA	2.87 (2.44–3.30)	2.21 (1.95–2.69)	0.024	1.5–2.5
4-moCA	2.48 (2.01–2.89)	2.07 (1.73–2.17)	0.037	
6-moCA	1.85 (1.67–2.25)	1.53 (1.39–1.63)	<0.001	
Vitamin A, IU/kg				
2-moCA	555.66 (294.81–779.81)	219.66 (165.33–357.06)	0.004	320–700
4-moCA	476.99 (301.20–665.91)	209.63 (185.04–238.95)	<0.001	
6-moCA	389.03 (227.10–521.58)	202.24 (191.11–221.02)	0.035	
Vitamin D, IU/kg				
2-moCA	107.98 (45.14–145.78)	50.00 (36.09–71.00)	0.007	60–160
4-moCA	91.19 (55.00–125.30)	42.72 (32.06–47.84)	<0.001	
6-moCA	73.23 (40.22–96.57)	40.78 (38.40–44.72)	<0.001	

Table 6. *Cont.*

Energy/Nutrient	Intervention Group (n = 22) Median (Q1–Q3)	Comparison Group (n = 22) Median (Q1–Q3)	p-Value	RDA
Calcium, mg/kg				
2-moCA	85.80 (63.95–88.95)	68.24 (63.17–69.86)	<0.001	60–120
4-moCA	94.64 (78.61–100.08)	54.20 (51.76–57.94)	<0.001	
6-moCA	66.01 (49.04–69.60)	48.75 (45.77–49.87)	0.016	
Phosphorus, mg/kg				
2-moCA	40.43 (31.31–59.31)	33.13 (30.00–36.92)	<0.001	35–60
4-moCA	71.31 (66.32–77.83)	32.29 (30.14–34.73)	<0.001	
6-moCA	44.35 (35.08–48.81)	30.30 (29.66–34.33)	0.018	
Zinc, mg/kg				
2-moCA	0.78 (0.70–0.84)	0.74 (0.70–0.78)	0.226	0.5–1
4-moCA	0.72 (0.64–0.79)	0.71 0.69–0.75)	0.451	
6-moCA	0.67 (0.59–0.72)	0.64 (0.59–0.69)	0.572	
Iron, mg/kg				
2-moCA	4.95 (4.30–5.72)	4.37 (3.99–5.16)	0.080	2–4
4-moCA	5.02 (3.64–5.47)	5.30 (4.16–5.49)	0.411	
6-moCA	4.73 (3.17–5.58)	4.51 (2.68–5.41)	0.231	

Q1 = the first quartile, Q3 = the third quartile, PIs = preterm infants, RDA = recommended dietary allowance, the upper limit is for PIs 37–40 weeks GA, the lower limit is for term infants at six months of age, no = number, moCA = months corrected age, IU = international unit.

3.4. *Infant Growth Outcomes*

Compared to the comparison group, the intervention group showed significantly greater body weight (p = 0.013) at 4- and 6-moCA and head circumference (p = 0.009) at 6-moCA (Figure 2). However, no significant difference in length and weight gain velocity were observed between two groups at any time point of age. Furthermore, a greater proportion of the intervention group reached body weight greater than −2SD (Z score) at 4-moCA (81.8% vs. 45.5%, p = 0.027) and 6-moCA (90.9% vs. 50.0%, p = 0.007) compared with their comparison counterpart. In addition, the intervention group reached head circumference greater than −2SD (Z score) at 6-moCA (95.5% vs. 54.5%, p = 0.004) compared to the comparison group (Table 7). On the other hand, no differences were observed for length. Also, there was no over-standard growth or growth with higher +2SD (Z score) for body weight, length, and head circumference in both groups. Moreover, there was no correlation between HM feeding duration and any growth outcomes.

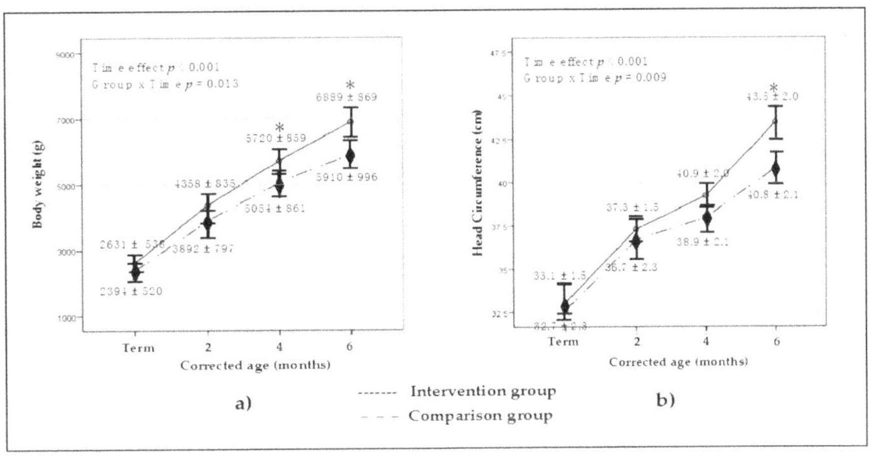

Figure 2. Anthropometric measurement of body weight, (**a**) and head circumference, (**b**) of the intervention and comparison group (n = 22). Data are reported as unadjusted mean ± SD. * denote a significant difference between groups at a specific time point with intervention greater than the comparison group (body weight at 4-moCA, p = 0.001, and 6-moCA, p < 0.001; head circumference at 6-moCA, p < 0.001).

Table 7. Comparisons of growth status of preterm infants between the groups.

Growth Status	Intervention Group (n = 22)	Comparison Group (n = 22)	p-Value
	n (%)		
2-moCA, higher−2SD (Z score) in			
Body weight	14 (63.6)	9 (40.9)	0.227
Length	15 (68.2)	8 (36.4)	0.069
Head circumference	17 (77.3)	10 (45.5)	0.062
4-moCA, higher−2SD (Z score) in			
Body weight	18 (81.8)	10 (45.5)	0.027 *
Length, n (%)	17 (77.3)	10 (45.5)	0.062
Head circumference, n (%)	18 (81.8)	11 (50.0)	0.055
6-moCA, higher−2SD (Z score) in			
Body weight	20 (90.9)	11 (50.0)	0.007 *
Length	17 (77.3)	11 (50.0)	0.116
Head circumference	21 (95.5)	12 (54.5)	0.004 *

moCA = months corrected age, −2SD (Z score) = −2SD line in Z score growth chart for newborn by World Health Organization. Data are expressed as number of cases (percentage). The difference between intervention and comparison group was determined by chi-square test. * refers to statistical significance.

4. Discussion

The current study found an increase in the proportion of infants who were underweight (after adjustment for gestational age) in both groups; 4.5% at birth and 86.3% at discharge for the intervention group and 9.1% at birth and 86.9% at discharge for the comparison group. The results may indicate that early protein and energy deficits were not recovered during hospital admission regardless of the groups. Our findings were consistent with previous studies [4,8,9,44,45] and the present study suggested a difficulty of preventing SGA among VLBW preterm infants during hospital admission.

The present study showed differences in anthropometric variables of fortified HM and/or EF fed versus HM alone and/or TF fed VLBW preterm infants from discharge to 6-moCA. The results indicated that the intervention group had significantly greater weight at 4- and 6-moCA and head circumference at 6-moCA compared to the comparison group. These results indicated the usefulness of the PIN program to compensate for energy and nutritional deficits which VLBW preterm infants experienced during their hospital stay and better recovery using fortified HM and/or EF. While there are controversies in beneficial effects of both fortified HM and enriched formula on growth parameters in preterm infants at post-discharge [7,18,46], the results from the current study were consistent with other studies that observed better recovery in infants who received energy and nutrient-enriched HM or formula at early hospital discharge [47–50].

In addition, the results showed significant differences in a proportion of infants reaching standard weight at 4- and 6-moCA, and head circumference at 6-moCA while no difference was observed at 2-moCA. This result showed that the PIN program may be effective in shortening the period of post-discharge growth restriction by 4-moCA without rapid acute effects. Casey, et al. [45] reported that achieving optimal catch-up growth during a post-natal period, especially by six months after term, will significantly result in better neurodevelopmental outcomes from 18 months to 6 years compared with those who achieved catch-up growth later. Considering suggestion by Casey, et al. [45], the PIN program that provides adequate nutrition to preterm infants during such a critical period may have beneficial impact on both short- and long-term health in this particular population.

Consistently, the nutrient intakes of infants with fortified HM and EF during study period were greater and more consistent with current dietary recommendations [15,23] than infants with unfortified HM and/or TF. These findings may attribute to the effect of enriching HM and formula to increase energy and protein intake. In addition, MVD, Ca, and P supplementation prescribed at a follow-up clinic according to the study protocol resulted in significantly higher intake of these nutrients. However, iron and zinc intakes did not differ between groups. This may be because of a similarity in iron and zinc supplementation practices in both groups. The results also showed a greater volume of human milk and the proportion of feed volume in the intervention group at 6-moCA. However, based on the obtained results, we interpreted the results as due to higher consumption of energy and protein that contained in enriched HM rather than increased volume.

While the PIN program included an education for mothers about benefits of breastfeeding before infant discharge, the present study did not show improvement in feeding duration between the groups and, in fact, was shorter than a previous study that reported a proportion and duration of exclusive HM feeding [20]. The results may indicate insufficient and inadequate lactation support of the PIN program to overcome problems that mothers experienced at post-discharge. Although the PIN program made more frequent home visits compared to the conventional service, the content including educational tools delivered prior to discharge and at each home visit should be adjusted as well as increasing involvement of lactation experts and frequencies of both on-site and distant counseling opportunities. In addition, the current study may indicate a presence of additional issues that prevent mothers from continuing HM feeding after discharge. As a result, further research may be warranted to evaluate factors that influence mothers to continue feeding HM to their child.

Study Limitations

Limitations of the current study included using the historical comparison group which contributed to slightly to differences in composition of TF formula intake. In addition, some data deviations might occur, such as an estimation of breast milk volume intake in some breastfed infants due to inadequate skill of test-weighing procedure in some mothers. Next, the currently applied inclusion and exclusion criteria also limited the extrapolation of the observations as documented in this cohort to all cases. Furthermore, except Hct, we cannot compare the nutritional status of biochemical blood test from 1- to 6-moCA. The main reason is that for the historical group, there were no regular biochemical blood tests after discharge at the follow-up clinic visit in the previous routine practice. The small sample size limits the interpretation and generalization of these results. Further studies are recommended in this area. Lastly, we use non-randomization to evaluate the program, resulting from a limitation of number of participants in a research setting.

5. Conclusions

Enlistment in a PIN program with enriched HM and formula feeding from hospital discharge to 6-moCA resulted in significantly reduced post-discharge growth restrictions for VLBW preterm babies compared to those who received unfortified HM and TF in conventional practices. Regular monitoring is needed to educate mothers or caregivers not to under- or overfeed their infants. Further lactation support and developed maternal education programs are needed to encourage continued HM feeding after discharge. Further studies are warranted with concurrent comparison groups and a longer follow-up period to analyze infant growth, neurodevelopment, and body composition.

Acknowledgments: We would like to thank the Director of Buddhasothorn Hospital for permission to conduct this study in the hospital and the NICU and hospital staff for coordination and assistance with providing the data. We also thank Dechavudh Nityasuddhi for attentive support and for his suggestions regarding statistical analysis. The study was partially funded by the Cerebos Health Research Foundation for Thai Society.

Author Contributions: S.J. was the principal investigator and carried out data collection. C.S. was responsible for overall supervision including the concept of the study, steps in the preterm infant nutrition program evaluation and data collection. S.J., C.S., U.S., B.C., M.K. and S.N. made contributions to the design of the study and the content validity of the nutrition program. U.S. invited and consulted with the experts on content validity of the protocol. S.N. provided substantial assistance with program implementation and research planning. J.S. was involved in the literature review and drafting of the manuscript. M.K. made contributions in coordination and program arrangements during S.J.'s Japan visit for conceptualization of the project proposal and assisted in editing the manuscript. C.S. revised the content and approved the final draft manuscript and all authors read and approved the final manuscript.

References

1. Afjeh, S.A.; Sabzehei, M.K.; Fallahi, M.; Esmaili, F. Outcome of very low birth weight infants over three years report from an Iranian center. *Iran. J. Pediatr.* **2013**, *23*, 579–587. [PubMed]
2. Fanaroff, A.A.; Stoll, B.J.; Wright, L.L.; Carlo, W.A.; Ehrenkranz, R.A.; Starh, A.R.; Bauer, C.R.; Donovan, E.F.; Korones, S.B.; Laptook, A.R.; et al. Trend in neonatal morbidity and mortality of very low birth weight infants. *Am. J. Obstet. Gynecol.* **2007**, *196*, 147–148. [CrossRef] [PubMed]
3. Ruegger, C.; Hegglin, M.; Adams, M.; The Swiss Neonatal Network. Population based trends in mortality, morbidity and treatment for very preterm and very low birthweight infants over 12 years. *BMC Pediatr.* **2012**, *12*. [CrossRef] [PubMed]
4. Euser, A.M.; de Wit, C.C.; Finken, M.J.; Rijken, M.; Wit, J.M. Growth of preterm born children. *Horm. Res. Paediatr.* **2008**, *70*, 319–328. [CrossRef] [PubMed]
5. De Curtis, M.; Rigo, J. Entrauterine growth restriction in very-low-birthweight infants. *Acta Pediatr.* **2004**, *93*, 1563–1568. [CrossRef]
6. Griffin, I.J.; Tancredi, D.J.; Bertino, E.; Lee, H.C.; Profit, J. Postnatal growth failure in very low birthweight infants born between 2005 and 2012. *Arch. Dis. Child. Fetal Neonatal Ed.* **2016**, *101*, F50–F55. [CrossRef] [PubMed]
7. McLeod, G.; Sherriff, J.; Patole, S. Post-discharge nutrition for high-risk preterm neonates. In *Nutrition for the Preterm Neonate: A Clinical Perspective*, 1st ed.; Patole, S., Ed.; Springer: Dordrecht, The Netherlands; Heidelberg, Germany; London, UK; New York, NY, USA, 2013; pp. 173–185.
8. Suppo, L.M.; Rugolo, S. Growth and developmental outcomes of the extremely preterm infant. *J. Pediatr.* **2005**, *81*, S101–S110.
9. Dusick, A.M.; Poindexter, B.B.; Ehrenkranz, R.A.; Lemons, J.A. Growth failure in the preterm infant: Can we catch up? *Semin. Perinatol.* **2003**, *27*, 302–310. [CrossRef]
10. Su, B.H. Optimizing nutrition in preterm infants. *Pediatr. Neonatol.* **2014**, *55*, 5–13. [CrossRef] [PubMed]
11. Morgan, C. Early amino acid administration in very preterm infants: Too little, too late or too much, too soon? *Semin. Fetal Neonatal Med.* **2013**, *18*, 160–165. [CrossRef] [PubMed]
12. Lee, B.S. Nutritional strategy of early amino acid administration in very low birth weight infants. *Korean J. Pediatr.* **2015**, *58*, 77–83. [CrossRef] [PubMed]
13. Yuen, D.E. Feeding premature infants after hospital discharge. *Paediatr. Child Health* **1998**, *3*, 307–308. [PubMed]
14. Menezes, M.A.; Garcia, D.C.; de Melo, E.V.; Cipolotti, R. Preterm newborns at Kangaroo Mother Care: A cohort follow-up from birth to six months. *Rev. Paul. Pediatr.* **2014**, *32*, 171–177. [CrossRef] [PubMed]
15. Authority, O.H. Nutrition Practice Care Guidelines for Preterm Infants in the Community. Available online: http://public.health.oregon.gov/HealthPeopleFamilies/wic/Documents/preterm.pdf (accessed on 16 January 2014).
16. Adamkin, D.H. *Nutritional Strategies for Very Low Birth Weight Infants*; Cambridge University Press: New York, NY, USA, 2009; pp. 101–108.
17. Dall'Agnola, A.; Beghini, L. Post-discharge supplementation of vitamins and minerals for preterm neonates. *Early Hum. Dev.* **2009**, *85*, S27–S29. [CrossRef] [PubMed]
18. Teller, I.C.; Embleton, N.D.; Griffin, I.J.; van Elberg, R.M. Post-discharge formula feeding in preterm infants: A systematic review mapping evedence about role of micronutrient enrichment. *Clin. Nutr.* **2016**, *35*, 791–801. [CrossRef] [PubMed]
19. Aimone, A.; Rovet, J.; Ward, W.; Jereries, A.; Campbell, D.M.; Asztalos, E.; Feldman, M.; Vaughan, J.; Westall, C.; Whyte, H.; et al. Growth and body composition of human milk-fed premature infants provided with extra energy and nutrients early after hospital discharge: 1-year follow-up. *J. Pediatr. Gastroenterol. Nutr.* **2009**, *49*, 456–466. [CrossRef] [PubMed]
20. Ors, R. The practical aspects of enteral nutrition in preterm infants. *J. Pediatr. Neonatal Individ. Med.* **2013**, *2*, 35–40.
21. Arthur, P.G.; Hartmann, P.E.; Smith, M. Measurement of the milk intake of breast-fed infants. *J. Pediatr. Gastroenterol. Nutr.* **1987**, *6*, 758–763. [CrossRef] [PubMed]

22. ESPGHAN Committee on Nutrition; Aggett, P.J.; Agostoni, C.; Axelsson, I.; De Curtis, M.; Goulet, O.; Hernell, O.; Koletzko, B.; Lafeber, H.N.; Michaelsen, K.F.; et al. Feeding preterm infants after hospital discharge. *J. Pediatr. Gastroenterol. Nutr.* **2006**, *42*, 596–603. [CrossRef] [PubMed]
23. Agostoni, C.; Buonocore, G.; Carnielli, V.P.; de Curtis, M.; Darmaun, D.; Decsi, T.; Domellof, M.; Embleton, N.D.; Fusch, C.; Genzel-Boroviczeny, O.; et al. Enteral nutrient supply for preterm infants: Commentary from the European Society of Paediatric Gastroenterology, Hepatology and Nutrition Committee on Nutrition. *J. Pediatr. Gastroenterol. Nutr.* **2010**, *50*, 85–91. [CrossRef] [PubMed]
24. Arslanoglu, S.; Bertino, E.; Coscia, A.; Tonetto, P.; Giuliani, F.; Moro, G.E. Update of adjustable fortification regimen for preterm infants: A new protocol. *J. Biol. Regul. Homeost. Agents* **2012**, *26*, 65–67. [PubMed]
25. Dutta, S.; Singh, B.; Chessell, L.; Wilson, J.; Janes, M.; McDonald, K.; Shahid, S.; Gardner, V.A.; Hjartarson, A.; Purcha, M.; et al. Guidelines for feeding very low birth weight infants. *Nutrients* **2015**, *7*, 423–442. [CrossRef] [PubMed]
26. Enrico, B.; Nicola, P.D.; Giuliani, F.; Peila, C.; Cester, E.; Vassia, C.; Pirra, A.; Tonetto, P.; Coscia, A. Benefits of human milk in preterm infant feeding. *J. Pediatr. Neonatal Individ. Med.* **2012**, *1*, 19–24.
27. Dewey, K.G. Energy and protein requirements during lactation. *Annu. Rev. Nutr.* **1997**, *17*, 19–36. [CrossRef] [PubMed]
28. Raiten, D.J.; Kalhan, S.C.; Hay, W.W., Jr. Maternal nutrition and optimal infant feeding practices: Executive summary. *Am. J. Clin. Nutr.* **2007**, *85*, S577–S583.
29. Turck, D. Safety Aspects in Preparation and Handling of Infant Food. *Ann. Nutr. Metab.* **2012**, *60*, 211–214. [CrossRef] [PubMed]
30. Agostoni, C.; Axelsson, I.; Goulet, O.; Koletzko, B.; Michaelsen, K.F.; Puntis, J.W.; Rigo, J.; Shamir, R.; Szajewska, H.; Turck, D.; et al. Preparation and handling of powdered infant formula: A commentary by the ESPGHAN Committee on Nutrition. *J. Pediatr. Gastroenterol. Nutr.* **2004**, *39*, 320–322. [CrossRef] [PubMed]
31. Thakur, S.K.; Roy, S.K.; Paul, K.; Khanam, M.; Khatun, W.; Sarker, D. Effect of nutrition education on exclusive breastfeeding for nutritional outcome of low birth weight babies. *Eur. J. Clin. Nutr.* **2012**, *66*, 376–381. [CrossRef] [PubMed]
32. Benzies, K.M.; Magill-Evans, J.E.; Hayden, K.A.; Ballantyne, M. Key components of early intervention programs for preterm infants and their parents: A systematic review and meta-analysis. *BMC Pregnancy Childbirth* **2013**, *13*, S10. [CrossRef] [PubMed]
33. Fanaro, S.; Borsari, G.; Vigi, V. Complementary feeding practices in preterm Infants: An observational study in a Cohort of Italian infants. *J. Pediatr. Gastroenterol. Nutr.* **2007**, *45*, S210–S214. [CrossRef] [PubMed]
34. Krebs, N.F.; Hambidge, K.M. Complementary feeding: Clinically relevant factors affecting timing and composition. *Am. J. Clin. Nutr.* **2007**, *85*, S639–S645.
35. Sanchez-Carrillo, C.; Padilla, B.; Marin, M.; Rivera, M.; Cercenado, E.; Vigil, D.; Sanchez-Luna, M.; Bouza, E. Contaminated feeding bottles: The source of an outbreak of *Pseudomonas aeruginosa* infections in a neonatal intensive care unit. *Am. J. Infect. Control* **2009**, *37*, 150–154. [CrossRef] [PubMed]
36. Suthutvoravut, U.; Tuntrachewathorn, S.; Khunsanong, S. *Manual of Complementary Feeding for Infants and Toddlers*; Beyond Enterprise: Bangkok, Thailand, 2009; pp. 5–36.
37. Anemia of Prematurity. Available online: http://emedicine.medscape.com/article/978238 (accessed on 23 August 2015).
38. Abrams, S.A. Calcium and vitamin D requirements of enterally fed preterm infants. *Pediatrics* **2013**, *131*, e1676–e1683. [CrossRef] [PubMed]
39. Gidrewicz, D.A.; Fenton, T.R. A systematic review and meta-analysis of the nutrient content of preterm and term breast milk. *BMC Pediatr.* **2014**, *14*, 216. [CrossRef] [PubMed]
40. Boyce, C.; Watson, M.; Lazidis, G.; Reeve, S.; Dods, K.; Simmer, K.; McLeod, G. Preterm human milk composition: A systematic literature review. *Br. J. Nutr.* **2016**, *116*, 1033–1045. [CrossRef] [PubMed]
41. Fenton, T.R.; Kim, J.H. A systematic review and meta-analysis to revise the Fenton growth chart for preterm infants. *BMC Pediatr.* **2013**, *13*, 59. [CrossRef] [PubMed]
42. Rao, S.C.; Tompkins, J.; World Health Organization. Growth curves for preterm infants. *Early Hum. Dev.* **2007**, *83*, 643–651. [CrossRef] [PubMed]
43. Bhatia, J. Growth curves: How to best measure growth of the preterm infant. *J. Pediatr.* **2013**, *162*, S2–S6. [CrossRef] [PubMed]

44. Cao, W.; Zhang, Y.H.; Zhao, D.Y.; Xia, H.P.; Zhu, T.W.; Xie, L.J. Risk factors for extrauterine growth restriction in preterm infants with gestational age less than 34 weeks. *Zhongguo Dang Dai Er Ke Za Zhi* **2015**, *17*, 453–458. [PubMed]
45. Casey, P.H. Growth of low birth weight preterm children. *Semin. Perinatol.* **2008**, *32*, 20–27. [CrossRef] [PubMed]
46. Young, L.; Embleton, N.D.; McCormick, F.M.; McGuire, W. Multinutrient fortification of human breast milk for preterm infants following hospital discharge. *Cochrane Database Syst. Rev.* **2013**, *28*, CD004866.
47. Young, L.; Morgan, J.; McCormick, F.M.; McGuire, W. Nutrient-enriched formula versus standard term formula for preterm infants following hospital discharge. *Cocharne Database Syst. Rev.* **2012**, *14*, CD004696.
48. Kuschel, C.A.; Harding, J.E. Multicomponent fortified human milk for promoting growth in preterm infants. *Cochrane Database Syst. Rev.* **2004**, *1*, CD000343.
49. Adamkin, D. Postdischarge nutritional therapy. *J. Perinat.* **2006**, *26*, S27–S30. [CrossRef] [PubMed]
50. Winston, W.K.; Koo, E.M.H. Posthospital discharge feeding for preterm infants: Effects of standard compared with enrinched milk formula on growth, bone mass and body composition. *Am. J. Clin. Nutr.* **2006**, *84*, 1357–1364.

9

Leptin Levels are Higher in Whole Compared to Skim Human Milk, Supporting a Cellular Contribution

Sambavi Kugananthan [1,2], Ching Tat Lai [2], Zoya Gridneva [2], Peter J. Mark [1], Donna T. Geddes [2,*] and Foteini Kakulas [2]

1 School of Anatomy, Physiology and Human Biology, The University of Western Australia, Perth 6009, Australia; 21141062@student.uwa.edu.au (S.K.); peter.mark@uwa.edu.au (P.J.M.)
2 School of Chemistry and Biochemistry, The University of Western Australia, Perth 6009, Australia; ching-tat.lai@uwa.edu.au (C.T.L.); zgridneva@gmail.com (Z.G.); foteini.kakulas@bigpond.com (F.K.)
* Correspondence: donna.geddes@uwa.edu.au

Abstract: Human milk (HM) contains a plethora of metabolic hormones, including leptin, which is thought to participate in the regulation of the appetite of the developing infant. Leptin in HM is derived from a combination of de novo mammary synthesis and transfer from the maternal serum. Moreover, leptin is partially lipophilic and is also present in HM cells. However, leptin has predominately been measured in skim HM, which contains neither fat nor cells. We optimised an enzyme-linked immunosorbent assay for leptin measurement in both whole and skim HM and compared leptin levels between both HM preparations collected from 61 lactating mothers. Whole HM leptin ranged from 0.2 to 1.47 ng/mL, whilst skim HM leptin ranged from 0.19 to 0.9 ng/mL. Whole HM contained, on average, 0.24 ± 0.01 ng/mL more leptin than skim HM ($p < 0.0001$, $n = 287$). No association was found between whole HM leptin and fat content ($p = 0.17$, $n = 287$), supporting a cellular contribution to HM leptin. No difference was found between pre- and post-feed samples (whole HM: $p = 0.29$, skim HM: $p = 0.89$). These findings highlight the importance of optimising HM leptin measurement and assaying it in whole HM to accurately examine the amount of leptin received by the infant during breastfeeding.

Keywords: leptin; human milk; whole human milk; skim human milk; appetite; obesity

---

1. Introduction

Human milk (HM) is a heterogeneous fluid composed of a combination of macro- and micro-nutrients, cells, and a plethora of biomolecules that provide the necessary elements to sustain infant growth, protection and development [1–3]. The developmental effects of breastfeeding extend to the programming of various organs and systems of the newborn, including that of appetite regulation [4]. This early developmental programming results in a reduction in obesity and other metabolic diseases not only in the short-term, but also in adulthood [5–9]. The complex system of breastfeeding-mediated appetite regulation is attributable to various factors associated with the practice of breastfeeding, such as feeding on demand, but also potentially to a host of appetite regulatory molecules present in HM [4]. These include whey and casein proteins, HM oligosaccharides, and recently discovered in HM appetite regulatory hormones, including the well-documented adipokine leptin, adiponectin, and many others [10–14].

Amongst these appetite molecules, leptin is the most widely studied, being primarily known for promoting satiety and energy expenditure in adults through binding to the full length leptin receptor (ObRb) expressed on the arcuate nucleus of the hypothalamus [15]. In addition, leptin stimulates cell proliferation, regulates blood pressure, and is also involved in the T-cell immune response, thus displaying pleiotropic roles [16,17]. White adipose tissue is one of the main sources of serum leptin, secreting leptin proportionally to the number of white adipocytes present in the body [18]. Further, gastric chief cells, the placenta, and the mammary epithelium also synthesise and secrete leptin in adults [19–22].

In infants, HM is believed to be a major source of leptin early in life, with the endogenous leptin-synthesising mechanisms being still immature [23]. Leptin in HM has been hypothesised to be involved both in the short-term control of appetite and in developmental programming of appetite and energy-signalling pathways, promoting efficient energy control and storage throughout life [9,24]. Leptin administered during the first 14 days of life has been shown to act as a neurotrophic agent, promoting neural growth from the arcuate nucleus of the hypothalamus to additional appetite control centres located in the central nervous system [25]. HM leptin may provide short-term appetite control in the infant also by up-regulating circulating melanocortins, potent anorexigenic agents that promote satiety [26]. Leptin in HM is sourced both endogenously from the mammary gland and from the maternal serum, following secretion from white adipocytes and gastric chief cells into the bloodstream [9]. In the lactating mammary gland, serum-derived leptin combines with locally-synthesised leptin by the mammary epithelium to yield the total leptin content of HM [22].

Leptin in HM has been predominately measured in skim HM, which does not contain the cellular and fat components of HM [26–28]. Considering that the leptin peptide is capable of lipophilic interactions [29,30], it is plausible it may associate with the fat globule in whole HM. Moreover, HM cells, which are predominantly of epithelial origin in mature HM of healthy mother/infant dyads [1,31], are also thought to contribute to the leptin concentration of whole HM [22]. Few previous studies have measured leptin in whole HM using a radioimmuno-assay (RIA) [21,32]. However, RIA is not considered appropriate for measuring leptin in a lipid-rich medium such as whole HM due to interference of triglycerides with the binding of radioactive-labelled antigens to antibodies, which compromises the sensitivity of the assay [33,34]. Given the lack of an optimised assay to detect leptin in whole HM and the absence of reliable comparisons of leptin levels between whole and skim HM, we developed an enzyme-linked immunosorbent assay (ELISA) as a more appropriate means of measuring leptin in HM, with two antibodies assisting in immobilising the leptin antigen, and compared the leptin concentration between pre- and post-feed samples, as well as whole and skim HM.

2. Materials and Methods

2.1. Study Participants

All procedures involving the recruitment of lactating mothers and HM sample collection and analyses were approved by, and conducted in accordance with, the guidelines of the Human Research Ethics Committee of The University of Western Australia (ethics approval number RA/4/1/4253). All mothers provided informed written consent in the form of a secure online questionnaire that was administered and securely stored by The University of Western Australia. A single sample of whole HM expressed by a mother in her first month of lactation was used for optimisation of the leptin assay. Following assay optimisation, 61 lactating mothers (38 Caucasian, 23 non-Caucasian) with a mean maternal age of 33.6 ± 4.39 years, of full-term healthy infants were recruited to assess leptin differences between whole and skim HM (Table 1). HM samples (~5 mL) were obtained at approximately 1100 h aseptically, as previously described by Hassiotou et al. [35], from each breast before and after the infant fed from a single breast session either by using a Medela Symphony (Medela AG, Baar, Zug, Switzerland) breast pump or by hand expression. Samples were stored at −20 °C prior to analysis. Samples were collected at the second, fifth, ninth, and 12th months of lactation (Table 1).

Table 1. Maternal and infant anthropometric and demographic characteristics (n = 61). Values are mean ± SD (range). Table includes mothers who provided samples for multiple months.

Stage of Lactation (Month)	2	5	9	12
Maternal age (years)	32.9 ± 4.21 (28–40)	33.4 ± 4.27 (24–40)	34.0 ± 4.57 (25–43)	34.1 ± 4.35 (26–44)
Maternal BMI	27.1 ± 7.15 (20.1–38.5)	23.5 ± 4.46 (18.0–35.2)	24.0 ± 5.15 (18.7–37.2)	24.8 ± 5.6 (18.2–34.6)
Parity	2.10 ± 0.75 (1–4)	2.13 ± 0.85 (1–4)	1.96 ± 0.94 (1–4)	2.05 ± 0.98 (1–4)
Infant sex (Male/Female)	12/9	16/16	17/13	12/12
Infant birth weight (kg)	3.58 ± 0.64 (2.66–4.23)	3.49 ± 0.45 (2.66–4.46)	3.49 ± 0.46 (2.82–4.46)	3.59 ± 0.46 (2.80–4.46)
Infant body length (cm)	57.6 ± 2.17 (54.2–61.3)	64.5 ± 2.09 (61.5–69.5)	70.9 ± 2.11 (68.0–74.5)	73.9 ± 2.38 (71.5–78.5)

BMI: body mass index.

2.2. Measurement of Leptin in Whole and Skim Human Milk by an Enzyme-Linked Immunosorbent Assay (ELISA)

Whole HM samples were thawed at room temperature, vortexed for 10 s and aliquoted (2 × 750 µL) into 1.5 mL microfuge tubes (Sarstedt, Numbrecht, Germany). One whole HM aliquot was centrifuged (05PR-22 Refrigerated Centrifuge, Hitachi, Tokyo, Japan) at 1500× g for 10 min at 4 °C and the resultant skim HM portion was aspirated. Both skim and whole HM aliquots were sonicated on ice at 100 Hz for three cycles of 5 s pulses, with a 20 s rest interval using an ultrasonic processor VCX130 (Sonics and Material, Newton, CT, USA). Eleven dilutions ranging from 1 to 50-fold were prepared from both milk preparations using 1% bovine serum albumin (BSA; Sigma-Aldrich, Castle Hill, NSW, Australia) in phosphate-buffered saline (PBS; Gibco Life Technologies, Paisley, Scotland).

Leptin concentration for each dilution was measured using the Human Leptin ELISA DuoSet (R&D Systems, Minneapolis, MN, USA). Capture antibody (4 ng/mL, diluted with PBS, pH 7.4) was pipetted (100 µL per well) to coat the bottom of the wells of flat bottom 96-well microtiter plates (Flow Laboratories, McLean, VA, USA). Plates were sealed and incubated overnight at room temperature. Wells were washed three times with PBS/Tween wash buffer (0.05% Tween 20; (Bio-Rad Laboratories, Gladesville, NSW, Australia) in PBS, pH 7.4), dispensed at 400 µL per well, using a plate washer (Immunowash 1575, Bio-Rad Laboratories, Hercules, CA, USA). Washed plates were inverted and blotted against absorbent paper to ensure no remaining solution was present inside the wells. Blocking buffer (1% *w/v* BSA in PBS, pH 7.4) was added (300 µL per well) to block non-specific binding sites. Plates were sealed and incubated for one hour at room temperature. Blocking buffer was washed according to the wash procedure described earlier. Diluted samples and standards (0–0.9 ng/mL) were added (100 µL per well) in duplicates and plates were sealed and incubated for 2 h at room temperature. Unbound components from samples and standards were washed, and biotinylated detection antibody (4 ng/mL, diluted in 1% *w/v* BSA in PBS, pH 7.4) was added (100 µL per well). Plates were sealed and incubated for 2 h at room temperature. Unbound detection antibody was washed, and streptavidin-horseradish peroxidase (HRP; R&D Systems, Minneapolis, MN, USA) (50 ng/mL in PBS, pH 7.4) was added (100 µL per well), and plates were sealed, wrapped in aluminium foil to avoid exposure to direct light, and incubated for 20 min at room temperature. Streptavidin-HRP was washed and substrate colour reagent (1:1 mixture of 12 mL/vial hydrogen peroxide and 4 mL/vial enhanced luminol, R&D Systems, Minneapolis, MN, USA) was added (100 µL per well). Plates were sealed and wrapped in aluminium foil and were incubated for 20 min at room temperature. Sulphuric acid (1 M, R&D Systems, Minneapolis, MN, USA) stop solution was added (50 µL per well) and absorbance was read at 450 nm by a plate spectrophotometer (Enspire Multimode Plate Reader, Waltham, MA, USA). Standard curves and leptin concentrations were calculated using linear regression (Figures 1 and 2).

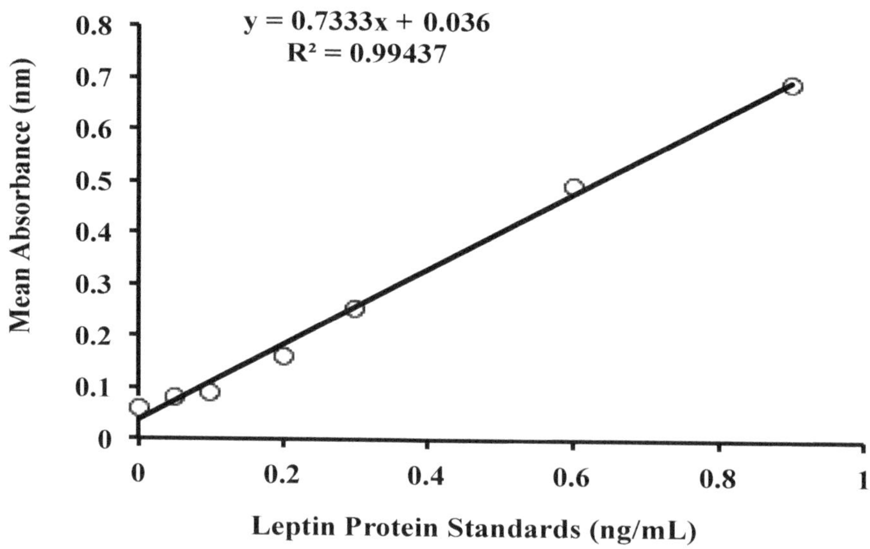

Figure 1. Standard curve for the leptin enzyme-linked immunoassay (ELISA) for whole and skim human milk. Standards were selected according to previous literature investigating levels of leptin in skim human milk, as well as recommendations provided by the leptin kit manufacturer [36].

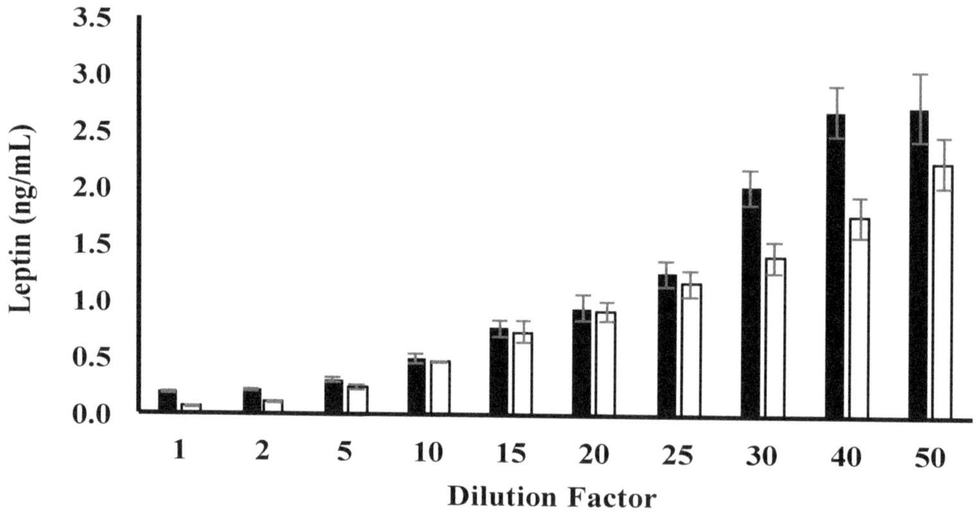

Figure 2. Leptin concentration for whole and skim human milk for each dilution tested. Values are mean ± SEM (n = 100 diluted human milk preparations). Leptin levels in whole and skim human milk are shown by black and white bars, respectively.

Recovery assays to discern the optimal dilution factor for leptin detection were conducted on dilutions reporting leptin concentrations within the range of the protein standards used (Table 2). Following optimisation of the dilution factor, leptin concentration in matched whole and skim HM samples from the study population was measured. All whole and skim HM samples were prepared according to the same centrifugation and sonication protocol used in the assay optimisation. Recovery of a known amount of the leptin protein when added to samples was 97.7% ± 9.7% (n = 10) (Table 2), with the leptin kit reporting an intra-assay variability of <5% and an inter-assay variability of <7.2%.

Table 2. Recovery percentages for each dilution factor for skim and whole human milk leptin measurement.

Dilution Factor	Skim Human Milk Leptin (%)	Whole Human Milk Leptin (%)
1	61.5 ± 2.09	17.1 ± 2.9
2	179.0 ± 0.82	14.0 ± 2.7
5	96.3 ± 1.2	14.0 ± 1.4
10	71.3 ± 1.6	97.1 ± 9.1

2.3. Measurement of Fat Content in Human Milk

The total fat content of HM samples was measured using the creamatocrit method [37,38]. Samples were placed in micro-haematocrit tubes, plugged with sealant and centrifuged at 12,000× g for ten min in a micro-haematocrit centrifuge (Hermle Z230H Labortechnik, Wehingen, Germany). The resultant milk column was placed on the creamatocrit analyser (Creamatocrit Plus, Medela Inc., McHenry, IL, USA) and the length of the fat layer and the total milk column was measured, from which the total fat content was calculated. It has been shown that Creamatocrit measurements strongly correlate with the biochemical spectroscopic esterified fatty acid assay [38–40].

2.4. Statistical Analyses

Statistical analyses were performed using Microsoft Excel 2013 (Microsoft Corporation, Redmond, WA, USA) and R 2.9.10 (R Core Team, Vienna, Austria) [41] for Windows 10, with the additional R package "nlme" (R Core Team, Vienna, Austria) used for linear mixed effects modelling [42]. Student's paired t-tests were conducted to assess leptin differences between matched skim and whole HM samples in the entire study population. Differences between whole and skim HM leptin concentrations were subsequently analysed within each month of breastfeeding, also using matched Student's t-test.

Linear mixed effects modelling was used to examine any associations between HM fat content and whole HM leptin concentration. Responses were modelled with and without controlling for the volume of milk that had been removed from the breast during the collection of the HM sample. To discern the significant random effects to use for each statistical model analysing the association between HM fat content and whole HM leptin concentration, three separate models were devised; one linear model with no random effects and two linear mixed effects models with the following random effects: the effect of general inter-individual variation present in the study population, and the effect of the stage of lactation in addition to inter-individual variation. Analysis of variance (ANOVA) tests were then used to compare each model with the same fixed effects, namely fat content and fat content when controlled for volume of milk removed from the breast. The final model for the association between whole HM leptin concentration and fat content accounted for inter-individual variation and the stage of lactation as random effects when volume removed was not controlled for in the model. Similarly, when volume of milk removed from the breast was controlled for in the linear mixed effects models, inter-individual variation and stage of lactation were also considered as significant random variables to include in the analysis of associations between fat content and whole HM leptin concentration.

Similarly, the association between leptin concentration in whole HM samples and the corresponding fat content was also analysed within each month of lactation. Given that the volume of HM removed during feeding was only collected for 74 samples out of the entire study population, the liner mixed effects models used for intra-month analysis did not control for volume of milk removed from the breast. As with the analysis between the association of leptin levels in whole HM samples and fat content for the entire population, for each month, three statistical models were devised; one linear model with no random effects, and two linear mixed effects models with the following random variables included: the effect of inter-individual variation present in the study population and the effect of the stage of lactation in addition to inter-individual variation. Analysis of variance (ANOVA) was then used to compare each model within each month. For each month of breastfeeding, the only significant random effect found was general inter-individual variation. $p < 0.05$ was considered statistically significant. All values presented are mean $\pm$ standard deviation (SD), unless stated otherwise. All R^2 values were generated from the linear regression line of best fit equations.

3. Results

3.1. Participants

The demographic characteristics of mothers and infants in the study population are shown in Table 2. All infants ($n = 61$) were born at term, healthy, and were growing appropriately for their age according to the World Health Organisation's (WHO) growth charts for exclusively-breastfed infants [43,44]. Mean maternal body mass index (BMI) was highest at 27.1 $\pm$ 7.15 kg/m^2 during the second month of lactation and lowest during the fifth month of lactation at 23.5 $\pm$ 4.46 kg/m^2 (Table 1). Compared to the second month of lactation, maternal BMI decreased by 2.30 $\pm$ 1.55 kg/m^2 over the first 12 months of breastfeeding ($p < 0.01$).

3.2. Leptin Optimisation

Measurement of leptin in whole and skim HM was optimised using an ELISA-based assay. One- to 20-fold dilutions for both skim and whole HM yielded leptin concentrations within the standard range of the assay (0–0.9 ng/mL), whilst dilutions above 20-fold reported values Redmond outside of the upper protein standard used (Figure 2). Mean leptin concentrations for 15-fold (whole HM: 0.8 $\pm$ 0.07 ng/mL, skim HM: 0.75 $\pm$ 0.09 ng/mL) and 20-fold (whole HM: 0.9 $\pm$ 0.11 ng/mL, skim HM: 0.9 $\pm$ 0.09 ng/mL) dilutions were close to the highest protein standard, thus further consideration was not given to these dilution factors (Figure 2). Ten-fold dilution of whole HM yielded the best recovery rates (97.7% $\pm$ 9.7%) (Table 2). Five-fold-diluted skim HM recovered 96.3% $\pm$ 1.2% of leptin (Table 2). Therefore, subsequent samples were diluted by 10-fold and five-fold with the diluent reagent for whole and skim HM samples, respectively, given these dilution factors recovered the highest percentage of leptin protein when the assay was performed for whole and skim HM.

3.3. Whole and Skim Human Milk Leptin

Leptin levels measured using the optimised assay were compared between whole and skim HM obtained during different stages of lactation from 61 lactating mothers. Whole HM leptin levels ranged from 0.2–1.47 ng/mL, whilst a 0.19–0.9 ng/mL range was obtained for skim HM leptin (Figure 3). Whole HM leptin was 0.24 $\pm$ 0.01 ng/mL higher than skim HM leptin across all samples ($p < 0.0001$, $n = 287$) (Figure 3). Leptin levels were also higher in whole HM compared to skim HM within each month of lactation (Table 3). Matched pre-feed whole HM samples contained 0.24 $\pm$ 0.07 ng/mL more leptin than pre-feed skim preparations ($p < 0.01$, $n = 157$), with 0.25 ng/mL $\pm$ 0.05 ng/mL more leptin measured in post-feed whole HM samples compared to paired skim post-feed aliquots ($p < 0.01$, $n = 137$).

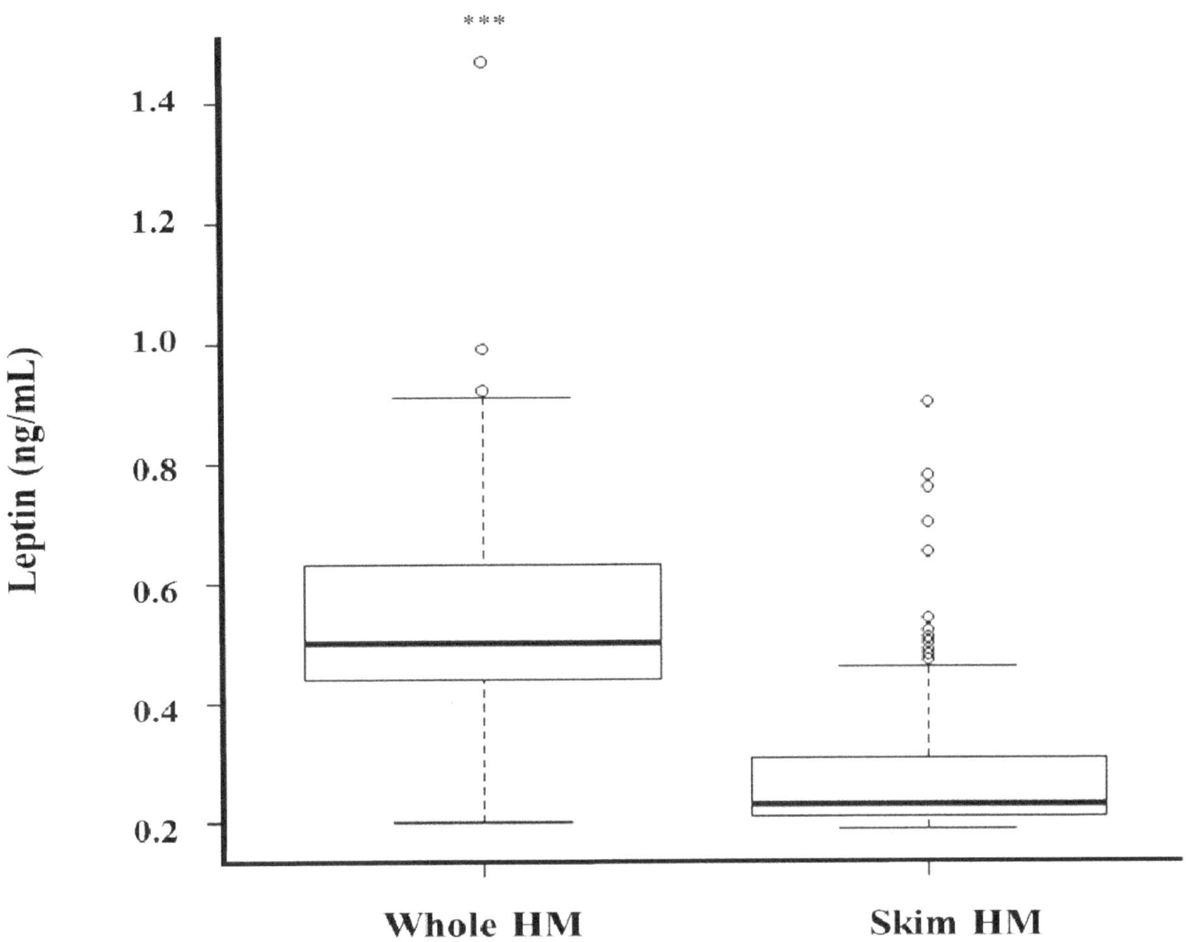

Figure 3. Comparison between whole and skim human milk (HM) leptin concentration ($n = 287$). *** Indicates significant difference between matched whole and skim human milk leptin values ($p < 0.001$).

No association was observed between whole and skim HM leptin ($p = 0.55$, $n = 287$) (Figure 4a). HM fat content was not related to leptin concentration in whole HM when the volume of milk removed from the breast during sample collection was not accounted for ($p = 0.52$, $n = 283$) (Figure 4b) or accounted for ($p = 0.24$, $n = 74$) in the analysis. Further, no association between leptin levels in whole HM samples and fat content were found within each stage of lactation (Table 4).

Table 3. Leptin concentrations for whole and skim human milk at each month of lactation. Values are mean ± SD.

Month of Lactation	Whole Human Milk Leptin (ng/mL)	Skim Human Milk Leptin (ng/mL)	*p*-Value *
2	0.50 ± 0.16	0.32 ± 0.16	$p < 0.0001$
5	0.48 ± 0.16	0.26 ± 0.07	$p < 0.0001$
9	0.56 ± 0.11	0.22 ± 0.03	$p < 0.0001$
12	0.54 ± 0.14	0.21 ± 0.02	$p < 0.0001$

* *p*-values indicate significant differences between whole and skim human milk leptin concentrations at given time points.

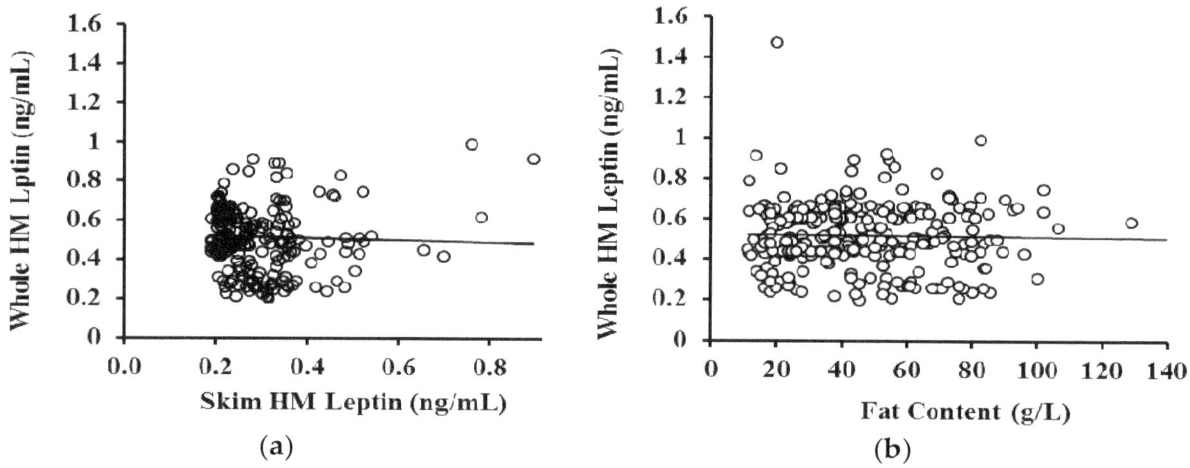

Figure 4. (**a**) Association between skim and whole human milk (HM) leptin ($n = 287$). No association was detected between skim and whole HM leptin levels in matched samples ($R^2 = 0.001$, $p = 0.552$); (**b**) no association was detected between fat content and leptin concentration in whole HM ($R^2 = 0.0004$, $p = 0.17$, $n = 284$). The solid black line is the line of best fit.

Table 4. Association between leptin levels in whole human milk and fat content at each stage of lactation.

Month of Lactation	*N* (Samples)	R^2	*p*-Value *
2	66	0.0013	0.782
5	72	0.018	0.686
9	83	0.069	0.577
12	66	0.153	0.889

* *p*-values indicate absence of associations between whole human milk leptin concentrations and fat concentrations at given time points.

No differences between pre- and post-feed whole ($p = 0.29$, $n = 74$) and skim ($p = 0.89$, $n = 74$) leptin levels were detected after accounting for the volume of milk consumed by the infant during the session (Figure 5). Post-feed samples contained 36.2 ± 2.82 g/L more fat compared to matched pre-feed samples ($p < 0.01$, $n = 74$).

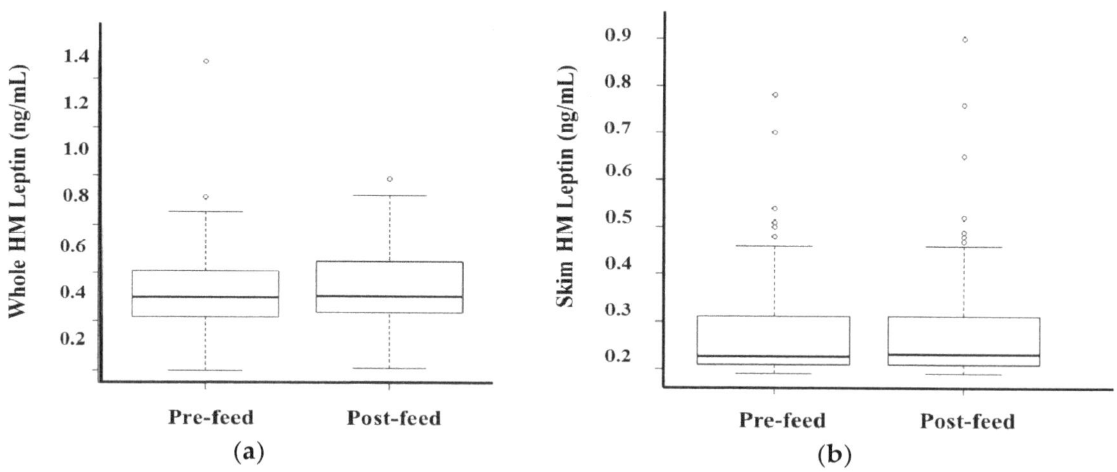

Figure 5. After accounting for the volume of milk consumed by the infant during the session, no differences in pre- and post-feed (**a**) whole and (**b**) skim human milk (HM) leptin values were detected in the study population.

4. Discussion

This study has shown that whole HM contains significantly higher levels of leptin compared to skim HM and that sampling either before or after a breastfeed does not influence this level.

Leptin has been previously shown to be present in HM and has been hypothesised to participate in the short- and long-term regulation of appetite in the breastfed infant [9,45]. In addition, HM leptin may be involved in other functions in the breastfed infant given its known pleiotropic properties, and in mammary development [46,47]. Although many studies have previously measured leptin in HM, optimisation of the methodology has not been well documented and most studies have focused on the levels of leptin in skim HM. However, leptin has been proposed to have lipophilic properties [29] and is also synthesised by mammary epithelial cells [22], which comprise the majority of cells in mature HM from healthy mother/infant dyads [1,48,49]. It is, therefore, conceivable that leptin in HM is associated with the fat and/or cells, which are not present in its skim fraction, suggesting that previous measurements of skim HM leptin have underestimated the concentration of leptin in HM. In this study, we performed a comparison of leptin levels between whole and skim HM and optimised an ELISA assay to accurately measure it in both HM preparations.

Leptin levels were found to be, on average, two-fold higher in whole HM compared to skim HM (Figure 3, Table 3). There are limited studies that have compared whole and skim HM leptin levels and they utilized RIA based methodologies. While results of our study are in agreement with two previous studies that found higher levels of leptin in whole than skim HM, the actual values are different. Houseknecht et al. [32] reported whole HM leptin levels (10.1 $\pm$ 2.6 ng/mL, n = 23) that were approximately seven times higher than in skim HM (1.5 $\pm$ 0.87 ng/mL, n = 23) and, on average, 20 times higher than levels found in this study (Figure 3). Moreover, Smith-Kirwin et al. [21] reported 56-fold higher leptin levels in whole HM (73.2 $\pm$ 39.0 ng/mL, n = 8) compared to skim HM (approximately 1.3 ng/mL), and a 130-fold higher mean whole HM leptin concentration compared to the present study. For skim HM both studies observed leptin levels 1.5–2.5 times greater than those found here [21]. The higher absolute leptin levels measured in these studies may be attributable to the analysis. Both studies used the RIA technique, which is not as reliable as ELISA in measuring leptin levels in whole HM due to its known inaccuracies of immune-reactive antibodies binding to the epitopes of antigens suspended in a lipid-rich medium, such as whole HM, or of interference of iron and emulsifiers with the assay [33,34]. In addition, differences in the technique optimisation between the two previous studies are apparent, as the whole HM leptin level in one study is seven times greater than the other. Both commercially available RIA and ELISA kits are originally designed to measure leptin in serum, not in HM; therefore, optimisation is critical. On the other hand, our results are comparable to leptin levels in many other studies that measured it in skim HM using ELISA, or whole and skim HM using RIA. ELISA in skim HM detected similar leptin levels (from 0.30 $\pm$ 0.04 ng/mL at 1 month to 0.10 $\pm$ 0.02 ng/mL at 12 months, n = 72) in a study by Bronsky et al. [50], (0.28 $\pm$ 0.38 ng/mL, n = 651) in a study by Weyermann et al. [27], and (0.16 $\pm$ 0.04 ng/mL, n = 28) in a study by Miralles et al. [26]. RIA in skim HM also detected close leptin levels: (0.18 $\pm$ 0.15 ng/mL, n = 23) in a study by Schuster et al. [28] and (1.00 $\pm$ 0.80 ng/mL, n = 13) in a study by Schueler et al. [51]. RIA results in whole HM (1.34 $\pm$ 0.14, n = 24) in a study by Bielicki et al. [52] were also comparable to our whole HM leptin levels.

Whilst it has been hypothesised that leptin may be associated with fat globules present in whole HM due to its lipophilic nature [21,29] this was not borne out in this study (Figure 4b, tab:nutrients-08-00711-t004) despite analysing pre- and post-feeding milk samples with a wide range of fat content of 11.0–128.8 g/L. The lack of an association between HM fat content and whole HM leptin levels suggests that fat may not have a strong contribution to HM leptin levels compared to the cellular fraction of HM. Lactocytes, myoepithelial cells, and stem cells present in HM have been previously shown to express the leptin gene [22]. Additionally, flow cytometric analysis of HM cells has revealed that the majority of lactocytes and stem cells contain the leptin protein [22]. Given that lactocytes are the dominant cell type in mature whole HM when both the mother and infant are healthy [1,48,49,53,54], it is likely that lactocytes contribute significantly to HM leptin levels. Indeed, the cellular fraction of HM can constitute a significant portion of milk, comparable to its skim and fat fractions [1,31]. This warrants investigation to further discern the cellular contribution to leptin levels in whole HM, and emphasises the need to assay whole HM for leptin and, potentially, for other appetite hormones, to obtain accurate measurements of the levels of these hormones in HM. Importantly, the procedures of whole HM preparation for such measurements must enable complete lysis of the milk cells for accurate results. This is also very important during sample preparation for whole HM ELISA, achieved in the present study by sonication.

Higher leptin levels in whole HM compared to the skim fraction indicate that infants ingest a larger dose of leptin than that calculated from skim HM. Whilst HM cells likely contribute to the increased leptin level in whole HM the bioavailability of this source is unknown. However, we speculate that the process of digestion would release leptin proteins from HM cells. It is also possible that these cells are absorbed through the stomach mucosa after ingestion and enter the circulation, as has been confirmed with HM leukocytes and stem cells [35,55].

The lack of an association between whole HM leptin and milk fat content may be also attributable to the biochemical properties of the leptin peptide. Although paradoxical to the notion that leptin is synthesised by white adipocytes which exhibit a lipophilic nature, leptin may also consist of hydrophilic regions, enabling it to primarily interact with aqueous fluids. The specific hydrophilic regions exhibited on the leptin peptide are hypothesised to be conserved cysteine residues tethered to disulphide bridges [29,56], which may form polar bonds with water molecules, given sulphide's strong electronegativity properties [57]. Leptin crystallization studies could further confirm its hydrophilic properties [56], providing insight into the lack of an association between the leptin protein and the fat component of whole HM.

Upon analysis, we also found no difference between the concentration of whole HM leptin in pre- and post-feed samples, indicating the small samples taken either pre- or post-feed provide the same levels of leptin despite differences in fat content. To measure the cellular contribution of leptin in HM, it may be possible to acquire larger pre- and post-feed sample volumes and examine the number of cells in the sample. Hassiotou et al. [1] has shown that cell content increases post-feed, as does fat, when larger sample volumes were attained or the breast was well drained of milk.

5. Conclusions

We describe the first standardised and optimised ELISA assay for the measurement of leptin in both skim and whole HM, demonstrating higher concentrations of leptin in whole HM preparations compared to skim HM samples. Further, we provide evidence supporting the lack of an association between the fat component of HM and its leptin content, suggesting a contribution of HM cells, which merits further investigation. Accurate analysis of whole HM leptin will assist in clarifying the biological role of this milk component for the breastfed infant, improving our understanding of early developmental programming of appetite and its implications for obesity prevention later in life.

Acknowledgments: This study was supported by an unrestricted research grant from Medela AG (Switzerland). Sambavi Kugananthan received a Margaret Lomann-Hall Scholarship from the School of Anatomy, Physiology and Human Biology, The University of Western Australia. Zoya Gridneva received an Australian Postgraduate Award from The University of Western Australia (Australia). Many thanks are extended to all mothers who participated in this study, and to the Australian Breastfeeding Association for assistance in recruitment of participants.

Author Contributions: Sambavi Kugananthan designed the study, conducted experiments and data analyses, interpreted results, and wrote the manuscript; Ching Tat Lai conducted experiments and data analyses, and critically reviewed the manuscript; Zoya Gridneva conducted experiments, collected the data, and critically reviewed the manuscript; Peter J. Mark designed the study, interpreted results, and critically reviewed the manuscript; Donna T. Geddes designed the study, interpreted results, and critically reviewed the manuscript; Foteini Kakulas designed the study, interpreted results and critically reviewed the manuscript.

Abbreviations

The following abbreviations are used in this manuscript:

HM	Human milk
ELISA	Enzyme linked immunosorbent assay
RIA	Radioimmunoassay
PBS	Phosphate-buffered solution
BMI	Body mass index
SD	Standard deviation
SEM	Standard error of the mean

References

1. Hassiotou, F.; Geddes, D.T.; Hartmann, P.E. Cells in Human Milk: State of the Science. *J. Hum. Lact.* **2013**, *29*, 171–182. [CrossRef] [PubMed]
2. Ballard, O.; Morrow, A.L. Human Milk Composition: Nutrients and Bioactive Factors. *Pediatr. Clin. N. Am.* **2013**, *60*, 49–74. [CrossRef] [PubMed]
3. Hamosh, M. Bioactive Factors in Human Milk. *Pediatr. Clin. N. Am.* **2001**, *48*, 69–86. [CrossRef]
4. Hassiotou, F.; Geddes, D.T. Programming of Appetite Control during Breastfeeding as a Preventative Strategy against the Obesity Epidemic. *J. Hum. Lact.* **2014**, *30*, 136–142. [CrossRef] [PubMed]
5. Von Kries, R.; Koletzko, B.; Sauerwald, T.; von Mutius, E.; Barnert, D.; Grunert, V.; von Voss, H. Breast feeding and obesity: cross sectional study. *BMJ* **1999**, *319*, 147–150. [CrossRef] [PubMed]
6. Gillman, M.W.; Rifas-Shiman, S.L.; Camargo, C.A., Jr.; Berkey, C.S.; Frazier, A.L.; Rockett, H.R.; Field, A.E.; Colditz, G.A. Risk of overweight among adolescents who were breastfed as infants. *JAMA* **2001**, *285*, 2461–2467. [CrossRef] [PubMed]
7. Armstrong, J.; Reilly, J.J. Breastfeeding and lowering the risk of childhood obesity. *Lancet* **2002**, *359*, 2003–4. [CrossRef]
8. Bouret, S.G.; Bates, S.H.; Chen, S.; Myers, M.G.; Simerly, R.B. Distinct Roles for Specific Leptin Receptor Signals in the Development of Hypothalamic Feeding Circuits. *J. Neurosci.* **2012**, *32*, 1244–1252. [CrossRef] [PubMed]
9. Pico, C.; Oliver, P.; Sanchez, J.; Miralles, O.; Caimari, A.; Priego, T.; Palou, A. The intake of physiological doses of leptin during lactation in rats prevents obesity in later life. *Int. J. Obes.* **2007**, *31*, 1199–1209. [CrossRef] [PubMed]
10. Savino, F.; Liguori, S.A.; Petrucci, E.; Lupica, M.M.; Fissore, M.F.; Oggero, R.; Silvestro, L. Evaluation of leptin in breast milk, lactating mothers and their infants. *Eur. J. Clin. Nutr.* **2010**, *64*, 972–977. [CrossRef] [PubMed]
11. Savino, F.; Lupica, M.M.; Benetti, S.; Petrucci, E.; Liguori, S.A.; Cordero Di Montezemolo, L. Adiponectin in breast milk: Relation to serum adiponectin concentration in lactating mothers and their infants. *Acta Paediatr.* **2012**, *101*, 1058–1062. [CrossRef] [PubMed]
12. Savino, F.; Sorrenti, M.; Benetti, S.; Lupica, M.M.; Liguori, S.A.; Oggero, R. Resistin and leptin in breast milk and infants in early life. *Early Hum. Dev.* **2012**, *88*, 779–782. [CrossRef] [PubMed]
13. Alderete, T.L.; Autran, C.; Brekke, B.E.; Knight, R.; Bode, L.; Goran, M.I.; Fields, D.A. Associations between human milk oligosaccharides and infant body composition in the first 6 mo of life. *Am. J. Clin. Nutr.* **2015**, *102*, 1381–1388. [CrossRef] [PubMed]
14. Alvarez, M. Proteins in human milk. *Breastfeed. Rev.* **2007**, *15*, 5–16.
15. Tartaglia, L.A.; Dembski, M.; Weng, X.; Deng, N.; Culpepper, J.; Devos, R.; Richards, G.J.; Campfield, L.A.; Clark, F.T.; Deeds, J.; et al. Identification and expression cloning of a leptin receptor, OB-R. *Cell* **1995**, *83*, 1263–1271. [CrossRef]
16. Bassi, M.; Furuya, W.I.; Zoccal, D.B.; Menani, J.V.; Colombari, E.; Hall, J.E.; do Carmo, J.M.; Colombari, D.S. Control of respiratory and cardiovascular functions by leptin. *Life Sci.* **2015**, *125*, 25–31. [CrossRef] [PubMed]
17. Magariños, M.P.; Sánchez-Margalet, V.; Kotler, M.; Calvo, J.C.; Varone, C.L. Leptin Promotes Cell Proliferation and Survival of Trophoblastic Cells. *Biol. Reprod.* **2007**, *76*, 203–210. [CrossRef] [PubMed]
18. Klein, S.; Coppack, S.W.; Mohamed-Ali, V.; Landt, M. Adipose Tissue Leptin Production and Plasma Leptin Kinetics in Humans. *Diabetes* **1996**, *45*, 984–987. [CrossRef] [PubMed]

19. Myers, M.G., Jr. Leptin receptor signaling and the regulation of mammalian physiology. *Recent Prog. Horm. Res.* **2004**, *59*, 287–304. [CrossRef] [PubMed]
20. Mix, H.; Widjaja, A.; Jandl, O.; Cornberg, M.; Kaul, A.; Goke, M.; Beil, W.; Kuske, M.; Brabant, G.; Manns, M.P.; et al. Expression of leptin and leptin receptor isoforms in the human stomach. *Gut* **2000**, *47*, 481–486. [CrossRef] [PubMed]
21. Smith-Kirwin, S.M.; O'Connor, D.M.; De Johnston, J.; Lancey, E.D.; Hassink, S.G.; Funanage, V.L. Leptin expression in human mammary epithelial cells and breast milk. *J. Clin. Endocrinol. Metab.* **1998**, *83*, 1810–1813. [CrossRef] [PubMed]
22. Hassiotou, F.; Savigni, D.; Hartmann, P.; Geddes, D. Mammary cells synthesize appetite hormones that may contribute to breastmilk. In Proceedings of the Bi-annual Conference of International Society for Research in Human Milk and Lactation, Charleston, SC, USA, 27 October 2014.
23. Oliver, P.; Pico, C.; De Matteis, R.; Cinti, S.; Palou, A. Perinatal expression of leptin in rat stomach. *Dev. Dyn. Off. Publ. Am. Assoc. Anat.* **2002**, *223*, 148–154. [CrossRef] [PubMed]
24. Bouret, S.G.; Draper, S.J.; Simerly, R.B. Formation of projection pathways from the arcuate nucleus of the hypothalamus to hypothalamic regions implicated in the neural control of feeding behavior in mice. *J. Neurosci. Off. J. Soc. Neurosci.* **2004**, *24*, 2797–2805. [CrossRef] [PubMed]
25. Proulx, K.; Richard, D.; Walker, C.D. Leptin regulates appetite-related neuropeptides in the hypothalamus of developing rats without affecting food intake. *Endocrinology* **2002**, *143*, 4683–4692. [CrossRef] [PubMed]
26. Miralles, O.; Sanchez, J.; Palou, A.; Pico, C. A physiological role of breast milk leptin in body weight control in developing infants. *Obesity (Silver Spring, MD)* **2006**, *14*, 1371–1377. [CrossRef] [PubMed]
27. Weyermann, M.; Beermann, C.; Brenner, H.; Dietrich, R. Adiponectin and Leptin in Maternal Serum, Cord Blood, and Breast Milk. *Clin. Chem.* **2006**, *52*, 2095–2102. [CrossRef] [PubMed]
28. Schuster, S.; Hechler, C.; Gebauer, C.; Kiess, W.; Kratzsch, J. Leptin in maternal serum and breast milk: association with infants' body weight gain in a longitudinal study over 6 months of lactation. *Pediatr. Res.* **2011**, *70*, 633–637. [CrossRef] [PubMed]
29. Kline, A.D.; Becker, G.W.; Churgay, L.M.; Landen, B.E.; Martin, D.K.; Muth, W.L.; Rathnachalam, R.; Richardson, J.M.; Schoner, B.; Ulmer, M.; et al. Leptin is a four-helix bundle: Secondary structure by NMR. *FEBS Lett.* **1997**, *407*, 239–242. [CrossRef]
30. Xie, X.; Steiner, S.H.; Bickel, M.H. Kinetics of distribution and adipose tissue storage as a function of lipophilicity and chemical structure. II. Benzodiazepines. *Drug Metab. Dispos.* **1991**, *19*, 15–19. [PubMed]
31. Hassiotou, F.; Hartmann, P.E. At the Dawn of a New Discovery: The Potential of Breast Milk Stem Cells. *Adv. Nutr. Int. Rev. J.* **2014**, *5*, 770–778. [CrossRef] [PubMed]
32. Houseknecht, K.L.; McGuire, M.K.; Portocarrero, C.P.; McGuire, M.A.; Beerman, K. Leptin Is Present in Human Milk and Is Related to Maternal Plasma Leptin Concentration and Adiposity. *Biochem. Biophys. Res. Commun.* **1997**, *240*, 742–747. [CrossRef] [PubMed]
33. Resto, M.; O'Connor, D.; Leef, K.; Funanage, V.; Spear, M.; Locke, R. Leptin Levels in Preterm Human Breast Milk and Infant Formula. *Pediatrics* **2001**, *108*, e15. [CrossRef] [PubMed]
34. Grundy, S.M.; Mok, H.Y.I.; Zech, L.; Steinberg, D.; Berman, M. Transport of Very Low Density Lipoprotein Triglycerides in Varying Degrees of Obesity and Hypertriglyceridemia. *J. Clin. Investig.* **1979**, *63*, 1274–1283. [CrossRef] [PubMed]
35. Hassiotou, F.; Beltran, A.; Chetwynd, E.; Stuebe, A.M.; Twigger, A.J.; Metzger, P.; Trengove, N.; Lai, C.T.; Filgueira, L.; Blancafort, P.; et al. Breastmilk is a novel source of stem cells with multilineage differentiation potential. *Stem Cells* **2012**, *30*, 2164–2174. [CrossRef] [PubMed]
36. Cannon, A.; Kakulas, F.; Hepworth, A.; Lai, C.; Hartmann, P.; Geddes, D. The Effects of Leptin on Breastfeeding Behaviour. *Int. J. Environ. Res. Public Health* **2015**, *12*, 12340. [CrossRef] [PubMed]
37. Khan, S.; Hepworth, A.R.; Prime, D.K.; Lai, C.T.; Trengove, N.J.; Hartmann, P.E. Variation in Fat, Lactose, and Protein Composition in Breast Milk over 24 Hours: Associations with Infant Feeding Patterns. *J. Hum. Lact.* **2013**, *29*, 81–89. [CrossRef] [PubMed]
38. Mitoulas, L.R.; Kent, J.C.; Cox, D.B.; Owens, R.A.; Sherriff, J.L.; Hartmann, P.E. Variation in fat, lactose and protein in human milk over 24 h and throughout the first year of lactation. *Br. J. Nutr.* **2002**, *88*, 29–37. [CrossRef] [PubMed]
39. Czank, C.; Simmer, K.; Hartmann, P.E. A method for standardizing the fat content of human milk for use in the neonatal intensive care unit. *Int. Breastfeed. J.* **2009**, *4*, 3. [CrossRef] [PubMed]

40. Hassiotou, F.; Hepworth, A.R.; Williams, T.M.; Twigger, A.-J.; Perrella, S.; Lai, C.T.; Filgueira, L.; Geddes, D.T.; Hartmann, P.E. Breastmilk Cell and Fat Contents Respond Similarly to Removal of Breastmilk by the Infant. *PLoS ONE* **2013**, *8*, 1–11. [CrossRef] [PubMed]
41. R Core Team. *A Language and Environment for Statistical Computing*; R Foundation for Statistical Computing: Vienna, Austria, 2014.
42. Pinheiro, J.; Bates, D.; DebRoy, S.; Sarkar, D. *Linear and Nonlinear Mixed Effects Models*; Foundation for Statistical Computing: Vienna, Austria, 2008.
43. World Health Organization. *Birth to 24 Months: Boys Head Circumference-for-Age and Weight-for-Length Percentiles*; Centres for Disease Control and Prevention: Atlanta, GA, USA, 2009.
44. World Health Organization. *Birth to 24 Months: Girls Head Circumference-for-Age and Weight-for-Length Percentiles*; Centres for Disease Control and Prevention: Atlanta, GA, USA, 2009.
45. Bouret, S.G.; Simerly, R.B. Developmental programming of hypothalamic feeding circuits. *Clin. Genet.* **2006**, *70*, 295–301. [CrossRef] [PubMed]
46. Lord, G.M.; Matarese, G.; Howard, J.K.; Baker, R.J.; Bloom, S.R.; Lechler, R.I. Leptin modulates the T-cell immune response and reverses starvation-induced immunosuppression. *Nature* **1998**, *394*, 897–901. [PubMed]
47. Lord, G.M.; Matarese, G.; Howard, J.K.; Bloom, S.R.; Lechler, R.I. Leptin inhibits the anti-CD3-driven proliferation of peripheral blood T cells but enhances the production of proinflammatory cytokines. *J. Leukoc. Biol.* **2002**, *72*, 330–338. [PubMed]
48. Ho, F.C.; Wong, R.L.; Lawton, J.W. Human colostral and breast milk cells. A light and electron microscopic study. *Acta Paediatr. Scand.* **1979**, *68*, 389–396. [CrossRef] [PubMed]
49. Boutinaud, M.; Jammes, H. Potential uses of milk epithelial cells: A review. *Reprod. Nutr. Dev.* **2002**, *42*, 133–147. [CrossRef] [PubMed]
50. Bronsky, J.; Mitrova, K.; Karpisek, M.; Mazoch, J.; Durilova, M.; Fisarkova, B.; Stechova, K.; Prusa, R.; Nevoral, J. Adiponectin, AFABP, and leptin in human breast milk during 12 months of lactation. *J. Pediatr. Gastroenterol. Nutr.* **2011**, *52*, 474–477. [CrossRef] [PubMed]
51. Schueler, J.; Alexander, B.; Hart, A.M.; Austin, K.; Larson-Meyer, D.E. Presence and dynamics of leptin, GLP-1, and PYY in human breast milk at early postpartum. *Obesity (Silver Spring, MD)* **2013**, *21*, 1451–1458. [CrossRef] [PubMed]
52. Bielicki, J.; Huch, R.; von Mandach, U. Time-Course of leptin levels in term and preterm human milk. *Eur. J. Endocrinol./Eur. Fed. Endocr. Soc.* **2004**, *151*, 271–276. [CrossRef]
53. King, B.L.; Crisi, G.M.; Tsai, S.C.; Haffty, B.G.; Phillips, R.F.; Rimm, D.L. Immunocytochemical analysis of breast cells obtained by ductal lavage. *Cancer Cytopathol.* **2002**, *96*, 244–249. [CrossRef] [PubMed]
54. Hassiotou, F.; Geddes, D.T. Immune cell-mediated protection of the mammary gland and the infant during breastfeeding. *Adv. Nutr. (Bethesda, MD)* **2015**, *6*, 267–275. [CrossRef] [PubMed]
55. Weiler, I.J.; Hickler, W.; Sprenger, R. Demonstration That Milk Cells Invade the Suckling Neonatal Mouse. *Am. J. Reprod. Immunol.* **1983**, *4*, 95–98. [CrossRef] [PubMed]
56. Imagawa, K.; Numata, Y.; Katsuura, G.; Sakaguchi, I.; Morita, A.; Kikuoka, S.; Matumoto, Y.; Tsuji, T.; Tamaki, M.; Sasakura, K.; et al. Structure-Function Studies of Human Leptin. *J. Biol. Chem.* **1998**, *273*, 35245–35249. [CrossRef] [PubMed]
57. Bergstrom, F.W. Solutions of the electronegative elements in liquid ammonia; the actions of selenium, tellurium, arsenic acid and a solution of sulfur in liquid ammonia upon cyanides. *J. Am. Chem. Soc.* **1926**, *48*, 2319–2327. [CrossRef]

Dietary Pattern Trajectories from 6 to 12 Months of Age in a Multi-Ethnic Asian Cohort

Geraldine Huini Lim [1,†], Jia Ying Toh [1,†], Izzuddin M. Aris [1], Ai-Ru Chia [2], Wee Meng Han [3], Seang Mei Saw [4], Keith M. Godfrey [5], Peter D. Gluckman [1,6], Yap-Seng Chong [1,2], Fabian Yap [7,8,9], Yung Seng Lee [1,10,11], Michael S. Kramer [2,12] and Mary Foong-Fong Chong [1,4,13,*]

[1] Singapore Institute for Clinical Sciences (SICS), Agency for Science, Technology and Research (A*STAR), Singapore 117609, Singapore; gerlimhn@gmail.com (G.H.L.); toh_jia_ying@sics.a-star.edu.sg (J.Y.T.); izzuddin_aris@sics.a-star.edu.sg (I.M.A.); pd.gluckman@auckland.ac.nz (P.D.G.); yap_seng_chong@nuhs.edu.sg (Y.-S.C.); yung_seng_lee@nuhs.edu.sg (Y.S.L.)

[2] Department of Obstetrics & Gynaecology, Yong Loo Lin School of Medicine, National University of Singapore, Singapore 119228; chiaairu@u.nus.edu (A.-R.C.); michael.kramer@mcgill.ca (M.S.K.)

[3] Department of Nutrition and Dietetics, KK Women's and Children's Hospital, Singapore 229899, Singapore; han.wee.meng@kkh.com.sg

[4] Saw Swee Hock School of Public Health, National University of Singapore, Singapore 117549, Singapore; seang_mei_saw@nuhs.edu.sg

[5] Medical Research Council Lifecourse Epidemiology Unit and National Institute for Health Research Southampton Biomedical Research Centre, University of Southampton and University Hospital Southampton National Health Service Foundation Trust, Southampton SO16 6YD, UK; kmg@mrc.soton.ac.uk

[6] Liggins Institute, University of Auckland, Auckland 1023, New Zealand

[7] Department of Paediatrics, KK Women's and Children's Hospital, Singapore 229899, Singapore; fabian.yap.kp@kkh.com.sg

[8] Department of Paediatrics, Duke-National University of Singapore Graduate Medical School, Singapore 169857, Singapore

[9] Lee Kong Chian School of Medicine, Nanyang Technological University, Singapore 308232, Singapore

[10] Departments of Paediatrics, Yong Loo Lin School of Medicine, National University of Singapore, Singapore 119228, Singapore

[11] Division of Paediatric Endocrinology and Diabetes, Khoo Teck Puat-National University Children's Medical Institute, National University Hospital, National University Health System, Singapore 119074, Singapore

[12] Departments of Pediatrics and of Epidemiology, Biostatistics and Occupational Health, McGill University Faculty of Medicine, Montreal, QC H3A 1A2, Canada

[13] Clinical Nutrition Research Centre, Singapore Institute for Clinical Sciences, Agency for Science, Technology and Research, Singapore 117609, Singapore

* Correspondence: ephmcff@nus.edu.sg

† These authors contributed equally to this work.

Abstract: Little is known about the dietary patterns of Asian infants in the first year of life, nor of their associations with maternal socio-demographic factors. Based on the Growing Up in Singapore towards healthy Outcomes (GUSTO) mother-offspring cohort, cross-sectional dietary patterns were derived by factor analysis using 24-h recalls and food diaries of infants at 6-, 9- and 12-months of age. Dietary pattern trajectories were modeled by mapping similar dietary patterns across each age using multilevel mixed models. Associations with maternal socio-demographic variables, collected through questionnaires during pregnancy, were assessed using general linear models. In n = 486 infants, four dietary pattern trajectories were established from 6- to 12-months. *Predominantly breastmilk:* mainly breastmilk and less formula milk, *Guidelines:* rice porridge, vegetables, fruits and low-fat fish and meat, *Easy-to-prepare foods:* infant cereals, juices, cakes and biscuits and *Noodles (in soup) and seafood*: noodle and common accompaniments. In adjusted models, higher maternal education attainment was correlated with higher start scores on *Predominantly breastmilk,* but lowest education attainment increased its adherence over time. Older mothers had higher start scores on *Easy-to-prepare foods*, but younger mothers had increased adherence over time. Chinese mothers had higher start scores on *Predominantly breastmilk* but greater adherence to *Guidelines* over time, while Indian mothers had higher start scores on *Easy-to-prepare foods* but greater adherence to *Predominantly breastmilk* with time ($p < 0.05$ for all). Changes in trajectories over time were small. Hence, dietary patterns established during weaning are strongly influenced by maternal socio-demographic factors and remain stable over the first year of life.

Keywords: infant dietary patterns; dietary pattern trajectories; first year of life; Asian; factor analysis; multilevel mixed models

---

1. Introduction

Tracking of eating habits through childhood and into adulthood has been observed in different populations [1–4], demonstrating the value of healthful dietary patterns early in life in setting the foundation for life-long eating habits [5]. Thus, besides ensuring an adequate supply of key nutrients and calories to achieve optimal growth, development and health during infancy, the establishment of healthful dietary patterns is also critical.

The importance of healthful dietary patterns during infancy is further supported by recent studies demonstrating associations in infant dietary patterns with growth [6–8] and cognitive outcomes [9,10]. For example, *Health conscious* and *Family foods* dietary patterns, comprising mainly family table foods, at 9-months of age have been related to lower body mass index (BMI) at the same time point [8], while *Discretionary* dietary pattern trajectories, comprising finger foods that are convenient to prepare, from 6 to 24-months appeared have been associated with lower IQ in adolescence [11]. Most of these studies, however, have examined infancy dietary patterns in Caucasian populations and less is known about dietary patterns in Asian infants.

The influence of maternal socio-demographic factors in shaping infancy dietary patterns is widely recognized. Dietary patterns that adhere to infant feeding guidelines are often adopted by mothers with higher educational levels [6,7,12–17], lower BMI [12–14], higher household income [7,14,15] and who are multiparous [8,12,14,17,18]. In contrast, unhealthy infant dietary patterns [19] are associated with younger mothers [6,12,13,15–19] and mothers who smoke [6,14,15,17]. The majority of these have been conducted in Caucasian populations [6,8,12–18,20] with the exception of one study in Japan [18] and another in a multi-ethnic population in America [7]. While it is well established that dietary patterns differ markedly between Asian and Caucasian adults [21,22], the extent to which dietary patterns in Asian infants differ from their Caucasian counterparts and whether maternal predictors of those patterns differ in an Asian infant population remains unexplored.

Weaning represents a transition period during which the diet undergoes rapid changes from milk-based to solid foods, increasing in variety to resemble an adult-like diet. Yet, most studies have limited their scope to a single time-point [7,8,12,17] and may not have adequately accounted for the transitory nature of weaning diets. The concept of modeling dietary patterns longitudinally across time points into dietary trajectories has recently been developed by Smithers *et al.* [11] to address this issue, but no study to date have explored predictors of infant dietary pattern trajectories using this model.

In this study, we aim to better understand the dietary patterns of Asian infants by longitudinally examining the dietary pattern trajectories of infants participating in a multi-ethnic Asian mother-offspring cohort study from 6- to 12-months of age. We also examined potential maternal socio-demographic predictors of these dietary pattern trajectories during this period.

2. Subjects and Methods

Our study is based on the Growing Up in Singapore Towards healthy Outcomes (GUSTO) cohort [23]. Between June 2009 and September 2010, pregnant women 18–50 years of age were recruited from Singapore's two major public maternity units: National University Hospital (NUH) and KK Women's and Children's Hospital (KKH). In brief, the participants were Singapore citizens or permanent residents with the intention to deliver in one of the above-named hospitals, reside in Singapore for the next 5 years, spouses were of the same race, and both parents had a homogenous parental background of Chinese, Malay, or Indian ethnicity. The exclusion criteria included receipt of chemotherapy treatment or psychotropic drugs or the presence of serious medical conditions such as type-1 diabetes mellitus. The study received ethical approval from the institutional review boards of the respective hospitals involved. Written consent was obtained from all participants.

2.1. Maternal and Infant Characteristics

Socio-demographic characteristics such as maternal age, ethnicity, marital and employment status, housing, monthly household income and education level were obtained from the participants during the first clinic visit upon recruitment (<14 weeks gestation). At 26–28 weeks of gestation, self-reported information on pre-pregnancy BMI, tobacco smoking and alcohol consumption were collected. Details on infant gender and birth order were obtained from birth delivery reports.

2.2. Infant Dietary Assessment

Mothers were sent 3-day food diaries to record dietary intakes of their children prior to their postnatal clinic visits at 6-, 9- and 12-months and the diaries were collected at the visits. Instructions and further information on food recording were indicated in the diaries. Mothers who did not complete the food diaries were interviewed by trained personnel at the clinic visits, where a 24-h recall was conducted using the 5-stage, multiple-pass interviewing technique [24]. A set of food pictures and household measurements were provided in the food diaries and during the 24-h recalls to aid in the description of portion size consumed. For the dietary analyses, data from 24-h recalls and 1-day record from the food diaries were used to increase the sample size of the study. Breastmilk consumption via direct breastfeeding was estimated as 780 mL for 6 month-old infants and 600 mL for 9- and 12-month-old infants, based on methods described by Ponza *et al.* [25]. For expressed breastmilk, consumption was quantified according to exact volumes recorded by mothers.

2.3. Identifying Dietary Patterns

Food items from the 24-h recalls (n = 295, 322, 249 at 6, 9 and 12 months, respectively) or 1-day record (chosen by a randomized order) from the food diaries (n = 191, 164, 237 at 6, 9 and 12 months, respectively) were grouped into pre-defined food groups. Food groups with low intakes among the infants (n < 3) were further combined based on similarity in culinary usage and nutrient profile [26,27]. A total of 493, 894 and 1137 food items were identified and subsequently grouped into 34, 44 and 61 food groups at 6, 9 and 12 months of age, respectively. Dietary patterns at each time point were extracted by exploratory factor analysis (EFA) using the principal factor method in SPSS version 22.0 (IBM) [28,29] (see Supplementary Materials). EFA solutions were assessed for the magnitude of loadings of food groups, and each pattern was named based on loadings of $\geqslant\pm0.30$ [9,12,13,15,16]. A dietary pattern score, standardized to a mean of zero and standard deviation of one, was calculated for each subject as a function of the contribution ("loading") that each food made to the pattern. Four dietary patterns were extracted at month-6 and -9 and five dietary patterns at month-12.

2.4. Construction of Dietary Pattern Trajectories

Using multi-level mixed models in Stata version 13.0 (Stata Corporation, College Station, Texas, TX, USA), dietary trajectories were empirically constructed by mapping the dietary patterns extracted by EFA at 6-, 9- and 12-months. This procedure accounts for the repeated measures of dietary pattern scores of each subject. The dietary patterns across the three time-points were examined for their similarity in the types of foods and their loadings to ascertain their suitability to be modeled as trajectories. The mapping of each pattern to a trajectory was based on similar key constituent foods (with high loadings) found in the dietary patterns across the three time-points and this correspondingly determined the name of each trajectory [11]. The model generates estimates of intercepts and slopes. The intercept reflects the trajectory score at the start point of each trajectory (6-months of age), while the slope denotes the rate of change in trajectory scores over time. Details have been previously described by Smithers *et al.* [11].

2.5. Statistical Analysis

Of the 1247 women recruited, 486 singleton subjects with complete birth measurements and dietary records at 6-, 9- and 12-months were included in the final subgroup (illustrated in Supplementary Materials Figure S1). Pearson's chi-square tests and independent sample t-tests were used to compare the characteristics of mothers included in this analysis and those with missing dietary records. Pearson's correlation coefficients were used to assess the correlation between dietary scores derived from 1-day record of the food diaries with the average of the other 2-day records in the subset of mothers who completed the food diaries at the 3 time-points. General linear models were performed to study the associations between dietary trajectory estimates and maternal socio-demographic factors (maternal age, education, ethnicity, employment, BMI at 26-weeks gestation, pre-pregnancy smoking and alcohol status, monthly household income, cohabitation status, parity and infant sex). Socio-demographic factors were stratified into categorical variables and imputations were performed on missing data using the mode. These models were adjusted for potential covariates as described above.

All statistical analyses were performed using the statistical software package SPSS version 22.0 (IBM Corp, New York, NY, USA). A 2-tailed p-value of <0.05 was considered to be statistically significant.

3. Results

Maternal and infant characteristics of participants with complete dietary records from 6- to 12-months ($n = 486$) were similar to those without complete dietary records ($n = 438$) (Supplementary Materials Table S1). Nonetheless, mothers who provided complete dietary records were more likely to live together with their spouses and had higher monthly household income compared with those who did not provide complete dietary records.

3.1. Dietary Pattern Trajectories

Four dietary pattern trajectories were observed from 6- to 12-months and were labeled *Predominantly breastmilk*, *Guidelines*, *Easy-to-prepare foods* and *Noodles (in soup) and seafood* (Figure 1). The *Predominantly breastmilk* trajectory was characterized by breastmilk feeding that exceeded formula milk, the addition of fresh fruits at 9-months, and bean curd (tofu), high-fat ethnic breads and starchy vegetables at 12-months. The *Guidelines* trajectory followed recommended weaning guidelines [30] and was characterized by rice porridge, low-fat fish and meat, a variety of vegetables and fresh fruits as core foods items throughout the 6–12-month period. This trajectory was also characterized by lower intakes of infant cereal at 9- and 12-months.

The *Easy-to-prepare foods* trajectory consisted of foods that require little preparation (infant cereals, juices, cakes and biscuits, as well as adult table foods such as white rice, green vegetables) at 6-months and progressed to easy-to-prepare foods such as breads, spreads, biscuit and confectionaries at 12-months. The *Noodles (in soup) and seafood* trajectory was pre-dominantly noodle-based and consisted of common accompaniments such as eggs, seafood products, dried preserved fruits and bean curd (tofu) found in noodle soup meals. An additional dietary pattern emerged at 12-months of age but did not fall into any of the dietary trajectories: the *Pulses and grains* pattern. This pattern was distinguished by high intakes of nuts and seeds, grains, legumes and lentils and high energy-dense confectionaries.

A complete list of food items and their loading scores for each dietary pattern and trajectory is provided in the supplementary file (Supplementary Materials Tables S2–S4). Examples of foods consumed in each item are also provided in Supplementary Materials Table S5. Dietary patterns scores derived from 1-day record of the food diaries were found to be significantly correlated with the other 2-days of the same diaries (correlation coefficient ranged from 0.43 to 0.82) for all dietary patterns and all time points except for the *Easy-to-prepare foods* dietary pattern at 9-months (correlation coefficient = 0.123) (Supplementary Materials Tables S6).

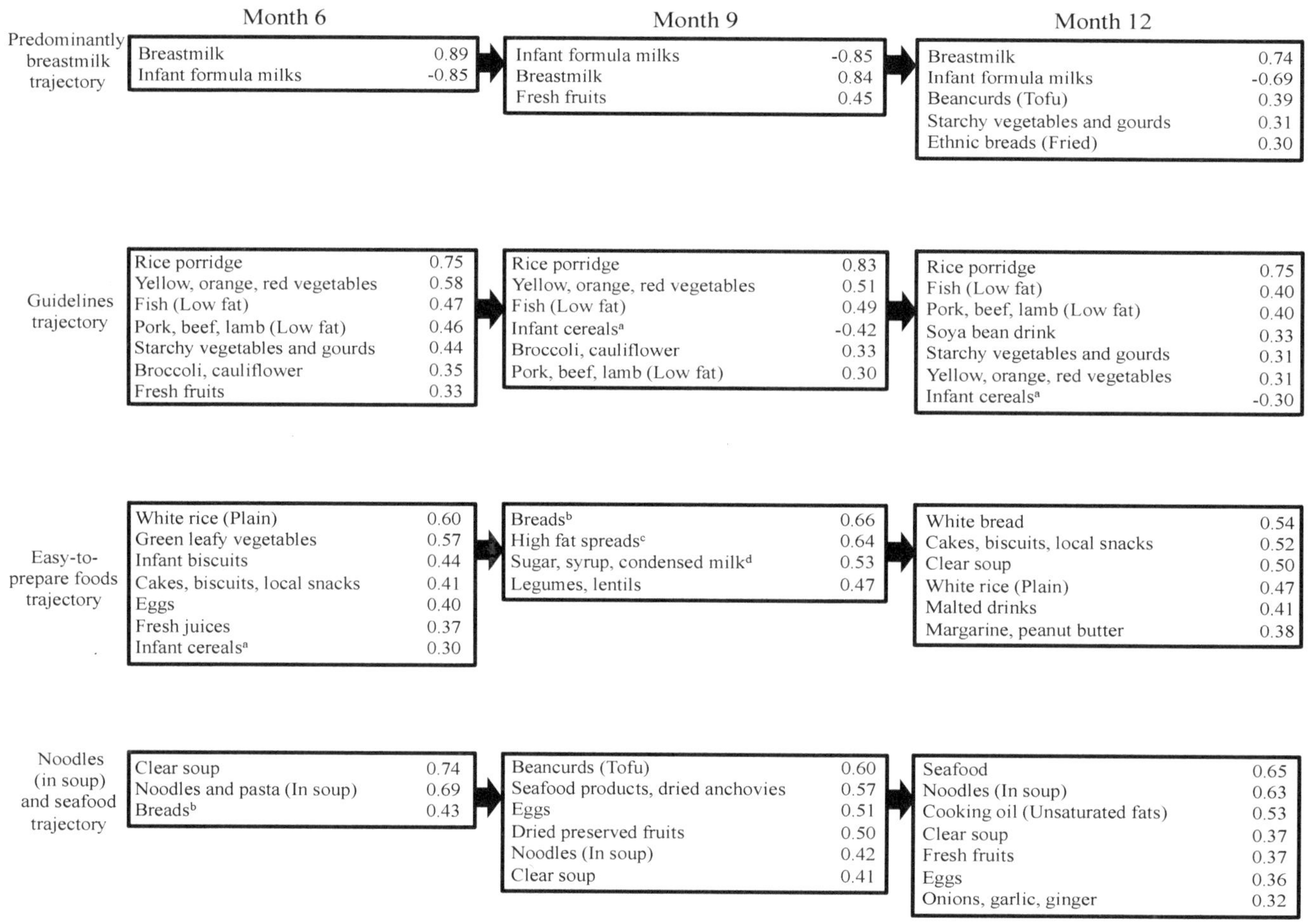

Figure 1. Mapping of dietary patterns at age 6, 9 and 12 months to trajectories. Only foods with loadings $\geqslant \pm 0.30$ are shown in the figure. A full list of food items and their loadings are provided in Supplementary Materials. [a] Includes rice, wheat and oat baby cereals; [b] Includes white and whole wheat breads, breads with fillings or toppings, and baked ethnic breads; [c] Includes butter, ghee, peanut butter and margarine; [d] Added to drinks and cereals.

3.2. *Characteristics of Study Population with Trajectory Estimates*

The dietary pattern trajectory estimates of 486 infants summarized with respect to their maternal and infant characteristics are shown in Supplementary Materials Tables S7 and S8. Ranges of intercepts and slopes are listed in the Supplementary Materials. In general, the slopes were small relative to the intercepts.

3.3. *Associations with Trajectory Intercepts*

The fully adjusted associations between the intercepts and maternal socio-demographic characteristics are shown in Table 1. Higher *Predominantly breastmilk* trajectory start scores for infants at 6 months were significantly associated with higher maternal education, higher income, Chinese ethnicity, not working outside the home and having more than one child at home. Higher *Guidelines* trajectory intercepts at 6 months were associated with post-secondary education. Male infants had higher *Easy-to-prepare foods* trajectory intercepts at 6 months, while their mothers were more likely to be older (>34 years old) and of Indian ethnicity. No significant maternal factors were associated with the *Noodles (in soup) and seafood* trajectory.

3.4. *Associations with Trajectory Slopes*

The fully adjusted associations between maternal socio-demographic characteristics and rates of change in dietary trajectory scores (slopes) over the period of 6 to 12-months are shown in Table 2. Mothers of Indian ethnicity, of lower education qualification and primiparous had higher positive slopes for the *Predominantly breastmilk* trajectory. Chinese infants had higher positive slopes for the *Guidelines* trajectory than Malay or Indian infants. Infants with higher slopes for the *Easy-to-prepare foods* trajectory had younger mothers. Chinese infants had higher slopes for the *Noodles (in soup) and seafood* trajectory.

The *Pulses and grain* dietary pattern emerged only at 12-months of age and was associated with Indian ethnicity and mothers with post-secondary education (Supplementary Materials Table S9).

Table 1. Adjusted associations between dietary pattern trajectory intercepts and sociodemographic characteristics ($n = 486$) [a].

Maternal and Child Characteristics	**β (95% CI)**			
	Predominantly Breastmilk	**Guidelines**	**Easy-to-Prepare Foods**	**Noodles (in Soup) and Seafood**
Maternal characteristics				
Ethnicity				
Indian	−0.245 (−0.463, −0.026) *	0.069 (−0.035, 0.173)	0.123 (0.063, 0.184) ***	0.028 (−0.015, 0.072)
Malay	−0.259 (−0.476, −0.042) *	−0.069 (−0.172, 0.034)	0.031 (−0.029, 0.091)	0.028 (−0.015, 0.071)
Chinese	*Reference*	*Reference*	*Reference*	*Reference*
Maternal Age				
18–29	0.084 (−0.123, 0.292)	−0.026 (−0.125, 0.073)	−0.088 (−0.145, −0.030) **	0.035 (−0.006, 0.076)
30–34	0.040 (−0.161, 0.241)	−0.006 (−0.102, 0.089)	−0.069 (−0.125, −0.014) *	0.034 (−0.005, 0.074)
>34	*Reference*	*Reference*	*Reference*	*Reference*
Maternal Education [b]				
Primary education	−0.781 (−1.021, −0.541) ***	0.081 (−0.033, 0.195)	−0.025 (−0.091, 0.041)	−0.003 (−0.051, 0.044)
Post-secondary	−0.480 (−0.683, −0.277) ***	0.174 (0.077, 0.270) ***	<0.001 (−0.056, 0.056)	−0.007 (−0.047, 0.033)
University and other	*Reference*	*Reference*	*Reference*	*Reference*
Household Income (SGD)				
<1999	−0.441 (−0.746, −0.137) **	−0.065 (−0.21, 0.080)	0.053 (−0.031, 0.137)	−0.013 (−0.073, 0.047)
2000–5999	−0.057 (−0.258, 0.145)	−0.034 (−0.13, 0.061)	0.019 (−0.037, 0.074)	0.029 (−0.010, 0.069)
>6000	*Reference*	*Reference*	*Reference*	*Reference*
Employment				
Unemployed	0.273 (0.096, 0.449) **	0.014 (−0.069, 0.098)	0.009 (−0.040, 0.058)	0.019 (−0.016, 0.054)
Employed	*Reference*	*Reference*	*Reference*	*Reference*
Maternal BMI at 26 weeks [c]				
<18.5–24.9	0.126 (−0.093, 0.344)	0.015 (−0.089, 0.119)	0.010 (−0.050, 0.070)	−0.022 (−0.065, 0.022)
25.0–29.9	0.214 (−0.005, 0.433)	0.059 (−0.045, 0.163)	0.015 (−0.046, 0.075)	−0.009 (−0.052, 0.034)
>30.0	*Reference*	*Reference*	*Reference*	*Reference*
Alcohol [d]				
Yes	0.080 (−0.095, 0.255)	0.030 (−0.053, 0.113)	−0.019 (−0.068, 0.029)	0.013 (−0.021, 0.048)
No	*Reference*	*Reference*	*Reference*	*Reference*
Smoking [d]				
Yes	−0.209 (−0.456, 0.038)	−0.005 (−0.123, 0.112)	0.039 (−0.030, 0.107)	−0.010 (−0.059, 0.039)
No	*Reference*	*Reference*	*Reference*	*Reference*

Table 1. *Cont.*

Maternal and Child Characteristics	β (95% CI)			
	Predominantly Breastmilk	**Guidelines**	**Easy-to-Prepare Foods**	**Noodles (in Soup) and Seafood**
Cohabitation [e]				
Not living together	0.022 (−0.719, 0.752)	0.021 (−0.331, 0.372)	−0.039 (−0.244, 0.165)	0.063 (−0.083, 0.209)
Living together	*Reference*	*Reference*	*Reference*	*Reference*
Infant characteristics				
Gender				
Female	0.027 (−0.122, 0.176)	0.012 (−0.059, 0.082)	−0.042 (−0.083, −0.001) *	−0.016 (−0.045, 0.013)
Male	*Reference*	*Reference*	*Reference*	*Reference*
Parity				
First child	−0.202 (−0.371, −0.033) **	0.014 (−0.066, 0.094)	0.032 (−0.015, 0.079)	0.005 (−0.029, 0.038)
Not first child	*Reference*	*Reference*	*Reference*	*Reference*

Abbreviations: BMI, body mass index. [a] Data shown are multivariable linear model β coefficients and their 95% confidence intervals (95% CIs) obtained from general linear models. Trajectory intercepts are the dependent variable for formed trajectories from age 6 to 12 months and each characteristic was assessed with adjustments for the other characteristics (covariates) [b] Maternal education categorized as primary and secondary education, post-secondary education, as well as university and others; [c] Mother's BMI recorded at 26 weeks of pregnancy (kg/m^2); [d] Status recorded prior to pregnancy; [e] Reflects the marital status; single, separated or divorced mothers as living separately; married mothers as living together. * p-value < 0.05; ** p-value < 0.01; *** p-value < 0.001.

Table 2. Adjusted associations between dietary pattern trajectory slopes and sociodemographic characteristics ($n = 486$) [a].

Maternal and Child Characteristics	β (95% CI)			
	Predominantly Breastmilk	**Guidelines**	**Easy-to-Prepare Foods**	**Noodles (in soup) and Seafood**
Maternal characteristics				
Ethnicity				
Indian	0.026 (0.013, 0.040) ***	−0.040 (−0.052, −0.028) ***	0.000 (−0.008, 0.008)	−0.013 (−0.020, −0.005) **
Malay	0.013 (−0.001, 0.026)	−0.014 (−0.026, −0.002) *	0.004 (−0.004, 0.012)	−0.013 (−0.021, −0.006) **
Chinese	*Reference*	*Reference*	*Reference*	*Reference*
Maternal Age				
18–29	-8.823×10^{-5} (−0.013, 0.013)	0.005 (−0.007, 0.016)	0.009 (0.001, 0.017) *	−0.005 (−0.012, 0.002)
30–34	0.003 (−0.010, 0.015)	0.007 (−0.004, 0.018)	0.006 (−0.002, 0.013)	−0.003 (−0.010, 0.004)
>34	*Reference*	*Reference*	*Reference*	*Reference*

Table 2. *Cont.*

Maternal and Child Characteristics	β (95% CI)			
	Predominantly Breastmilk	**Guidelines**	**Easy-to-Prepare Foods**	**Noodles (in soup) and Seafood**
Maternal Education [b]				
Primary education	0.029 (0.014, 0.044) ***	0.001 (−0.012, 0.015)	0.008 (−0.001, 0.017)	−0.002 (−0.010, 0.007)
Post-secondary	0.013 (0.000, 0.026) *	−0.004 (−0.015, 0.007)	0.003 (−0.004, 0.011)	0.004 (−0.003, 0.011)
University and other	*Reference*	*Reference*	*Reference*	*Reference*
Household Income (SGD)				
<1999	0.002 (−0.017, 0.021)	−0.013 (−0.030, 0.004)	−0.001 (−0.013, 0.010)	−0.001 (−0.011, 0.010)
2000–5999	−0.009 (−0.022, 0.004)	−0.004 (−0.015, 0.007)	−0.001 (−0.009, 0.006)	−0.002 (−0.009, 0.005)
>6000	*Reference*	*Reference*	*Reference*	*Reference*
Employment				
Unemployed	0.007 (−0.004, 0.018)	0.001 (−0.009, 0.011)	0.001 (−0.005, 0.008)	0.002 (−0.004, 0.008)
Employed	*Reference*	*Reference*	*Reference*	*Reference*
Maternal BMI at 26 weeks [c]				
<18.5–24.9	−0.010 (−0.023, 0.004)	0.003 (−0.009, 0.015)	−0.004 (−0.012, 0.004)	0.003 (−0.004, 0.011)
25.0–29.9	−0.008 (−0.022, 0.006)	−0.007 (−0.020, 0.005)	−0.002 (−0.010, 0.006)	0.001 (−0.006, 0.009)
>30.0	*Reference*	*Reference*	*Reference*	*Reference*
Alcohol [d]				
Yes	−0.002 (−0.013, 0.009)	−0.002 (−0.011, 0.008)	0.001 (−0.006, 0.007)	−0.004 (−0.010, 0.002)
No	*Reference*	*Reference*	*Reference*	*Reference*
Smoking [d]				
Yes	0.005 (−0.010, 0.020)	−0.004 (−0.017, 0.010)	−0.002 (−0.012, 0.007)	−0.001 (−0.009, 0.008)
No	*Reference*	*Reference*	*Reference*	*Reference*
Cohabitation [e]				
Not living together	0.011 (−0.035, 0.058)	−0.002 (−0.042, 0.039)	0.018 (−0.010, 0.045)	−0.013 (−0.038, 0.013)
Living together	*Reference*	*Reference*	*Reference*	*Reference*
Infant characteristics				
Gender				
Female	−0.003 (−0.012, 0.006)	−0.005 (−0.014, 0.003)	0.004 (−0.002, 0.009)	−0.001 (−0.006, 0.004)
Male	*Reference*	*Reference*	*Reference*	*Reference*
Parity				
First child	0.014 (0.004, 0.025) **	0.006 (−0.003, 0.016)	−0.006 (−0.012, 0.001)	−0.004 (−0.010, 0.002)
Not first child	*Reference*	*Reference*	*Reference*	*Reference*

Abbreviations: BMI, body mass index. [a] Data shown are multivariable linear model β coefficients and their 95% confidence intervals (95% CIs) obtained from general linear models. Dietary pattern trajectory slopes as the dependent variable for patterns that formed trajectories from age 6 to 12 months and each characteristic was assessed with adjustments for the other characteristics; [b] Maternal education categorized as primary and secondary education, post-secondary education, as well as university and others; [c] Mother's BMI recorded at 26 weeks of pregnancy (kg/m^2); [d] Status recorded prior to pregnancy; [e] Reflects the marital status; single, separated or divorced mothers as living separately; married mothers as living together. * p-value < 0.05; ** p-value < 0.01; *** p-value < 0.001.

4. Discussion

Using multi-level modeling, we integrated food intakes at 6-, 9- and 12-months of age and identified four well-defined dietary patterns and their trajectories over that time period. A key observation was that the rates of change (slopes) of the trajectory scores were much smaller than the differences in the start scores (intercepts) in groups defined by maternal socio-demographic characteristics. This suggests that the maternal characteristics that predict dietary patterns at 6-months of age also largely determine the adherence to the same dietary patterns trajectories for the first year of life. To our knowledge, this is the first study to examine these dietary patterns and associations in an Asian population.

4.1. Dietary Patterns

In our study, the *Predominantly breastmilk* pattern resembles the "breastfeeding" pattern and "longer breastfeeding, late contemporary food introduction and use of home-made foods" reported in the ALSPAC [12] and EDEN studies [8,13], respectively. This pattern was characterized by higher intake of breastmilk and lower intake of formula milk and was accompanied by intakes of fruits and vegetables. The *Guidelines* pattern in our study corresponds to the healthy/prudent eating pattern [7,8,14–17,20] and was characterized by higher intakes of fruits, vegetables, whole grains, poultry and fish. While continued breastfeeding is encouraged during complementary feeding (6–12 months of age), the emphasis in current guidelines for this period is to offer infants a variety of food groups, rather than the type of milk taken [31,32]. The *Easy-to-prepare foods* pattern corresponds to an unhealthy eating pattern characterized by intakes of sugary desserts, high-fat foods and refined grains [6,15,17,18]. Lastly, the *Noodles (in soup) and seafood* pattern, which has not been observed in other studies, appears to reflect Asian adult eating patterns. It resembles the "use of adults' foods" in the EDEN study [8,13].

4.2. Associations between Maternal Factors and Trajectory Intercepts

The trajectory intercept values obtained from the mixed models represents the start point of each dietary pattern trajectory (at 6-months of age). To our knowledge, only three cohort studies to date have reported results for infant dietary patterns at 6-months of age [7,12,17]. Similar to the ALSPAC study [12], higher start scores of our *Predominantly breastmilk* trajectory at 6-months was associated with higher maternal education attainment. The IFPS II study reported that a higher "formula" dietary pattern (reverse of breastmilk) at 6-months of age was negatively associated with maternal education [7]. The relationship we observed with household income is not surprising, as income is closely linked to educational attainment. Its effect on breastfeeding status tends to attenuate when adjusted for education attainment [33,34]. The relationship we observed between higher start scores on the *Predominantly breastmilk* trajectory and unemployment is supported by evidence from studies showing that women working part-time or unemployed are more likely than their counterparts to breastfeed [35–37]. In Singapore, working mothers are entitled to 16 weeks of government-paid maternity leave or 12 weeks of maternity leave depending on citizenship, marriage status and duration of employment, but can choose to consume leave non-consecutively [38]. This may in part explain the lower start scores at 6 months on the *Predominantly breastmilk* trajectory for employed mothers when they return to work. Similarly, we found higher educational attainment to be associated with higher start scores of the *Guidelines* trajectory. Mothers with higher education are probably more aware of recommended practices and guidelines for weaning diets. A similar finding was also observed in the IFPS II study [7].

Maternal ethnicity was strongly associated with the start scores of our diet trajectories. Chinese mothers tended to start their infants on the *Predominantly breastmilk* pattern, while Indian ethnicity was associated with the *Easy-to-prepare foods* pattern. Ethnic differences in dietary patterns has also been observed in the American population, where White and African-American mothers scored higher on "guidelines" and "easy-to-prepare foods" patterns compared to their Hispanic counterparts [7], suggesting the importance of culture on diet and weaning practices.

We observed that higher start scores on the *Easy-to-prepare foods* trajectory were also associated with older mothers. In contrast, previous findings suggest that younger mothers tend to provide their children with more convenient foods, perhaps owing to time constraints [39]. Differences in childcare practices among different populations may explain these contrasting findings. For example, young Singaporean couples tend to live with their parents and leave their infants under the grandparents' supervision. Those infants are more likely to be fed traditional, home-prepared weaning meals than ready-to-eat meals.

No key maternal determinant emerged in the full model analyses for the *Noodles (in soup) and seafood* trajectory, suggesting it may be less influenced by cultural or socioeconomic factors.

4.3. Associations between Maternal Factors and Trajectory Slopes

The trajectory slopes represent the rate of change of each dietary pattern trajectory between 6- and 12-months. The means and standard deviations of the trajectory slopes were small ($<0.05 \pm 0.10$) compared to the intercepts ($<0.51 \pm 1.04$), suggesting that infants tend to maintain their dietary patterns over time. The range of the slopes we observed is similar to that reported by Smithers *et al* [11].

Mothers with lowest educational attainment and primiparous had higher slopes for the *Predominantly breastmilk* trajectory, suggesting a greater adherence to this pattern over time. This may not be ideal as the World Health Organization (WHO) recommends that solid foods be introduced shortly after 6-months of age [31] to ensure that infants obtain adequate micronutrients that breastmilk may not supply in sufficient quantity [30,40]. In addition, the variety of food and food textures provided to infants are believed to facilitate the development of oral motor skills and taste preferences and thereby help build a foundation for healthy eating habits [31,32,41].

Mothers in the youngest age group (18–29) tended to have greater adherence to the *Easy-to-prepare foods* trajectory with time, possibly owing to limited knowledge and experience with infant nutrition [39].

Maternal ethnicity continues to be a prevailing determinant of the slope of the dietary pattern trajectories. We observed that while Indian mothers have greater adherence to the *Predominantly breastmilk* trajectory over time, Chinese mothers adhere more to the *Guidelines* and *Noodles (in soup) and seafood* trajectories over time, reflecting a transition to an increasing pattern of table and adult foods. We also observed a *Pulses and grain* dietary pattern emerging at 12-months, particularly in Indian mothers of higher education status.

4.4. Strengths and Limitations

Our study captures the important time points of an infant's weaning diet and fills an important data gap on early feeding patterns. The modeling of dietary pattern trajectories has enabled us to take a longitudinal approach to assessing the overall diet. Compared to conventional cross-sectional analyses, this technique allows us to observe the introduction of new foods through time and the dietary transition during the weaning period. Furthermore, the representation of dietary pattern scores as intercepts and slopes has enabled us to explore the extent to which changes in diet over time are influenced by socio-demographic variables. While the trajectory intercepts signify the cross-sectional dietary pattern scores at 6-months of age, the slopes illuminate the dynamic changes in dietary patterns over time, which cannot be observed in the cross-sectional studies.

Limitations of our study also merit comment. First, single 24-h recalls or 1-day dietary records may not be a good representative of an infant's usual diet due to day-to-day variation in intakes. However, we have demonstrated high correlation of dietary pattern scores across the 3-days of the food diaries, reflecting good reproducibility of the single day dietary records. Second, GUSTO participants were not randomly sampled from the general population, with deliberate over-sampling of Malay and Indian mothers, and were recruited from two maternity hospitals in Singapore. However, these recruitment sites are the two largest maternity hospitals in Singapore and consist of both private and subsidized patients.

5. Conclusions

We examined trajectories of four distinct dietary patterns across three time points between 6- and 12-months. The trajectories were largely determined at the start points (intercepts), and changes over time (slopes) were small. This suggests the importance of establishing the "right" diet at the start of complementary feeding, as dietary changes are more difficult once habits are established. By understanding the key maternal socio-demographic factors that influence dietary patterns during complementary feeding, health professionals and policy-makers can provide more targeted and culturally-appropriate support and advice for mothers and their infants.

Acknowledgments: This study acknowledges the contribution of the rest of the GUSTO study group, which includes the following: Allan Sheppard, Amutha Chinnadurai, Anne Eng Neo Goh, Anne Rifkin-Graboi, Anqi Qiu, Arijit Biswas, Bee Wah Lee, Birit F.P. Broekman, Boon Long Quah, Borys Shuter, Chai Kiat Chng, Cheryl Ngo, Choon Looi Bong, Christiani Jeyakumar Henry, Cornelia Yin Ing Chee, Yam Thiam Daniel Goh, Doris Fok, Fabian Yap, George Seow Heong Yeo, Helen Chen, Hugo P S van Bever, Iliana Magiati, Inez Bik Yun Wong, Ivy Yee-Man Lau, Jeevesh Kapur, Jenny L. Richmond, Jerry Kok Yen Chan, Joanna D. Holbrook, Joshua J. Gooley, Keith M. Godfrey, Kenneth Kwek, Kok Hian Tan, Krishnamoorthy Niduvaje, Leher Singh, Lin Lin Su, Lourdes Mary Daniel, Lynette Pei-Chi Shek, Marielle V. Fortier, Mark Hanson, Mary Foong-Fong Chong, Mary Rauff, Mei Chien Chua, Michael Meaney, Mya Thway Tint, Neerja Karnani, Ngee Lek, Oon Hoe Teoh, P. C. Wong, Peter D. Gluckman, Pratibha Agarwal, Rob M. van Dam, Salome A. Rebello, Seang-Mei Saw, Shang Chee Chong, Shirong Cai, Shu-E Soh, Sok Bee Lim, Chin-Ying Stephen Hsu, Victor Samuel Rajadurai, Walter Stunkel, Wee Meng Han, Wei Wei Pang, Yap-Seng Chong, Yin Bun Cheung, Yiong Huak Chan and Yung Seng Lee. This study is supported by the Singapore National Research Foundation under its Translational and Clinical Research (TCR) Flagship Programme and administered by the Singapore Ministry of Health's National Medical Research Council (NMRC), Singapore- NMRC/TCR/004-NUS/2008; NMRC/TCR/012-NUHS/2014. Additional funding is provided by the Singapore Institute for Clinical Sciences, Agency for Science Technology and Research(A*STAR), Singapore. Keith M. Godfrey is supported by the National Institute for Health Research through the NIHR Southampton Biomedical Research Centre.

Author Contributions: Geraldine Huini Lim: designed the study, contributed to data collection, performed the statistical analyses, wrote the manuscript, and had primary responsibility for final content. Jia Ying Toh: designed the study, contributed to data collection, wrote the manuscript, and had primary responsibility for final content. Izzuddin M. Aris: contributed to statistical analyses of dietary patterns data. Ai-Ru Chia: contributed to statistical analyses of dietary patterns data. Wee Meng Han: contributed to the conception and design of the study and the acquisition of data. Seang Mei Saw: designed and led the GUSTO study. Keith M. Godfrey: designed and led the GUSTO study, and revised the manuscript for important intellectual content. Peter D. Gluckman: designed and led the GUSTO study; Yap-Seng Chong: designed and led the GUSTO study. Fabian Yap: designed and led the GUSTO study. Yung Seng Lee: designed and led the GUSTO study, and revised the manuscript for important intellectual content. Michael S. Kramer: contributed to statistical analyses of dietary patterns data and revised the manuscript for important intellectual content. Mary Foong-Fong Chong: designed the study, revised the manuscript for important intellectual content, and had primary responsibility for final content. All authors have read and approved the final manuscript.

References

1. Oellingrath, I.M.; Svendsen, M.V.; Brantsaeter, A.L. Tracking of eating patterns and overweight—A follow-up study of Norwegian schoolchildren from middle childhood to early adolescence. *Nutr. J.* **2011**, *10*, 106. [CrossRef] [PubMed]
2. Mikkila, V.; Räsänen, L.; Raitakari, O.T.; Pietinen, P.; Viikari, J. Consistent dietary patterns identified from childhood to adulthood: The cardiovascular risk in Young Finns Study. *Br. J. Nutr.* **2005**, *93*, 923–931. [CrossRef] [PubMed]
3. Bjelland, M.; Brantsæter, A.L.; Haugen, M.; Meltzer, H.M.; Nystad, W.; Andersen, L.F. Changes and tracking of fruit, vegetables and sugar-sweetened beverages intake from 18 months to 7 years in the Norwegian Mother and Child. Cohort Study. *BMC Public Health* **2013**, *13*, 793. [CrossRef] [PubMed]
4. Grieger, J.A.; Scott, J.; Cobiac, L. Dietary patterns and breast-feeding in Australian children. *Public Health Nutr.* **2011** *14*, 1939–1947. [CrossRef] [PubMed]

5. Birch, L.; Savage, J.S.; Ventura, A. Influences on the Development of Children's Eating Behaviours: From Infancy to Adolescence. *Can. J. Diet. Pract. Res.* **2007**, *68*, s1–s56. [PubMed]
6. Bell, L.K.; Golley, R.K.; Daniels, L.; Magarey, A.M. Dietary patterns of Australian children aged 14 and 24 months, and associations with socio-demographic factors and adiposity. *Eur. J. Clin. Nutr.* **2013**, *67*, 638–645. [CrossRef] [PubMed]
7. Wen, X.; Kong, K.L.; Eiden, R.D.; Sharma, N.N.; Xie, C. Sociodemographic differences and infant dietary patterns. *Pediatrics* **2014**, *134*, e1387–e1398. [CrossRef] [PubMed]
8. Andersen, L.B.; Mølgaard, C.; Michaelsen, K.F.; Carlsen, E.M.; Bro, R.; Pipper, C.B. Indicators of dietary patterns in Danish infants at 9 months of age. *Food Nutr. Res.* **2015**, *59*, 27665. [PubMed]
9. Smithers, L.G.; Golley, R.K.; Mittinty, M.N.; Brazionis, L.; Northstone, K.; Emmett, P.; Lynch, J.W. Dietary patterns at 6, 15 and 24 months of age are associated with IQ at 8 years of age. *Eur. J. Epidemiol.* **2012**, *27*, 525–535. [CrossRef] [PubMed]
10. Gale, C.R.; Martyn, C.N.; Marriott, L.D.; Limond, J.; Crozier, S.; Inskip, H.M.; Godfrey, K.M.; Law, C.M.; Cooper, C.; Robinson, S.M.; *et al.* Dietary patterns in infancy and cognitive and neuropsychological function in childhood. *J. Child. Psychol. Psychiatr.* **2009**, *50*, 816–823. [CrossRef] [PubMed]
11. Smithers, L.G.; Golley, R.K.; Mittinty, M.N.; Brazionis, L.; Northstone, K.; Emmett, P.; Lynch, J.W. Do dietary trajectories between infancy and toddlerhood influence IQ in childhood and adolescence? Results from a prospective birth cohort study. *PLoS ONE* **2013**, *8*, e58904.
12. Smithers, L.G.; Brazionis, L.; Golley, R.K.; Mittinty, M.N.; Northstone, K.; Emmett, P.; McNaughton, S.A.; Campbell, K.J.; Lynch, J.W. Associations between dietary patterns at 6 and 15 months of age and sociodemographic factors. *Eur. J. Clin. Nutr.* **2012**, *66*, 658–666. [CrossRef] [PubMed]
13. Betoko, A.; Charles, M.A.; Hankard, R.; Forhan, A.; Bonet, M.; Saurel-Cubizolles, M.J.; Heude, B.; de Lauzon-Guillain, B. EDEN mother-child cohort study group. Infant feeding patterns over the first year of life: Influence of family characteristics. *Eur. J. Clin. Nutr.* **2013**, *67*, 631–637. [CrossRef] [PubMed]
14. Kiefte-de Jong, J.C.; de Vries, J.H.; Bleeker, S.E.; Jaddoe, V.W.; Hofman, A.; Raat, H.; Moll, H.A. Socio-demographic and lifestyle determinants of "Western-like" and "Health conscious" dietary patterns in toddlers. *Br. J. Nutr.* **2013**, *109*, 137–147. [CrossRef] [PubMed]
15. Ystrom, E.; Niegel, S.; Vollrath, M.E. The impact of maternal negative affectivity on dietary patterns of 18-month-old children in the Norwegian Mother and Child. Cohort Study. *Matern. Child. Nutr.* **2009**, *5*, 234–242. [CrossRef] [PubMed]
16. Lioret, S.; Betoko, A.; Forhan, A.; Charles, M.A.; Heude, B.; de Lauzon-Guillain, B. EDEN Mother–Child Cohort Study Group. Dietary patterns track from infancy to preschool age: Cross-sectional and longitudinal perspectives. *J. Nutr.* **2015**, *145*, 775–782. [CrossRef] [PubMed]
17. Robinson, S.; Marriott, L.; Poole, J.; Crozier, S.; Borland, S.; Lawrence, W.; Law, C.; Godfrey, K.; Cooper, C.; Inskip, H.; *et al.* Dietary patterns in infancy: The importance of maternal and family influences on feeding practice. *Br. J. Nutr.* **2007**, *98*, 1029–1037. [CrossRef] [PubMed]
18. Okubo, H.; Miyake, Y.; Sasaki, S.; Tanaka, K.; Murakami, K.; Hirota, Y. Osaka Maternal and Child Health Study Group. Dietary patterns in infancy and their associations with maternal socio-economic and lifestyle factors among 758 Japanese mother-child pairs: The Osaka Maternal and Child. *Health Study Matern. Child. Nutr.* **2014**, *10*, 213–225. [CrossRef] [PubMed]
19. Oddy, W.H.; Herbison, C.E.; Jacoby, P.; Ambrosini, G.L.; O'Sullivan, T.A.; Ayonrinde, O.T.; Olynyk, J.K.; Black, L.J.; Beilin, L.J.; Mori, T.A.; *et al.* The Western dietary pattern is prospectively associated with nonalcoholic fatty liver disease in adolescence. *Am. J. Gastroenterol.* **2013**, *108*, 778–785. [CrossRef] [PubMed]
20. Brazionis, L.; Golley, R.K.; Mittinty, M.N.; Smithers, L.G.; Emmett, P.; Northstone, K.; Lynch, J.W. Characterization of transition diets spanning infancy and toddlerhood: A novel, multiple-time-point application of principal components analysis. *Am. J. Clin. Nutr.* **2012**, *95*, 1200–1208. [CrossRef] [PubMed]
21. Smith, Z.; Knight, T.; Sahota, P.; Kernohan, E.; Baker, M. Dietary patterns in Asian and Caucasian men in Bradford: Differences and implications for nutrition education. *J. Hum. Nutr. Diet.* **1993**, *6*, 323–333. [CrossRef]
22. Vergne, S.; Sauvant, P.; Lamothe, V.; Chantre, P.; Asselineau, J.; Perez, P.; Durand, M.; Moore, N.; Bennetau-Pelissero, C. Influence of ethnic origin (Asian v. Caucasian) and background diet on the bioavailability of dietary isoflavones. *Br. J. Nutr.* **2009**, *102*, 1642–1653. [PubMed]

23. Soh, S.E.; Tint, M.T.; Gluckman, P.D.; Godfrey, K.M.; Rifkin-Graboi, A.; Chan, Y.H.; Stünkel, W.; Holbrook, J.D.; Kwek, K.; Chong, Y.S.; *et al.* Cohort profile: Growing Up in Singapore Towards healthy Outcomes (GUSTO) birth cohort study. *Int. J. Epidemiol.* **2014**, *43*, 1401–1409. [CrossRef] [PubMed]
24. Conway, J.M.; Ingwersen, L.A.; Vinyard, B.T.; Moshfegh, A.J. Effectiveness of the US Department of Agriculture 5-step multiple-pass method in assessing food intake in obese and nonobese women. *Am. J. Clin. Nutr.* **2003**, *77*, 1171–1178. [PubMed]
25. Ponza, M.; Devaney, B.; Ziegler, P.; Reidy, K.; Squatrito, C. Nutrient intakes and food choices of infants and toddlers participating in WIC. *J. Am. Diet. Assoc.* **2004**, *104*, s71–s79. [CrossRef] [PubMed]
26. Gao, X.; Chen, H.; Fung, T.T.; Logroscino, G.; Schwarzschild, M.A.; Hu, F.B.; Ascherio, A. Prospective study of dietary pattern and risk of Parkinson disease. *Am. J. Clin. Nutr.* **2007**, *86*, 1486–1494. [PubMed]
27. Crozier, S.R.; Robinson, S.M.; Borland, S.E.; Inskip, H.M.; SWS Study Group. Dietary patterns in the Southampton Women's Survey. *Eur. J. Clin. Nutr.* **2006**, *60*, 1391–1399. [CrossRef] [PubMed]
28. Joliffe, I.T.; Morgan, B.J. Principal component analysis and exploratory factor analysis. *Stat. Methods Med. Res.* **1992**, *1*, 69–95. [CrossRef] [PubMed]
29. Michels, K.B.; Schulze, M.B. Can dietary patterns help us detect diet-disease associations? *Nutr. Res. Rev.* **2005**, *18*, 241–248. [CrossRef] [PubMed]
30. Foote, K.D.; Marriott, L.D. Weaning of infants. *Arch. Dis. Child.* **2003**, *88*, 488–492. [CrossRef] [PubMed]
31. World Health Organization. WHO Guidelines Approved by the Guidelines Review Committee. In *Infant and Young Child. Feeding: Model. Chapter for Textbooks for Medical Students and Allied Health Professionals*; World Health Organization: Geneva, Switzerzland, 2009.
32. Health Promotion Board. *Healthy Start for Your Baby*; Health Promotion Board: Singapore, Singapore, 2012.
33. Heck, K.E.; Braveman, P.; Cubbin, C.; Chávez, G.F.; Kiely, J.L. Socioeconomic status and breastfeeding initiation among California mothers. *Public Health Rep.* **2006**, *121*, 51–59. [PubMed]
34. Celi, A.C.; Rich-Edwards, J.W.; Richardson, M.K.; Kleinman, K.P.; Gillman, M.W. Immigration, race/ethnicity, and social and economic factors as predictors of breastfeeding initiation. *Arch. Pediatr. Adolesc. Med.* **2005**, *159*, 255–260. [CrossRef] [PubMed]
35. Hawkins, S.S.; Griffiths, L.J.; Dezateux, C.; Law, C. Millennium Cohort Study Child Health Group. Maternal employment and breast-feeding initiation: Findings from the Millennium Cohort Study. *Paediatr. Perinat. Epidemiol.* **2007**, *21*, 242–247. [CrossRef] [PubMed]
36. Khoury, A.J.; Moazzem, S.W.; Jarjoura, C.M.; Carothers, C.; Hinton, A. Breast-feeding initiation in low-income women: Role of attitudes, support, and perceived control. *Womens Health Issues* **2005**, *15*, 64–72. [CrossRef] [PubMed]
37. Barton, S.J. Infant feeding practices of low-income rural mothers. *MCN Am. J. Matern Child. Nurs.* **2001**, *26*, 93–97. [CrossRef] [PubMed]
38. Ministry of Manpower. Maternity Leave Eligibility and Entitlement, 2016. Available online: http://www.mom.gov.sg/employment-practices/leave/maternity-leave/eligibility-and-entitlement (accessed on 1 June 2016).
39. Bava, C.M.; Jaeger, S.R.; Park, J. Constraints upon food provisioning practices in "busy" women's lives: trade-offs which demand convenience. *Appetite* **2008**, *50*, 486–498. [CrossRef] [PubMed]
40. Dewey, K.G. Nutrition, growth, and complementary feeding of the breastfed infant. *Pediatr. Clin. N. Am.* **2001**, *48*, 87–104. [CrossRef]
41. WHO. Report by the Secretariat. In *Infant and Young Children Nutrition; Global Strategy for Infant and Young Child Feeding*; WHA55.25 Geneva: Fifty-fifth World Health Assembly; WHO: Geneva, Switerzland, 2002.

11

Retinol and α-Tocopherol in the Breast Milk of Women after a High-Risk Pregnancy

Reyna Sámano [1], Hugo Martínez-Rojano [2,3,*], Rosa M. Hernández [1], Cristina Ramírez [1], María E. Flores Quijano [1], José M. Espíndola-Polis [4] and Daniela Veruete [5]

1 Departamento de Nutrición y Bioprogramación, Instituto Nacional de Perinatología, Secretaría de Salud Montes Urales 800, Miguel Hidalgo, Lomas Virreyes, Ciudad de México CP. 11000, Mexico; ssmr0119@yahoo.com.mx (R.S.); rmh080868@yahoo.com (R.M.H.); crisra07@yahoo.com.mx (C.R.); maru_fq@yahoo.com (M.E.F.Q.)

2 Departamento de Posgrado e Investigación, Escuela Superior de Medicina del Instituto Politécnico Nacional, Plan de San Luis y Díaz Mirón s/n, Colonia Casco de Santo Tomas, Delegación Miguel Hidalgo, Ciudad de México CP. 11340, Mexico

3 Coordinación de Medicina Laboral, Instituto de Diagnóstico y Referencia Epidemiológicos (InDRE) "Dr. Manuel Martínez Báez", Secretaría de Salud Francisco de P. Miranda 177, Lomas de Plateros, Ciudad de México CP. 01480, Mexico

4 Departamento de Nutrición Humana, Universidad del Altiplano, Mirasol 1, Tlacomulco, Tlaxcala de Xicohténcatl CP. 90102, Mexico; jjmartinezr@yahoo.com

5 Universidad del Valle de México, campus Chapultepec Av. Constituyentes No. 151, Miguel Hidalgo, San Miguel Chapultepec I Secc, Ciudad de México CP. 11850, Mexico; analilia_000@hotmail.com

* Correspondence: hmartinez_59@yahoo.com.mx or hugo.martinezr@salud.gob.mx

Abstract: Background: There is scant information about whether, after a high-risk pregnancy, breast milk provides enough vitamins for assuring satisfactory bodily reserves in newborns. Objective: To comparatively evaluate, in women with high-risk and normal pregnancy, the concentration of retinol and α-tocopherol in breast milk. Methods: This cross-sectional, analytical study was evaluated with reverse-phase high-performance liquid chromatography (HPLC). Informed consent was signed by 95 mothers with a high-risk pregnancy and 32 mothers with a normal pregnancy. From the mothers with a high-risk pregnancy were obtained: 23 samples of colostrum, 24 of transitional milk, and 48 of mature milk. From the normal pregnancy group, 32 mature milk samples were collected. Pregestational Body Mass Index (BMI) and the gestational weight gain were noted. Models of logistic regression were constructed to identify the variables related to a low concentration of either retinol or α-tocopherol in breast milk. Results: The concentration of retinol and α-tocopherol in mature milk was 60 (interquartile range (IQR), 41–90) and 276 (103–450) μg/dL, respectively, for the high-risk pregnancy group, and 76 (65–91) and 673 (454–866) μg/dL, respectively, for the normal pregnancy group ($p = 0.001$). The concentration of retinol and α-tocopherol was similar in the subgroups of mothers with different disorders during gestation. A clear correlation was found between a greater pregestational weight and a lower concentration of retinol ($Rho = -0.280$, $p = 0.006$), and between α-tocopherol and retinol in all cases ($Rho = 0.463$, $p = 0.001$). Among women having a high-risk pregnancy, those delivering prematurely rather than carrying their pregnancy to term had a reduced concentration of retinol (54 (37–78) vs. 70 (49–106) μg/dL; $p = 0.002$) and a tendency to a lower concentration of α-tocopherol in breast milk (185 (75–410) vs. 339 (160–500) μg/dL; $p = 0.053$). Compared to mothers with a normal pregnancy, those with a high-risk pregnancy (whether carried to term or ending in preterm delivery) exhibited a reduced concentration of retinol in mature milk ($p = 0.003$), as well as a tendency to a lower concentration of α-tocopherol ($p = 0.054$). Conclusion: Even though the women in the high-risk pregnancy group showed a deficiency of vitamins A and E in their breast milk, the unique biological benefits of this milk justify the promotion of breast feeding as the optimal method of nourishing neonates and infants. In these cases, it should be recommended that the woman increase her consumption of certain nutrients during pregnancy. Additionally, after childbirth mothers should consider the use of supplements to produce milk of adequate quality and thus meet the needs of the baby and prevent any deficiency in micronutrients.

Keywords: breast milk; liposoluble vitamins; high-performance liquid chromatography; pregestational obesity

1. Introduction

Approximately 22% of all pregnancies are high-risk in Mexico each year [1]. One of the risk factors for complications during pregnancy is being overweight, leading to a higher prevalence of gestational diabetes, hypertension, pre-eclampsia, asthma, and thromboembolic disease [2]. Around 60% of Mexican women in reproductive age are overweight [3]. Additionally, excessive weight gain during pregnancy also increases the risk of adverse outcomes for both mother and child [4], and a high percentage of Mexican women gain more weight than recommended [5].

Similarly, gestational diabetes is a risk factor for the increased incidence today of teratogenicity, which has been observed more frequently in fetuses of diabetic versus healthy mothers. These malformations are the result of tissue injury caused by the activity of free radicals [6]. Natural antioxidants reduce the adverse effects of these radicals, since they can capture and neutralize reactive oxygen species, thus preventing lipid peroxidation. This neutralization is essential, especially in situations where oxidative stress is elevated, such as gestational diabetes and preeclampsia [7]. One of the essential natural antioxidants is vitamin E, which comprises a group of eight fat-soluble compounds that are classified as α-, β-, γ-, and δ-tocopherol or tocotrienol. Of these, α-tocopherol is the most active compound [8].

The variation of glycaemia during pregnancy leads to serious complications for the mother-child binomial [7,8]. Although there is currently little evidence of the association between the concentration of retinol and diabetes in pregnant women [9], this disease makes such women more prone to a marginal or poor biochemical status of vitamin A [9]. In addition to potentiating the complications caused by diabetes in pregnant women, low levels of vitamin A leave their children vulnerable to developing a deficiency of the same [10,11].

An adequate nutritional status during the first 2–3 years of life is necessary for subsequent health and well-being. Deficient development cannot be reversed after passing this critical window [12]. In this sense, a study in Egypt stressed that vitamin E is a key micronutrient for development, with its deficiency leading to a delay in growth [13]. The authors also noted that 78.2% of children showing a delay in their growth were deficient in vitamin E, having plasma concentrations of α-tocopherol at 7.7 mmol/L versus 14.1 mmol/L for the group of control children [13]. Fares et al. [14] revealed that deficiencies of vitamins A, E, and D were very common among infants with very low birth weight in Tunisia, and were associated with preeclampsia. However, the risk of preeclampsia did not diminish after the administration of vitamin C and E in a series of studies in Western countries [15,16].

The results of administering vitamin E supplements have been variable. One reason is that the appropriate status of α-tocopherol during pregnancy has not yet been defined. Moreover, in the various global reports on the usefulness of vitamin E supplements during pregnancy, the plasma concentration of α-tocopherol is often not even determined. In situations where a low concentration of α-tocopherol was documented, the administration of supplements of vitamin E has proven beneficial. In a Hungarian population, for instance, supplementation of vitamin E in women was associated with a decreased incidence of premature babies [17]. The establishment of a clear criteria for adequate levels of vitamin E deserves further investigation.

It is also known that placental transfer of vitamins A and E during pregnancy is limited and that the reserve of these micronutrients in the newborn is low, especially in the case of premature babies. Consequently, exclusive breastfeeding is the only way to meet their nutritional needs [8]. Since exposure to hyperoxia at birth increases the risk of free radical formation [18], it is essential that the mother provide the infant a sufficient supply of vitamin E through breastfeeding.

Due to the importance of vitamins A and E for the mother and child, the aim of the present study was to determine the concentration of retinol and α-tocopherol in the breast milk of mothers after undergoing a high-risk versus normal pregnancy, as well as after giving birth preterm versus carrying their pregnancy to term. Associations were examined between low levels of vitamins A and E in breast milk and maternal characteristics.

2. Material and Methods

2.1. Study Design and Population

A cross-sectional and analytical study was conducted to determine the presence of retinol and α-tocopherol in the breast milk of 95 mothers with a high-risk pregnancy (and whose newborns were confined in the neonatal intensive care unit during the first and second month after birth) and 32 mothers with a normal pregnancy and healthy newborns. The study took place from January 2013 to October 2016. It was conducted at the Instituto Nacional de Perinatología (National Institute of Perinatology) and the School of Medicine, National Polytechnic Institute, in Mexico City.

The sample size was calculated with a 95% confidence interval, utilizing information from previous reports that estimated the mean content of vitamin A in breast milk [19]. After the mothers had agreed to participate and signed informed consent, they were asked to fill out a survey to provide data about their obstetrical background.

The manner of sampling mothers was not probabilistic or based on consecutive cases. Inclusion criteria were that the women lived in the metropolitan area of Mexico City, agreed to provide all data requested through a survey (maternal age, sociodemographic characteristics, medical and obstetrical history, course of current pregnancy and term, mode of delivery, pregnancy-related complications, weight, and complications of the neonates), were breastfeeding their newborns/infants and secreting breast milk in adequate quantities, were 18–45 years old, and were not taking medications or vitamin/multivitamin supplements. All participating mothers had been eating customary Mexican food during pregnancy and none had adopted special diets.

The 127 mothers that participated in the study were recruited by the nutrition team of the National Perinatology Institute (all women in this unit who consented were included). In the high-risk pregnancy group, all the newborns and some of the women were hospitalized. Contrarily, in the normal pregnancy group, none of the infants were hospitalized. Among the 95 mothers with a high-risk pregnancy, 48 delivered preterm and 47 carried their pregnancy to term. All 32 mothers with a history of normal pregnancy carried their pregnancy to term.

Preterm childbirth was defined as a gestation lasting less than 37 weeks. A normal pregnancy was defined as the lack of complications or disorders before and/or during gestation. When there were pregnancy-related complications, illnesses, or events that represented a health risk, the situation was considered high risk. Especially important was any appearance of the woman or an increase in complications that could have caused maternal/perinatal morbidity/mortality. The following conditions were examined for any possible association with low levels of retinol or α-tocopherol: (i) multiple gestation (involving twins, triplets, etc.), which increases the risk of infants being born prematurely (before 37 weeks of pregnancy); (ii) pregnancy with triplets or quadruplets, which implies a greater the probability of delivery by cesarean section; (iii) pregnancy after age 30 and/or after taking fertility drugs (both related to multiple births); and (iv) gestational diabetes, preeclampsia or eclampsia.

Preeclampsia, a syndrome marked by a sudden rise in the blood pressure of a pregnant woman after the 20th week of pregnancy, can affect the kidneys, liver, and brain. When left untreated, the condition may result in long term health problems or be fatal for the mother and/or the fetus. Eclampsia is a more severe form of preeclampsia, marked by anemia, seizures, and coma in the mother (implying an increased risk for a first-time pregnancy in women over 35 years of age). Preeclampsia and gestational diabetes were based on the criteria of the American College of Obstetricians and Gynecologists [20,21].

2.2. Milk Sampling

Samples of breast milk were aseptically obtained from the mothers, either at home or in the hospital, during the morning (08:00–10:00) and after 8–10 h of fasting. The first sample of breast milk from mothers with a history of high-risk pregnancy was obtained in the hospital during the 48 h immediately after birth. These samples were considered as colostrum. Transitional milk was obtained from these same mothers at eight days postpartum. Mature milk samples were obtained from both groups of women between the first and second month postpartum. Breast milk was delivered by mothers to the hospital milk bank with the high-risk pregnancy group, because the newborns were in the Neonatal Intensive Care. This milk was deposited in sterile polypropylene bottles and stored at 4 °C or colder. The women with a history of normal pregnancy delivered their sample of breast milk to the nutritionist when they brought their healthy child to the hospital. From each recipient, an aliquot of 15 mL was filled without leaving any air pockets (to avoid oxygenation). This aliquot was taken from a full breast sample, previously homogenized. Each aliquot was protected from ultraviolet light with aluminum foil and placed in refrigeration at –20 °C.

2.3. Type of Milk

From the high-risk pregnancy group, 23 of the breast milk samples obtained were considered as colostrum, 24 transitional milk, and 48 mature milk. From the normal pregnancy group, 32 mature milk samples were obtained. Colostrum is considered as the breast milk from delivery to approximately five days postpartum, transitional milk from day 6–15 postpartum, and mature milk from day 15 onwards.

2.4. Laboratory Methods

The procedure for determining the concentration of vitamins A and E (as retinol and α-tocopherol) was based on high-performance liquid chromatography (HPLC) in the reverse phase. The internal standard was all-trans-retinyl-acetate (800-Across-01, Software Total Chrome, version 6.3.2.0646, Whippany, NJ, USA). This determination was carried out on all of the breast milk samples from the 127 participating mothers.

Retinol and α-tocopherol levels were determined in breast milk by using a binary HPLC pump (Flexar model, Perkin-Elmer, Naperville, IL, USA) with an injector (loop size 100 μL, Flexar model), a sensitive UV7 detector (Flexar model, Norwalk, CT, USA), a three-column microbondapak rp-18 Pecosphere C-18 of 3 μm and 33.46 mm (Perkin-Elmer), and an acrodisc CR-13 mm syringe filter with a 0.2 μm PTFE (polytetrafluoroethylene) membrane (Teflon).

After the extraction, vitamins A and E were isolated from the samples of breast milk. First the matrix was saponified, followed by extraction of the analytes of interest. The esters of retinal were hydrolyzed to retinol by saponification. To 15 mL of breast milk was added 24 mL of potassium hydroxide in a solution of 16% methanol (weight per volume). This alkaline mixture was heated to 75 °C and maintained at that temperature for 30 min, then cooled for 5 min. For the extraction of the vitamins, 16 mL of petroleum ether was added in a separatory funnel, and then the solution was stirred and left to stand for 30 min. The aqueous phase was drained and disposed of three times. The etheric dissolution was washed with deionized water to eliminate the alkaline excess, reaching pH 7 (measured with pH paper). The solvent was recovered in Falcon tubes of 50 mL, to be evaporated in a steam bath at 70 °C. The residue was dissolved with 2 mL of ethanol, then filtered with acrodisk CR 13 mm syringe filters with a 0.2 μm PTFE membrane. An injection volume was taken from this solution for the chromatography with 50 μL, which was run for 10 min. To obtain the target of the reactives, a process of saponification and extraction was carried out in the absence of breast milk. All samples were processed in duplicate and each replicate was injected twice [22].

Microbondapak columns with a UV/visible detector were utilized to establish the conditions for the chromatographic system, with methanol/water (96:4) for the mobile phase and a wavelength of 325 nm for retinol and 290 nm for α-tocopherol. The analytic parameters for linearity were $R^2 = 0.9955$ for retinol and $R^2 = 0.9808$ for α-tocopherol, while the detection and quantification limits were 1.1 μg/dL and 2.7 μg/dL for retinol and 0.9 μg/dL and 2.3 μg/dL for α-tocopherol. Regarding accuracy, relative standard deviation (RSD) was 4.5% for the same day and RSD 4.8% between days for retinol, and 4.9% for the same day and 4.1% between days for α-tocopherol. The recovery was 85.8 ± 7.8% μg/dL for retinol and 98 ± 1.9% μg/dL for α-tocopherol. Once validated, the method was applied to the quantification of retinol and α-tocopherol in samples of breast milk [23].

2.5. Evaluating Maternal Body Mass Index (BMI) and Morbidity in Mothers and Newborns/Infants

The pregestational weight and height of the mother was obtained from the clinical history. The BMI was calculated considering ≤18.49 kg/m^2 as underweight, 18.50–24.99 kg/m^2 as normal, 25–29.9 kg/m^2 as overweight and ≥30 kg/m^2 as obese. The evaluation of the gestational weight was based on both the pregestational BMI and the tables of the Institute of Medicine (IOM, Washington, DC, USA). The increase in gestational weight was calculated by subtracting the pregestational weight from the maximum gestational weight, and the result was classified as adequate or below/above the recommended level, according to the guidelines of the IOM [24]. The absence or presence of morbidity in mothers and newborns/infants was determined by reviewing the corresponding clinical history.

3. Statistical Analysis

For clinical data, anthropometric and sociodemographic characteristics of the mothers and newborns were reported as the mean ± Standard Deviation (SD) and the median with an interquartile range (IQR) of p25–p75. Due to the nature of the variables, a parametric analysis was performed with the Student's *t*-test and a non-parametric analysis with the Mann-Whitney *U* test and the Kruskal-Wallis test. Additionally, frequency and percentages for categorical variables were analyzed with the Pearson's X^2 test. For qualitative variables, such as marital status, occupation, level of education, and pregnancy outcome, frequency measurements were calculated. For numerical variables, including the age of the mother and pregestational weight and height, measurements of central tendency and dispersion were utilized. With the Kruskal-Wallis test, analysis was made of the difference between the concentration of retinol and α-tocopherol between groups and in relation to the pregestational BMI of the mother. For the concentration of the vitamins and the outcome of the pregnancy, the Mann-Whitney *U* test was employed. We used the median value for women with high-risk or normal pregnancy as a comparison group. The two values used in the logistic regression model were considered risk variables when they were below these medians. A statistical significance was considered at $p < 0.05$. Data entry and analysis were performed with the statistical program SPSS version 20 for Windows (SPSS Inc., Chicago, IL, USA).

4. Ethical Aspects

Data gathering and analysis was confidential, taking such ethical questions as autonomy and security into account. The guidelines of the Helsinki Declaration were followed. The project protocol was approved by the Scientific and Ethics Committee of our institution. All women participating in this study were given medical attention at the highest level of medical specialties in a health center in Mexico City (with ethical approval code number 212250-49501).

5. Results

Of the 95 mothers with a high-risk pregnancy and 32 with a normal pregnancy, the median age was 28 years (IQR = 20–34 years), cohabitation was the most common marital status, and homemaker was the most common occupation. Regarding educational level, nearly 90% had finished middle school. Concerning obstetric background, 44% of the participants were primigravida, 98% of the births took place by caesarean section, and the average weight of the neonates was 1686 g (Table 1).

Table 1. Clinical, anthropometric and sociodemographic characteristics of the mothers and newborns (n = 127).

Clinical and Anthropometric Characteristics			
	High-risk pregnancy n = 95	Normal pregnancy n = 32	
	Mean ± SD		p
Age (years) [a]	28 ± 5	27 ± 8	0.456
Pregestational weight (kg) [a]	62.2 ± 10	59.9 ± 10	0.253
Maximum gestational weight (kg) [a]	70.4 ± 13	67 ± 13	0.239
Height (cm) [a]	156 ± 6	156 ± 5	0.632
Pregestational BMI [a]	25.5 ± 4	24.5 ± 3	0.176
Number of prenatal check-ups [a]	4 ± 2	4 ± 0.5	0.211
Gynecological age (years) [a]	15 ± 8	16.5 ± 5	0.890
Menarche (age in years) [a]	12 ± 2	12 ± 1	0.878
Weight of the newborn (g) [a]	1686 ± 843	2167 ± 689	0.004
Length of the newborn (cm) [a]	40 ± 5	48.2 ± 5	0.006
Sociodemographic characteristics [b]	Frequency (%)		
Marital status			
Single	23 (24)	4 (13)	
Married	35 (37)	11 (34)	0.556
Cohabitation	37 (39)	17 (53)	
Occupation			
Homemaker	73 (77)	24 (75)	0.883
Working outside the home	22 (23)	8 (25)	
Level of education			
Primary or less	10 (11)	2 (6)	
Middle school	40 (42)	14 (44)	0.823
High school	33 (35)	13 (41)	
Professional	12 (12)	3 (9)	
Socioeconomic level			
Lower to lower-middle class	95 (100)	31 (96)	0.983

Data expressed as the [a] mean ± standard deviation—Student's t; [b] frequency (%)—Pearson's X^2.

There were differences between the two groups of mothers (normal versus high-risk pregnancy) in relation to the concentration of retinol and α-tocopherol in mature breast milk (Figures 1 and 2), as well as in neonate weight and length. Concerning anthropometric characteristics, women with a high-risk pregnancy had an average pregestational BMI of 25.5 kg/m^2 and those with a normal pregnancy 24.5 kg/km^2, while the average gestational weight gain was 8.2 kg for both groups (Table 1).

For the women with a high-risk pregnancy, the most common disorder or condition related to risk was preeclampsia (40/95), followed by anemia (29/95), advanced maternal age (14/95), and gestational diabetes (12/95). The complications of the neonates born of these women were preterm birth or low birth weight (62/95), infant respiratory distress syndrome or gastroschisis (18/95), and lesions related to the birth canal (6/95). The rest showed no complications (9/95).

When comparing the distinct subgroups of women with different disorders during gestation, there were similar concentrations of retinol and α-tocopherol in breast milk (Table 2). However, the concentration of retinol and α-tocopherol in breast milk was lower in women that gave preterm birth compared to those who carried their pregnancy to term. Considering the women with a high-risk pregnancy, the concentration of retinol was higher in the mature milk of women with normal pregestational weight, while no significant difference was found in the concentration of α-tocopherol among those having adequate gestational weight gain.

Table 2. Concentrations of retinol and α-tocopherol in breast milk, in relation to some perinatal data of the women with a high-risk pregnancy (n = 95).

			Retinol			α-Tocopherol		
		n	Colostrum µg/dL Median (IQR)	Transition Milk µg/dL Median (IQR)	Mature Milk µg/dL Median (IQR)	Colostrum µg/dL Median (IQR)	Transition Milk µg/dL Median (IQR)	Mature Milk µg/dL Median (IQR)
Maternal age (years)	≤19	21	73 (37–93)	57 (52–70)	67 (49–70)	500 (103–654)	276 (55–445)	207 (48–270)
	20–29	29	67 (35–128)	84 (64–103)	60 (49–82)	298 (127–492)	204 (103–321)	321 (68–436)
	30–34	23	42 (33–50)	93 (64–120)	42 (35–56)	500 (405–597)	654 (348–727)	103 (46–255)
	≥35	22	79 (52–106)	62 (39–81)	67 (49–70)	275 (192–570)	201 (167–475)	339 (180–423)
p [a]			0.225	0.340	0.173	0.632	0.407	0.330
Pregestational BMI	Normal weight	41	60 (47–96)	80 (66–97)	60 (42–80)	575 (154–654)	180 (131–410)	321 (55–448)
	Overweight	40	60 (38–94)	64 (41–93)	45 (34–64)	321 (130–540)	249 (90–450)	190 (54–340)
	Obesity	14	33 (33–33)	42 (32–52)	49 (38–55)	455 (410–500)	295 (146–445)	146 (103–423)
p [a]			0.209	0.095	0.003	0.575	0.945	0.620
Gestational weight increase	Adequate	19	31 (29–33)	72(44–120)	50 (34–60)	270 (130–410)	549 (323–727)	340 (61–423)
	Low	35	60 (42–93)	73 (70–110)	62 (49–90)	470 (120–654)	180 (107–433)	218 (63–339)
	Excessive	41	61 (45–94)	64 (53–89)	55 (40–79)	400 (253–602)	249 (103–372)	180 (103–423)
p [a]			0.090	0.136	0.337	0.802	0.911	0.951
Gestational age	To term	47	60 (46–102)	103 (73–120)	59 (49–91)	470 (275–654)	445 (160–676)	330 (63–441)
	Preterm	48	41 (33–89)	62 (47–77)	48 (38–70)	400 (125–525)	132 (233–371)	135 (61–276)
p [b]			0.069	0.005	0.058	0.260	0.290	0.118
Complication during pregnancy	Gestational diabetes	12	49 (44–93)	94 (70–119)	47 (35–99)	400 (321–500)	433 (189–676)	38 (18–431)
	Preeclampsia	40	60 (41–92)	62 (40–76)	59 (46–76)	343 (230–654)	233 (115–445)	218 (104–450)
	Anemia, myomas	29	49 (32–83)	93 (70–103)	47 (35–67)	545 (125–654)	321 (160–450)	205 (59–416)
	Advanced maternal age	14	90 (62–96)	76 (52–100)	68 (49–85)	360 (183–500)	274 (103–445)	180 (103–321)
p [a]			0.690	0.260	0.378	0.905	0.906	0.661

[a] Kruskal-Wallis; [b] Mann-Whitney U; IQR, interquartile ranges.

Women with normal pregestational BMI had a higher concentration of retinol compared to those who were overweight or obese (see Table 2). The Spearman correlation revealed that the greater the pregestational weight (relative to normal), the lower the concentration of retinol ($Rho = -0.280$, $p = 0.006$). Moreover, there was a correlation between α-tocopherol and retinol ($Rho = 0.463$, $p = 0.001$).

Compared to women with a normal pregnancy, the mature breast milk of those with a high-risk pregnancy who delivered at full term showed a similar concentration of retinol but a lower concentration of α-tocopherol. Compared to the mature milk of women with a normal pregnancy, in contrast, the breast milk of those with a high-risk pregnancy who delivered preterm had a reduced concentration of retinol and α-tocopherol in the diverse types of milk (colostrum, transition milk, and mature milk) (Figures 1 and 2).

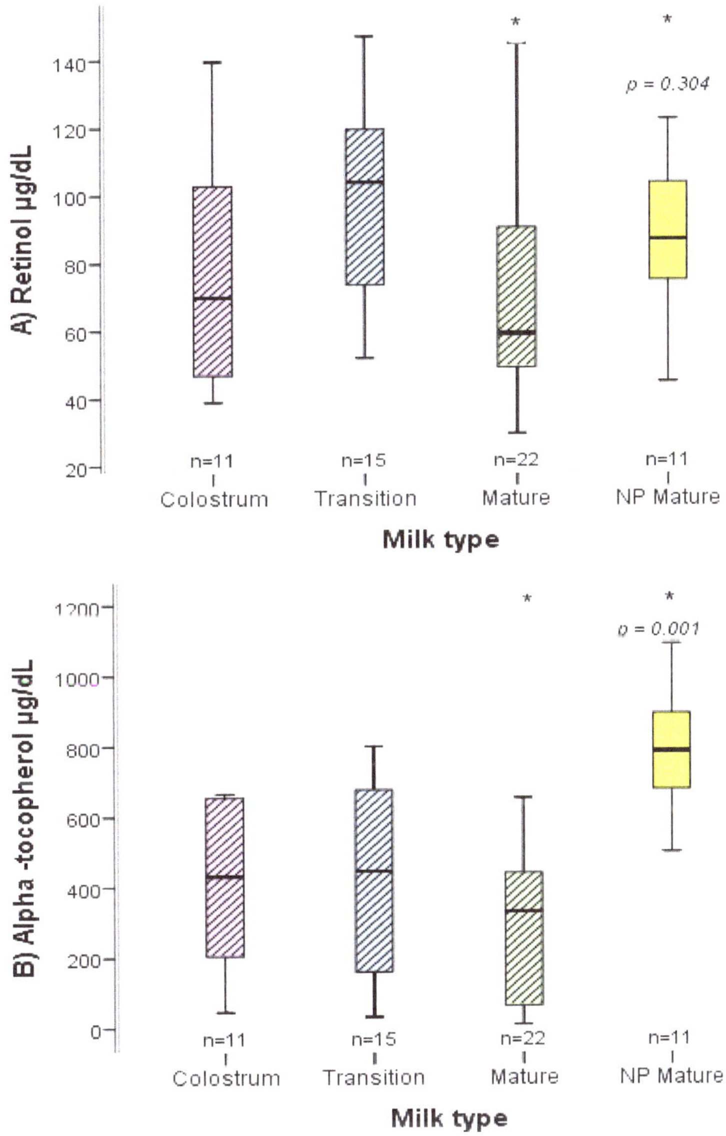

Figure 1. Box plot distribution of the concentration of retinol (**A**) and α-tocopherol (**B**) in breast milk, comparing the women with a full-term, high-risk pregnancy to those with a normal pregnancy. For the high-risk pregnancy, the distinct types of breast milk are shown (colostrum, transition milk, and mature milk). * *p*; Mann-Whitney *U*. The bottom and top of the box represent the first and third quartiles (IQR), and the band inside the box the median. The ends of the whiskers denote the lowest and highest values still within 1.5 IQR. Outlier values are not displayed. NP, normal pregnancy.

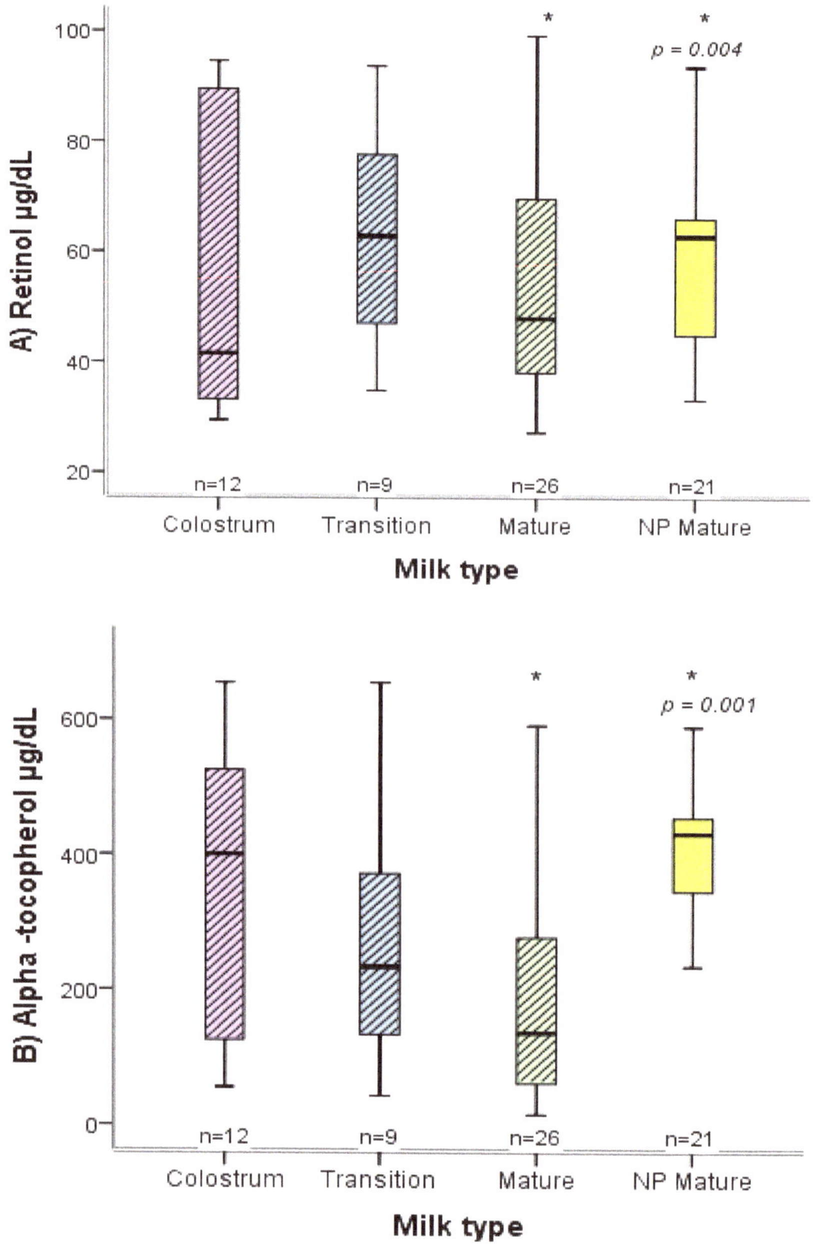

Figure 2. Box plot distribution of the concentration of retinol (**A**) and α-tocopherol (**B**) in breast milk, comparing women with a preterm, high-risk pregnancy to those with a normal pregnancy. For the high-risk pregnancy, the distinct types of breast milk (colostrum, transition milk and mature milk) are shown. * *p*; Mann-Whitney *U*. The bottom and top of the box represent the first and third quartiles (IQR), and the band inside the box the median. The ends of the whiskers denote the lowest and highest values still within 1.5 IQR. Outlier values are not displayed. NP, normal pregnancy.

When the logistic regression model included variables that corresponded to a high-risk pregnancy, it was observed that in all cases the concentration of both vitamin precursors was lower with high-risk versus normal pregnancy. However, no particular risk factors were associated with these lower concentrations. Hence, the following model was performed.

For the regression model, we utilized the median values for concentrations of retinol below 60 µg/dL and for α-tocopherol below 276 µg/dL in the group high-risk pregnancy, while using these values below 76 and 673 µg/dL for retinol and α-tocopherol, respectively, in the group with a history of normal pregnancy. For the high-risk pregnancy group, the variables associated with a low concentration of retinol in breast milk were preterm childbirth and pregestational overweight or obesity. For the normal pregnancy group, only pregestational overweight or obesity was significant. Meanwhile, for all the women (whether having a high-risk pregnancy or a history of normal pregnancy), a significant risk of a low concentration of α-tocopherol was correlated with preterm childbirth and a tendency was associated with preeclampsia (Table 3).

Table 3. Variables associated with low concentrations of retinol and α-tocopherol in mothers that underwent a high-risk pregnancy (n = 95).

Maternal variables	The Median Concentration in Mature Milk of Mothers Who Underwent a High-Risk Pregnancy			The Median Concentration in Mature Milk of Mothers Who Experienced a Normal Pregnancy		
	OR	CI 95%	p *	OR	CI 95%	p *
	Retinol concentration (≤60 μg/dL)			(≤76 μg/dL)		
Preterm childbirth	2.618	1.111–6.169	0.028	2.112	0.858–5.856	0.112
Preeclampsia	1.512	0.429–5.450	0.512	0.992	0.992–1.138	0.102
Gestational diabetes	0.879	0.277–3.122	0.575	0.272	0.023–3.249	0.273
Anemia	0.877	0.281–3.629	0.258	0.955	0.906–1.006	0.331
Maternal age: under 19 or over 29 years	0.818	0.364–1.838	0.390	2.189	0.858–5.586	0.101
Pregestational overweight or obesity	1.179	1.822–2692	0.039	3.563	1.422–8.927	0.007
	α-tocopherol concentration (≤276 μg/dL) [a]			(≤673 μg/dL) [b]		
Preterm childbirth	2.243	0.985–5.111	0.039	2.091	1.689–2.588	0.038
Preeclampsia	1.304	0.567–3.001	0.532	1.063	0.992–1.138	0.051
Gestational diabetes	0.892	0.228–3.483	0.869	0.289	0.023–2.951	0.336
Anemia	0.914	0.252–3.319	0.892	0.955	0.906–1.006	0.331
Maternal age: under 19 or over 29 years	1.879	0.459–2.484	0.879	0.402	0.035–4.591	0.441
Pregestational overweight or obesity	1.056	0.447–2.494	0.870	0.772	0.064–9.302	0.838

CI 95%: 95% confidence interval. OR: odds ratio. Low concentrations of retinol and α-tocopherol: value below the median in mothers after a high-risk pregnancy and those with a history of a normal pregnancy. * p Value in logistic regression model.

Regarding the different types of breast milk (Table 4), the concentration of both α-tocopherol and retinol were lower among women who gave preterm childbirth. A positive correlation existed in all cases between the concentration of retinol and that of α-tocopherol in the different types of milk, with *Rho* values of 0.325 for colostrum, 0.375 for transition milk, and 0.300 for mature milk ($p \leq 0.001$).

Table 4. Concentration of retinol and α-tocopherol in relation to the type of breast milk.

Pregnancy Length	Colostrum	Transition	Mature
	Retinol, median (IQR), μg/dL		
Preterm (n = 48)	36 (32–63)	60 (39–81)	43 (36–66)
Full term (n = 47)	49 (39–86)	73 (49–115)	52 (37–72)
p [a]	0.010	0.020	0.032
	α-tocopherol, median (IQR), μg/dL		
Preterm (n = 48)	405 (109–676)	233 (90–372)	175 (59–465)
Full term (n = 47)	654 (205–2313)	676 (174–1884)	285 (55–477)
p [a]	0.004	0.001	0.012

Data expressed as the median (IQR). [a] *Mann Whitney U*; IQR, interquartile range.

There was a reduced level of retinol and α-tocopherol in mothers giving preterm birth or having low birth-weight neonates compared to those that carried their pregnancy to term. However, the concentration of retinol (p = 0.244) and α-tocopherol (p = 0.090) did not show a significant difference in relation to complications of the newborn. Likewise, no significant difference existed for the concentration of retinol (p = 0.243) or α-tocopherol (p = 0.897) in regard to the history of pregnancies.

When comparing women with preterm delivery to those who carried their pregnancy to term, the concentration of retinol was 54 (IQR; 37–78) vs. 70 (IQR; 49–106) μg/dL (p = 0.002), while that of α-tocopherol was 155 (IQR; 74–410) vs. 445 (IQR; 160–500) μg/dL ($p = 0.053$). On the other hand, compared to women with a high-risk pregnancy, those with a normal pregnancy had a higher level of both vitamin precursors in mature milk.

6. Discussion

There was an association between a lower concentration of retinol and α-tocopherol in mature breast milk and two risk factors: pregestational overweight or obesity and preterm delivery. This significance was established with the original statistical analysis and confirmed by the logistic regression model. No significant difference in the concentration of retinol or α-tocopherol was found in relation to either of the morbidities existing among women in the high-risk pregnancy group. Although no direct association was detected between preeclampsia and lower levels of these vitamin precursors, this morbidity is related to overweight and obesity, a condition that, in turn, may cause preterm delivery.

6.1. Concentration of Retinol and α-Tocopherol

Considering that breast milk is the only source of nutrition for newborns, it is important to determine whether the content of vitamins A and E are adequate, especially when the neonate is premature or of very low weight [25,26]. In the majority of reports, the concentration of α-tocopherol in the colostrum of women is two to three times higher than that detected presently in Mexican women after a high-risk pregnancy. For the women with a normal evolutive pregnancy, some of the current results are similar to those described for women from Bangladesh and Poland [27,28].

Concerning retinol, for the group of mothers in this study with a history of normal pregnancy and having a normal delivery, the average concentration of this vitamin precursor is close to that commonly reported. In contrast, the women in the present study with a high-risk pregnancy had, on the average, about half the concentration of retinol previously found for women with a normal pregnancy, and a third of this concentration in the cases of preterm childbirth. These values are close to those observed in a group of women in Bangladesh [27,29,30].

The similarities in the concentration of these two vitamins between Mexico and Bangladesh [27] may be due to the characteristics of the particular populations under study. That is, the women in both studies had a low socioeconomic status and poor health indicators, which makes them more prone to the development of nutritional deficiencies. Although the nutrient concentrations found in the women are low, Ahmed et al. demonstrated that this amount is sufficient to satisfy the nutritional needs of infants.

In relation to transitional milk, the concentration of retinol and α-tocopherol described in diverse populations [31–35] is higher than that evidenced in the present study after a high-risk pregnancy. Kodentsova and Vrzhesinskaya reported a mean concentration for each of these vitamin precursors in Russian women that was very similar to the present high-risk pregnancy group. This similarity is likely due to the fact that approximately 50% of Russian women who participated in the study experienced a preterm pregnancy [36].

Regarding mature milk in the current contribution, the mean concentration of α-tocopherol and retinol for both groups of women (with a normal pregnancy and high-risk pregnancy) is very similar to most reports on these micronutrients. However, for women who, herein, had a high-risk pregnancy, the median concentration of α-tocopherol was higher than that detected in Polish women [37–43] and in a group of adolescent mothers in Brazil [44]. In another study by Tokusoglu et al. [45], the concentration of α-tocopherol in the mature milk of Turkish women was similar to that commonly observed in colostrum. Quiles et al. [26] found higher than average values for mature milk in Spain, but this was based on only 15 women. The small sample size likely influenced the results.

The level of α-tocopherol and retinol in breast milk is normally greater in colostrum and thereafter exhibits a downward trend during the different stages of lactation. In this study, the women with a high-risk pregnancy showed this downward trend. We compared the average concentration of α-tocopherol previously reported for different groups of women, mostly with a normal evolutive pregnancy, to that found presently for women with a high-risk pregnancy. This concentration was herein found to be 2–3 times lower in colostrum, approximately two times lower in transitional milk, and very similar in mature milk [31,32,46–48].

Although an inverse correlation has been reported between the concentration of retinol and α-tocopherol in colostrum [49], the current results evidence a positive correlation between these two vitamins, which implies the existence of suboptimal concentrations. This manifests the need for supplementation [50] to prevent deficiencies in any given population.

6.2. Preterm Childbirth

For women in the present study with preterm birth, the median concentration of 405 (IQR; 109–676) μg/dL of α-tocopherol in colostrum was lower than that detected in the colostrum of some other groups of women having the same gestational age. For example, there were 1450 μg/dL in a group of German women [51], 1292.1–1722.8 μg/dL in Spanish women [26], and 1222 ± 772 μg/dL in Tunisian women [14]. Nevertheless, the current findings coincide with the concentration of α-tocopherol in the colostrum of women in other studies that gave preterm birth, such as the 250 μg/dL detected in Canadian women [52] and the 260.0 ± 30.0 μg/dL for Russian women [31]. In the case of retinol in the colostrum of women having given preterm birth, the median value of 36 (32–63) μg/dL observed herein is lower than the 57.5 ± 50.1 μg/dL described by Fares et al. [14]. This suggests the need to focus on reinforcing vitamin levels in women with preterm births and their neonates.

The hypothesis that the concentration of vitamin E depends on gestational age is still very controversial [49,53]. Nonetheless, this idea is supported by the current findings. Similar results were reported for a group of Spanish women by Quiles et al. [26], who found significantly higher concentrations of vitamin E at all stages of lactation in women who had carried their pregnancy to term compared to those giving preterm birth.

Compared to the women that carried their pregnancy to term in the present study, those that gave preterm birth had lower concentrations of retinol and α-tocopherol. The greatest deficiency was detected for the latter vitamin precursor. These results coincide with the findings of Souza et al. [54]. To compensate for this deficiency, supplementation of these vitamins should be provided during pregnancy (especially when involving high-risk) and breastfeeding. Unlike the current results, a Brazilian study reported variable concentrations of α-tocopherol, without any difference between women giving premature birth and those carrying their pregnancy to term. It has been postulated that the concentration of this vitamin is associated with birth weight more than prematurity [53]. However, this idea was not corroborated presently, evidencing multifactorial causes for the deficiency of this vitamin.

The current findings emphasize the fact that the neonate of a preterm birth requires special care, such as optimal nutrition. Not only does the prematurity of birth imply low reserves of vitamins A and E, but also the poor nutritional status of the mother indicates a limited transfer of the same through the placenta. For these reasons, liposoluble vitamins (e.g., retinol and α-tocopherol) should be assimilated by women with high-risk pregnancies [55] to avoid complications such as a delay in intrauterine growth or in neurodevelopment. A deficiency of these vitamins can even induce miscarriage [29].

Furthermore, it is recommended that preterm neonates immediately begin enteral feeding with breast milk and, if possible, vitamin supplementation [55]. Indeed, clinical assays have been conducted in which pregnant women were given a supplement of RRR α-tocopherol acetate, resulting in a significantly elevated concentration of this vitamin in transition milk and mature milk, as well as in the mothers themselves who gave preterm birth [50].

6.3. Does the BMI Affect the Concentrations of Retinol and α-Tocopherol?

The current results reveal that the higher the pregestational BMI (relative to normal) and the greater the gap between the real and recommended gestational weight gain, the lower the concentration of retinol tends to be. In this sense, the simple fact of having a high BMI is a risk factor for increased production of proinflammatory cytokines, a problem that can be counteracted if women are protected by adequate concentrations of two antioxidant substances, retinol and α-tocopherol. Perhaps it was the deficiency of retinol and α-tocopherol that, in large part, caused the relatively high frequency of preeclampsia among the women presently studied, considering that this deficiency (as well as others) can lead to greater oxidative stress [37] which, in turn, when coupled with other factors, tends to trigger this disorder [56,57].

A negative correlation was observed herein between pregestational BMI and the concentration of retinol and α-tocopherol. Like any population with overweight and obesity, pregnant women lack antioxidants and are exposed to cytokines that can harm their health and that of their offspring, thus affecting fetal programming and the first 1000 days of life [58–60].

The results suggest that the present participants showed no association between gestational diabetes (or other morbidities correlated with pregnancy) and low concentrations of retinol and α-tocopherol in breast milk, in agreement with another report that found no such association [11]. Since breast milk is the only source of these vitamins, however, there may be a greater risk, especially in the case that the newborn is premature or suffers from complications that increase oxidative stress.

The current results, like the vast majority of studies on liposoluble vitamins in breast milk [61–63], evidence a wide range in the concentration of vitamins A and E (especially vitamin E) among participants. This variation could be related to differences in lifestyle, in the consumption of nutrients and/or enrichment of food, and in the use of vitamin and food supplements. Some methodological factors, such as the day and time of collecting samples or the time elapsed since the last breastfeeding and the last meal, could contribute to this variability. Additionally, differences in methods of analysis also represent an important factor of variation. Finally, the methods employed for hydrolysis and extraction of an organic matrix of vitamins can affect the concentration of the same in breast milk [62].

Nourishing an infant with milk from his or her own mother results in better growth and nutritional status (including the level of vitamins A and E) than that observed in infants fed formula. Moreover, breast milk composition may be affected by obstetric characteristics, such as a premature delivery. In the present study, the composition of retinol and α-tocopherol in breast milk was negatively affected by premature birth and pregestational overweight and obesity. Furthermore, the concentration of these vitamin precursors was lower in the breast milk of women that had undergone a high-risk pregnancy compared to those having had a normal pregnancy.

Studies that explore the association between neonatal/maternal characteristics and the concentration of retinol and α-tocopherol in breast milk are important for determining the subgroups of newborns at risk for a vitamin A and E deficiency. This information should lead to strategies (e.g., vitamin supplementation) to target the subgroups at risk. Moreover, this approach can broaden the understanding of the influence of maternal factors such as gestational age on the adaptation capacity of mechanisms for transferring retinol and α-tocopherol to the mammary gland.

Certain elements of this study could be considered as limitations, including the lack of an evaluation of the nutritional state and diet of the participants. Another limitation is that a determination of fat in breast milk samples was not made. However, in other populations a high negative correlation has been shown between the concentration of serum cholesterol, the BMI, and the level of tocopherol and retinol. In addition, it must be kept in mind that all of the women participating in this study were of a low socioeconomic level, meaning that the results obtained cannot be generalized to all Mexican women during the period of breastfeeding.

7. Conclusions

Since the nutritional needs of a woman are sharply increased during pregnancy, it can be a challenge to meet these needs if careful attention is not paid to an adequate consumption of nutrients. Any inadequate dietary alteration can affect the health of the mother-fetus binomial. Deficiencies in micronutrients are related to gestational diabetes, preeclampsia, eclampsia, delayed intrauterine growth, low birth weight of the neonate, premature separation of the placenta, premature childbirth, spontaneous abortion, and congenital anomalies. Moreover, maternal nutrition determines the quality of breast milk. The concentration of vitamins A and E in breast milk depend on the concentration of the same in the mother. Hence, a maternal deficiency translates into the same problem for the neonate.

Even though the women in the high-risk pregnancy group showed a deficiency of vitamins A and E in their breast milk, the unique biological benefits of this milk justify the promotion of breast feeding as the optimal method of nourishing neonates. In these cases, it should be recommended that the woman increase her consumption of certain nutrients during pregnancy. Additionally, after childbirth, she should consider the use of supplements to produce milk of adequate quality and, thus, meet the needs of the baby and prevent a deficiency of micronutrients.

When the concentration of vitamins A and E are low in the breast milk of mothers after a high-risk pregnancy, we also recommend supplements for a child who receives nutrition exclusively from the mother. This supplementation should begin during the first days of life and continue until the infant initiates a complementary diet. Some studies have demonstrated that a deficiency in vitamins A and E in newborns, above all those with premature birth, increases the frequency of cases of bronchopulmonary dysplasia, intraventricular hemorrhage, periventricular leukomalacia, retinopathy, and necrotizing enterocolitis. Currently, there is not enough information to evaluate the possible benefits or adverse effects of supplementation during pregnancy.

In the current study, maternal overweight and obesity, as well as preterm birth, were associated with a low concentration of vitamins A and E in breast milk. It is necessary to determine whether the level of physical activity and the individual metabolism influence the quantity of food that each woman needs to achieve an optimal nutritional state and an adequate production of milk. The length and intensity of lactation also significantly affects the nutritional needs of the mother, although this is rarely considered.

Finally, during the period of breast feeding both the mother and child are at risk for a deficiency of vitamins A and E, especially in developing countries like Mexico and, thus, represent a public health problem. Moreover, if the concentration of vitamins A and E are low in the mother, the child is susceptible to suffering a like deficiency.

This study improves the knowledge about the content of vitamins A and E in breast milk from mothers after a high-risk pregnancy. Future research could include other nutrients that are also important for the development of the breast-fed child, as well as evaluate the nutritional intake of women during a high-risk pregnancy.

Acknowledgments: We are grateful to all of the mothers that participated in this study, as well as to all of the nursing personnel of the Neonatal Intensive Care Unit for the help provided in carrying out the present research.

Author Contributions: RS and HMR conceived and designed the experiments; RS, HMR, RMH, JMEP, and MEFQ performed the experiments; RS, HMR, CR, MEFQ and DV analyzed the data; HMR, RMH, DV, and CR, contributed reagents/materials/analysis tools; RS, HMR wrote the paper, all authors reading and approved this paper.

Abbreviations

HPLC	High-performance liquid chromatography
BMI	Body mass index
WHO	World Health Organization
PAHO	Pan American Health Organization
IQR	Interquartile range

References

1. Simmons, H.A.; Goldberg, L.S. 'High-risk' pregnancy after perinatal loss: Understanding the label. *Midwifery* **2011**, *27*, 452–457. [CrossRef] [PubMed]
2. Aune, D.; Saugstad, O.D.; Henriksen, T.; Tonstad, S. Maternal body mass index and the risk of fetal death, stillbirth, and infant death: A systematic review and meta-analysis. *JAMA* **2014**, *311*, 1536–1546. [CrossRef] [PubMed]
3. Secretaría de Salud. *Encuesta Nacional de Salud y Nutrición 2012, Resultados Nacionales*; Instituto Nacional de Salud Pública: Cuernavaca, Mexico, 2012.
4. Institute of Medicine Report Brief. *Weight Gain during Pregnancy: Reexamining the Guidelines*; National Academies Press: Washington, DC, USA, 2009.
5. Langford, A.; Joshu, C.; Chang, J.J.; Myles, T.; Leet, T. Does gestational weight gain affect the risk of adverse maternal and infant outcomes in overweight women? *Matern. Child Health J.* **2011**, *15*, 860–865. [CrossRef] [PubMed]
6. Surapaneni, K.M. Oxidant–antioxidant status in gestational diabetes patients. *J. Clin. Diagn. Res.* **2007**, *1*, 235–238.
7. Resende, F.B.; Clemente, H.A.; Bezerra, D.F.; Grilo, E.C.; de Melo, L.R.; Bellot, P.E.; Dantas, R.C.; Dimenstein, R. Alpha-tocopherol concentration in serum and colostrum of mothers with gestational diabetes mellitus. *Rev. Paul. Pediatr.* **2014**, *32*, 178–186. [CrossRef] [PubMed]
8. Debier, C.; Larondelle, Y. Vitamins A and E: Metabolism, roles and transfer to offspring. *Br. J. Nutr.* **2005**, *93*, 153–174. [CrossRef] [PubMed]
9. Lira, L.Q.; Dimenstein, R. Vitamin A and gestational diabetes. *Rev. Assoc. Med. Bras.* **2010**, *56*, 355–359. [CrossRef] [PubMed]
10. Krzyzanowska, K.; Zemany, L.; Krugluger, W.; Schernthaner, G.H.; Mittermayer, F.; Schnack, C.; Rahman, R.; Brix, J.; Kahn, B.B.; Schernthaner, G. Serum concentrations of retinol-binding protein 4 in women with and without gestational diabetes. *Diabetologia* **2008**, *51*, 1115–1122. [CrossRef] [PubMed]
11. Resende, F.B.; De Lira, L.Q.; Grilo, E.C.; Lima, M.S. Dimenstein, R. Gestational diabetes: A risk of puerperal hypovitaminosis A? *An. Acad. Bras. Cienc.* **2015**, *87*, 463–470. [CrossRef] [PubMed]
12. Dewey, K.G.; Begum, K. Long-term consequences of stunting in early life. *Matern. Child Nutr.* **2011**, *7* (Suppl. 3), 5–18. [CrossRef] [PubMed]
13. Ibrahim, S.A.; Abd el-Maksoud, A.; Nassar, M.F. Nutritional stunting in Egypt: Which nutrient is responsible? *East. Mediterr. Health J.* **2002**, *8*, 272–280. [PubMed]
14. Fares, S.; Sethom, M.M.; Khouaja-Mokrani, C.; Jabnoun, S.; Feki, M.; Kaabachi, N. Vitamin A, E, and D deficiencies in Tunisian very low birth weight neonates: Prevalence and risk factors. *Pediatr. Neonatol.* **2014**, *55*, 196–201. [CrossRef] [PubMed]
15. Weissgerber, T.L.; Gandley, R.E.; McGee, P.L.; Spong, C.Y.; Myatt, L.; Leveno, K.J.; Thorp, J.M., Jr.; Mercer, B.M.; Peaceman, A.M.; Ramin, S.M.; et al. Haptoglobin phenotype, preeclampsia risk and the efficacy of vitamin C and E supplementation to prevent preeclampsia in a racially diverse population. *PLoS ONE* **2013**, *8*, e60479. [CrossRef] [PubMed]
16. Weissgerber, T.L.; Gandley, R.E.; Roberts, J.M.; Patterson, C.C.; Holmes, V.A.; Young, I.S.; McCance, D.R. Haptoglobin phenotype, pre-eclampsia, and response to supplementation with vitamins C and E in pregnant women with type-1 diabetes. *BJOG* **2013**, *120*, 1192–1199. [CrossRef] [PubMed]
17. Bártfai, L.; Bártfai, Z.; Nedeczky, I.; Puho, E.H.; Bánhidy, F.; Czeizel, A.E. Rate of preterm birth in pregnant women with vitamin E treatment: A population-based study. *J. Matern. Fetal Neonatal Med.* **2012**, *25*, 575–580. [CrossRef] [PubMed]
18. Schmölz, L.; Birringer, M.; Lorkowski, S.; Wallert, M. Complexity of vitamin E metabolism. *World J. Biol. Chem.* **2016**, *7*, 14–43. [CrossRef] [PubMed]
19. Stam, J.; Sauer, P.J.J.; Boelm, G. Can we define an infant's need from the composition of human milk? *Am. J. Clin. Nutr.* **2013**, *98*, 521S–528S. [CrossRef] [PubMed]

20. American College Obstetrician and Gynecologists Committee on Practice bulletin–Obstetrics. ACGO Practice Bulletin. Clinical Management Guidelines for Obstetrician-Gynecologists, No. 30, September 2001 (replaces Technical Bulletin No. 200, December 1994); Gestational diabetes. Available online: http://c.ymcdn.com/sites/chronicdisease.site-ym.com/resource/resmgr/Womens_Health_Council_GDM/pb030_gestational_diabetes_r.pdf (accessed on 1 July 2016).
21. American College Obstetrician and Gynecologists Committee on Practice bulletin–Obstetrics. ACGO Practice Bulletin. Diagnosis and Management of Preeclampsia and Eclampsia, No. 33, January 2002; American College Obstetrician and Gynecologists. Available online: https://www.scribd.com/document/116952914/No-33-Diagnosis-and-Management-of-Preeclampsia-and-Eclampsia (accessed on 1 July 2016).
22. Xue, X.; You, J.; He, P. Simultaneous determination of five fat-soluble vitamins in feed by high-performance liquid chromatography following solid-phase extraction. *J. Chromatogr. Sci.* **2008**, *46*, 345–350. [CrossRef] [PubMed]
23. Rish, L.; Yaqoob, M.; Waseem, A.; Nabi, A. Vitamin A determination in milk sample based on the luminol-periodate chemiluminescence system. *J. Nutr. Sci. Vitaminol.* **2014**, *60*, 9–16. [CrossRef]
24. IOM (Institute of Medicine) and NRC (National Research Council). *Weight Gain During Pregnancy: Reexamining the Guidelines*; The National Academies Press: Washington, DC, USA, 2009.
25. Schweigert, F.J.; Bathe, K.; Chen, F.; Büscher, U.; Dudenhausen, J.W. Effect of the stage of lactation in humans on carotenoid levels in milk, blood plasma and plasma lipoprotein fractions. *Eur. J. Nutr.* **2004**, *43*, 39–44. [CrossRef] [PubMed]
26. Quiles, J.L.; Ochoa, J.J.; Ramirez-Tortosa, M.C.; Linde, J.; Bompadre, S.; Battino, M.; Narbona, E.; Maldonado, J.; Mataix, J. Coenzyme Q concentration and total antioxidant capacity of human milk at different stages of lactation in mothers of preterm and full-term infants. *Free Radic. Res.* **2006**, *40*, 199–206. [CrossRef] [PubMed]
27. Ahmed, L.; Nazrul Islam, S.; Khan, M.N.; Huque, S.; Ahsan, M. Antioxidant micronutrient profile (Vitamin E, C, A, copper, zinc, iron) of colostrum: Association with maternal characteristics. *J. Trop. Pediatr.* **2004**, *50*, 357–358. [CrossRef] [PubMed]
28. Szlagatys-Sidorkiewicz, A.; Zagierski, M.; Jankowska, A.; Łuczak, G.; Macur, K.; Baczek, T.; Korzon, M.; Krzykowski, G.; Martysiak-Żurowska, D.; Kamińska, B. Longitudinal study of vitamins A, E and lipid oxidative damage in human milk throughout lactation. *Early Hum. Dev.* **2012**, *88*, 421–424. [CrossRef] [PubMed]
29. De Lira, L.Q.; Ribeiro, P.P.; Grilo, E.C.; Lima, M.S.; Dimenstein, R. Alpha-tocopherol level in serum and colostrum of breastfeeding women and association with maternal variables. *Rev. Bras. Ginecol. Obstet.* **2012**, *34*, 362–368. (In Portuguese) [PubMed]
30. Shi, Y.D.; Sun, G.Q.; Zhang, Z.G.; Deng, X.; Kang, X.H.; Liu, Z.D.; Ma, Y.; Sheng, Q.H. The chemical composition of human milk from Inner Mongolia of China. *Food Chem.* **2011**, *127*, 1193–1198. [CrossRef] [PubMed]
31. Martysiak-Zurowska, D.; Szlagatys-Sidorkiewicz, A.; Zagierski, C. Concentrations of alpha- and gamma-tocopherols in human breast milk during the first months of lactation and in infant formulas. *Matern. Child Nutr.* **2013**, *9*, 473–482. [CrossRef] [PubMed]
32. Garcia, L.R.; Ribeiro, K.D.; Araújo, K.F.; Azevedo, G.M.; Pires, J.F.; Batista, S.D.; Dimenstein, R. Níveis de alfa-tocoferol no soro e leite maternos de puérperas atendidas em maternidade pública de Natal. *Rio Grande do Norte Rev. Bras. Saude. Matern. Infant.* **2009**, *9*, 423–428. [CrossRef]
33. Sakurai, T.; Furukawa, M.; Asha, M.; Kanno, T.; Kojima, T.; Yonekubo, A. Fat-soluble and water-soluble vitamin contents of breast milk from Japanese women. *J. Nutr. Sci. Vitaminol.* **2005**, *5*, 239–247. [CrossRef]
34. Engle-Stone, R.; Haskell, M.J.; Nankap, M.; Ndjebayi, A.O.; Brown, K.H. Breast milk retinol and plasma retinol-binding protein concentrations provide similar estimates of vitamin A deficiency prevalence and identify similar risk groups among women in Cameroon but breast milk retinol underestimates the prevalence of deficiency among young children. *J. Nutr.* **2014**, *144*, 209–217. [PubMed]
35. Tanumihardjo, S.A.; Russell, R.M.; Stephensen, C.B.; Gannon, B.M.; Craft, N.E.; Haskell, M.J.; Lietz, G.; Schulze, K.; Raiten, D.J. Biomarkers of nutrition for development (BOND)-vitamin A Review. *J. Nutr.* **2016**, *146*, 1816S–1848S. [CrossRef] [PubMed]
36. Kodentsova, V.M.; Vrzhesinskaya, O.A. Evaluation of the vitamin status in nursing women by vitamin content in breast milk. *Bull. Exp. Biol. Med.* **2006**, *141*, 323–327. [CrossRef] [PubMed]

37. Kamao, M.; Tsugawa, N.; Suahra, Y.; Okano, T. Determination of fat-soluble vitamins in human plasma, breast milk, and food samples: Application in nutrition survey for establishment of "Dietary Reference Intakes for Japanese". *J. Health Sci.* **2007**, *53*, 257–262. [CrossRef]
38. Tijerina-Sáenz, A.; Innis, S.M.; Kitts, D.D. Antioxidant capacity of human milk and its association with vitamins A and E and fatty acid composition. *Acta Paediatr.* **2009**, *98*, 1793–1798. [CrossRef] [PubMed]
39. Antonakou, A.; Chiou, A.; Andrikopoulos, N.K.; Bakoula, C.; Matalas, A.L. Breast milk tocopherol content during the first six months in exclusively breastfeeding Greek women. *Eur. J. Nutr.* **2011**, *50*, 195–202. [CrossRef] [PubMed]
40. Szlagatys-Sidorkiewicz, A.; Zagierski, M.; Luczak, G.; Macur, K.; Baczek, T.; Kaminska, B. Maternal smoking does not influence vitamin A and E concentrations in mature breastmilk. *Breastfeed. Med.* **2012**, *7*, 285–289. [CrossRef] [PubMed]
41. Wallingford, J.; Underwood, B. Vitamin A deficiency in pregnancy, lactation and the nursing child. In *Vitamin A deficiency and Its Control*; Bauernfeind, J., Ed.; Academic Press: Orlando, FL, USA, 1986; pp. 101–152.
42. Agne-Djigo, A.; Idohou-Dossou, N.; Kwadjode, K.M.; Tanumihardjo, S.A.; Wade, S. High prevalence of vitamin A deficiency is detected by the modified relative dose-response test in six-month-old Senegalese breast-fed infants. *J. Nutr.* **2012**, *142*, 1991–1996. [CrossRef] [PubMed]
43. Tyndall, J.A.; Okoye, V.; Elumelu, F.; Dahiru, A.; Pariya, H.B. Vitamin A and iron deficiency in pregnant women, lactating mothers and their infants in Adamawa State, Nigeria: A prospective cohort study. *Am. J. Food Nutr.* **2012**, *2*, 14–20. [CrossRef]
44. Azeredo, V.B.; Trugo, N.M. Retinol, carotenoids, and tocopherols in the milk of lactating adolescents and relationships with plasma concentrations. *Nutrition* **2008**, *24*, 133–139. [CrossRef] [PubMed]
45. Tokusoglu, O.; Tansug, N.; Aksit, S.; Dinc, G.; Kasirga, E.; Ozcan, C. Retinol and α-tocopherol concentrations in breast milk of Turkish lactating mothers under different socio-economic status. *Int. J. Food Sci. Nutr.* **2008**, *59*, 166–174. [CrossRef] [PubMed]
46. Debier, C. Vitamin E during pre- and postnatal periods. *Vitam. Horm.* **2007**, *76*, 357–373. [PubMed]
47. Sziklai-László, I.; Majchrzak, D.; Elmadfa, I.; Cser, M.A. Selenium and vitamin E concentrations in human milk and formula milk from Hungary. *J. Radioanalytical Nuclear Chem.* **2009**, *279*, 585–590. [CrossRef]
48. Fujita, M.; Shell-Ducan, B.; Ndemwa, P.; Brindle, E.; Lo, Y.J.; Kombe, Y.; O'Connor, K. Vitamin A Dynamics in breastmilk and liver stores: A life history perspective. *Am. J. Hum. Biol.* **2011**, *23*, 664–673. [CrossRef] [PubMed]
49. De Lira, L.Q.; Lima, M.S.; de Medeiros, J.M.; da Silva, I.F.; Dimenstein, R. Correlation of vitamin A nutritional status on alpha-tocopherol in the colostrum of lactating women. *Matern. Child Nutr.* **2013**, *9*, 31–40. [CrossRef] [PubMed]
50. Pires Medeiros, J.F.; Ribeiro, K.D.; Lima, M.S.; das Neves, R.A.; Lima, A.C.; Dantas, R.C.; da Silva, A.B.; Dimenstein, R. α-tocopherol in breast milk of women with preterm delivery after a single postpartum oral dose of vitamin E. *Br. J. Nutr.* **2016**, *115*, 1424–1430. [CrossRef] [PubMed]
51. Haug, M.; Laubach, C.; Burke, M.; Harzer, G. Vitamin E in human from mothers of preterm and term infants. *J. Pediatr. Gastroenterol. Nutr.* **1987**, *6*, 605–609. [CrossRef] [PubMed]
52. Bishara, R.; Dunn, M.S.; Merko, S.E.; Darling, P. Nutrient composition of hindmilk produced by mothers of very low mothers of very low birth weight infants born at less than 28 weeks gestation. *J. Hum. Lact.* **2008**, *24*, 159–167. [CrossRef] [PubMed]
53. Grilo, E.C.; Lira, L.Q.; Dimenstein, R.; Ribeiro, K.D. Influence of prematurity and birth weight on the concentration of α-tocopherol in colostrum milk. *Rev. Paul. Pediatr.* **2013**, *31*, 473–479. [CrossRef] [PubMed]
54. Souza, G.; Dolinsky, M.; Matos, A.; Chagas, C.; Ramalho, A. Vitamin A concentration in human milk and its relationship with liver reserve formation and compliance with the recommended daily intake of vitamin A in preterm and full term infants in exclusive breastfeeding. *Arch. Gynecol. Obstet.* **2015**, *291*, 319–325. [CrossRef] [PubMed]
55. Ho, M.Y.; Yen, Y.H. Trend of nutritional support in preterm infants. *Pediatr. Neonatol.* **2016**, *57*, 365–370. [CrossRef] [PubMed]
56. Shamim, A.A.; Schulze, K.; Merrill, R.D.; Kabir, A.; Christian, P.; Shaikh, S.; Wu, L.; Ali, H.; Labrique, A.B.; Mehra, S.; et al. First-trimester plasma tocopherols are associated with risk of miscarriage in rural Bangladesh. *Am. J. Clin. Nutr.* **2015**, *101*, 294–301. [CrossRef] [PubMed]

57. Cohen, J.M.; Kramer, M.S.; Platt, R.W.; Basso, O.; Evans, R.W.; Kahn, S.R. The association between maternal antioxidant levels in midpregnancy and preeclampsia. *Am. J. Obstet. Gynecol.* **2015**, *213*, 695.e1–695.e13. [CrossRef] [PubMed]
58. Wei, X.; Peng, R.; Cao, J.; Kang, Y.; Qu, P.; Liu, Y.; Xiao, X.; Li, T. Serum vitamin A status is associated with obesity and the metabolic syndrome among school-age children in Chongqing, China. *Asia Pac. J. Clin. Nutr.* **2016**, *25*, 563–570. [PubMed]
59. Hrolfsdottir, L.; Schalkwijk, C.G.; Birgisdottir, B.E.; Gunnarsdottir, I.; Maslova, E.; Granström, C.; Strøm, M.; Olsen, S.F.; Halldorsson, T.I. Maternal diet, gestational weight gain, and inflammatory markers during pregnancy. *Obesity (Silver Spring)* **2016**, *24*, 2133–2139. [CrossRef] [PubMed]
60. McCurdy, C.E.; Schenk, S.; Hetrick, B.; Houck, J.; Drew, B.G.; Kaye, S.; Lashbrook, M.; Bergman, B.C.; Takahashi, D.L.; Dean, T.A.; et al. Maternal obesity reduces oxidative capacity in fetal skeletal muscle of Japanese macaques. *JCI Insight* **2016**, *1*, e86612. [CrossRef] [PubMed]
61. Lima, M.S.R.; Dimenstein, R.; Ribeiro, K.D.S. Vitamin E concentration in human milk and associated factors: A literature review. *J. Pediatr. (Rio J.)* **2014**, *90*, 440–448. [CrossRef] [PubMed]
62. Fares, S.; Sethom, M.M.; Kacem, S.; Ksibi, I.; Feki, M.; Jebnoun, S.; Kaabachi, N. Retinol and alpha-tocopherol in the colostrum of lactating Tunisian women delivering prematurely: Associations with maternal characteristics. *Pediatr. Neonatol.* **2016**, *57*, 120–126. [CrossRef] [PubMed]
63. Debier, C.; Pottier, J.; Goffe, C.H.; Larondelle, Y. Present knowledge and unexpected behaviors of vitamins A and E in colostrum and milk. *Liviest. Prod. Sci.* **2005**, *98*, 135–147. [CrossRef]

12

Introduction of Complementary Foods in a Cohort of Infants in Northeast Italy: Do Parents Comply with WHO Recommendations?

Claudia Carletti, Paola Pani, Lorenzo Monasta, Alessandra Knowles * and Adriano Cattaneo

Clinical Epidemiology and Public Health Research Unit, Institute for Maternal and Child Health IRCCS "Burlo Garofolo", Via dell'Istria 65/1, Trieste 34137, Italy; claudiaveronica.carletti@burlo.trieste.it (C.C.); paola.pani@burlo.trieste.it (P.P.); lorenzo.monasta@burlo.trieste.it (L.M.); adriano.cattaneo@gmail.com (A.C.)

* Correspondence: alessandra.knowles@burlo.trieste.it

Abstract: Timing and type of complementary food in infancy affect nutritional status and health later in life. The objective of this paper was to assess complementary feeding practices, looking at timing, type, and compliance with World Health Organization (WHO) recommendations. Data were obtained from a birth cohort of 400 infants, enrolled in Trieste (Italy) between July 2007 and July 2008 and followed up for three years, using a "food introduction timing table". Five WHO recommendations standards were used to assess parental compliance and associated factors. Thirty seven percent of mothers returned the completed "timing table" up until the child was three years of age. Eighty six percent of infants were already receiving complementary foods at six months. The first food type to be introduced was fresh fruit (170 days from birth, median). Overall, infants shared a very similar diet, which was different from the family diet and characterized by delayed introduction of certain food types. Five percent of parents complied with either all five or only one of the WHO recommendations, 34% with three, and 35% with four. The parents' partial compliance with WHO recommendations is probably due to conflicting information received from different sources. This advocates for national evidence-based guidelines, supported and promoted by health professionals.

Keywords: complementary feeding; compliance with WHO recommendation; timing of introduction of complementary food; infant nutrition; Italy

1. Introduction

Complementary feeding is a process that, according to World Health Organization (WHO) [1], should take place between the ages of around six months and two years, this being a crucial period for child growth, development, and health. Studies conducted in low and high-income countries show that inadequate nutrition during this period increases the risk of becoming underweight or overweight, with potentially serious life-long health effects [2–5]. Under- and over-nutrition can coexist in the same country, regardless of the country's economic status, and tend to affect the poorest population groups [6]. The time of introduction of complementary foods, as well as their type, are crucial not only to ensure that nutritional needs are met in the short term, but also to promote good health later in life and to prevent overweight and obesity [7–10].

The WHO recommends, as a public health measure, exclusive breastfeeding up to six months of age, followed by adequate, safe and appropriate complementary foods with breastfeeding continuing up to two years and beyond [1]. This recommendation has been adopted in many countries, including Italy [11]. In conflict with the WHO recommendation, the European Society for Pediatric Gastroenterology Hepatology and Nutrition (ESPGHAN) recommends the introduction of complementary foods no earlier than 17 and no later than 26 weeks of age [12]. This commentary triggered a debate [13], and in 2011 the WHO released a statement reaffirming that exclusive breastfeeding for six months has several advantages over exclusive breastfeeding for three to four months, and should be followed by gradual introduction of solid food alongside breastfeeding [14]. WHO also recommends that, between the ages of 6 and 12 months, the infant's diet should be progressively integrated into a healthy family diet, without restrictions on the types of food that are offered. There is no evidence to support the practice of delaying the introduction of potentially allergenic foods (e.g., tomatoes, fish, eggs), with the exception of the replacement of breast milk or formula with cow milk, which is not recommended before 12 months of age due to its low content in iron [15]. This recommendation is shared by ESPGHAN [12]. Finally, WHO warns against the use of honey in the first 12 months due to the risk of botulism, and recommends that, from six months onwards, infants should make a gradual transition to eating family foods limiting the consumption of commercial complementary foods [1,16] as these may delay the infant's acceptance of the family's normal diet [15].

In spite of these recommendations, data on current feeding practices suggest that the introduction of complementary foods before six months is common in many countries [17,18], including Italy [19,20], where there are no Ministry of Health guidelines on complementary feeding. The national guidelines on the protection, promotion, and support of breastfeeding simply state that "after six months, breast milk, with appropriate complementary feeding, provides an important contribution to the nutrition, health and development of the child" [11]. What "appropriate complementary feeding" means is not clearly explained.

The cohort study aimed at investigating the transition from milk to family foods, and its association with overweight, in a birth cohort of 400 children followed up for 36 months. The prevalence and duration of breastfeeding, the data on nutrient intake at six month of age and on the mothers' socioeconomic status, have already been reported in previous papers [20,21]. The specific objective of the present research was to assess complementary feeding practices, focusing on timing, characteristics, and compliance with the WHO recommendations. Considering that there is very little national data [19,22] describing complementary feeding practices, a better understanding of parents' approach to the introduction of complementary foods could support the development of evidence-based national guidelines on infant feeding.

2. Materials and Methods

Data were obtained from a cohort study conducted at the maternity hospital of Trieste (Institute for Maternal and Child Health Burlo Garofolo), Italy, between July 2007 and July 2011. A cohort of 400 mother-infant pairs was followed up for three years, using telephone interviews and self-reported diaries to investigate feeding practices and attitudes of mothers. The study was approved by the ethics committee of the Institute. The study design, methods, and sampling procedures have already been reported [21]. In brief, mother-infant pairs were enrolled at birth according to the following eligibility criteria: birth weight ≥2000 g, no congenital malformation nor severe diseases that required hospital admission, gestational age of 36 completed weeks or more, and residence in the province of Trieste. Upon enrolment, mothers were checked for eligibility and asked to give their informed consent. During the first contact, they were given a feeding diary with instructions on how to record type and quantity of foods over a 24-h period on three separate non-consecutive days at 3, 6, 9, 12, 18, 24, and 36 months of age of the infant [23,24].

At the same time, mothers were also given a "timing of introduction of food timetable" ("food timetable") in which they were asked to record information on the characteristics, preparation and date of introduction of the first food type for each of 17 set food categories. The food timetable was handed back to the researchers when the child was 36 months old, together with the last feeding diary and the data on weight and length/height of the child recorded by the paediatricians at 1, 3, 6, 9, 12, 18, 24 and 36 months, on the occasion of periodic health checks.

The food timetable was divided into food categories: fresh fruit, vegetables (with a separate category for tomatoes because of their potential allergenicity), cereals (with a focus on gluten free pasta and bread), cow milk, milk products, meat, legumes, fish, eggs, cured meats, industrial fruit juice, tubers, honey, sugar (added to drinks or foods), sweets, creamy porridge, and nuts and seeds. For each food category, mothers were asked to record the date of the first tasting and the date from which the food type was fully incorporated in the infant's diet, if different from the date of the first tasting. Mothers were also asked to record the method of preparation (e.g., raw or cooked, homogenized or lyophilized) and the characteristics (e.g., commercial baby food or homemade) of each food item.

WHO recommends appropriate complementary feeding starting from the age of six months, with continued breastfeeding up to two years and beyond. Appropriate complementary feeding is: timely, adequate, safe, and properly fed. On the basis of these indications we derived from the WHO recommendations five standards to assess compliance:

1. introduction at or after 6 months;
2. "minimum dietary diversity";
3. use of homemade vs. commercial baby food;
4. introduction of cow's milk at 12 months or more;
5. introduction of honey at 12 months or more.

Recommendation 1 describes the concept of "timeliness", recommendations 2, 3, and 4 cover "adequateness", meaning that food provides sufficient energy, protein, and micronutrients to meet a growing child's nutritional needs. "Safety" is represented by recommendation 5. With regards to "propriety of feeding" the timing questionnaire did not assess either meal frequency or feeding methods.

The second recommendation is based on a slightly modified version of WHO's "minimum dietary diversity" indicator, by which infants are defined as "compliant" if their diet incorporates four to seven different food categories by the age of 12 months. [25]. The seven food groups used by WHO to codify this indicator are: "grains, roots, and tubers"; "flesh foods (meat and fish)"; "dairy (milk) products"; "legumes and nuts"; "vitamin-A rich fruits and vegetables"; "other fruits and vegetables"; and "eggs". In the present study, "vitamin-A rich fruits and vegetables" were not assessed as an independent group because Italy is considered to be free from vitamin A deficiency [26]. Instead, we chose to allocate to fruits and vegetables two separate categories with the aim of evaluating their independent contribution to the daily diet. Because our timing questionnaire covered a period of three years, we also extracted an index of "maximum dietary diversity" to determine how many children had introduced all seven food categories into their diet by the age of 12 months.

For the third recommendation, we analyzed the consumption of homemade vs. commercial complementary baby food defining the use of the latter as 'high' if it covered at least three out of five food groups (fruit, vegetables, meat, fish, cereals, and milk products) at six months of age. Almost 38% of infants fell into this category.

Differences between groups were examined with Fisher exact two-tailed test for categorical variables and with Mann-Whitney rank-sum test for continuous variables.

In order to perform the logistic regression analyses described below, the sample was divided into two groups based on the timing of the first introduction of complementary food. The cut-off was set at 21 weeks, which was the median of the distribution curve (Figure 1). The 21 weeks value had the additional advantage of falling in the middle of the ESPGHAN recommended window (17 to 26 weeks). This timing distribution was used as dependent variable.

The independent variables reflected the objective of the study to assess compliance with WHO recommendations both as stand-alone variables and as overall compliance with any three out of five. The relation between these independent variables and timing was analyzed using stratified and simultaneous univariate and multivariate logistic regression analyses. The variables included in the simultaneous models are presented in Supplementary Materials Tables S1–S6.

The stratified analysis was carried out considering each of the following variables: mothers' characteristics, including age (≥34 years), body mass index (BMI) before pregnancy (≥25), place of birth (Italy vs. other), level of education (degree or higher vs. lower), occupation, whether she was breastfeeding or had breastfed, if she had allergies or a family history of allergies, if she was or had been a smoker, and type of professional figure (paediatrician or midwife) who provided counselling on complementary feeding.

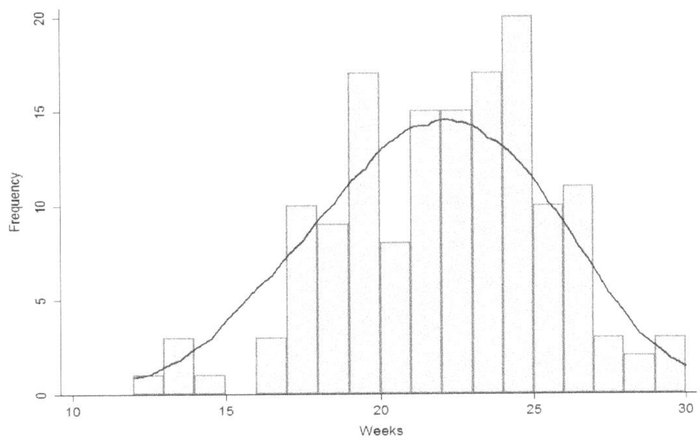

Figure 1. Distribution curve of the timing of first introduction of complementary foods in weeks. The probability density function was estimated with a non-parametric Kernel density estimation (KDE).

The characteristics of the mothers were selected based on literature data. The information on which professional figures were providing counselling on complementary feeding was based on the hypothesis, formulated by the authors but also supported by literature [27,28], that this may influence mothers' behavior.

All the analyses were carried out using Stata IC 14.1 (StataCorp LP, College Station, TX, USA).

3. Results

3.1. Population Characteristics

Four hundred mother-infant pairs were enrolled in the study, but only 148 (37%) completed and returned the food timetable when the child reached 36 months of age. The participation rate declined during the study: after three months 34% (135/400) of mothers had withdrawn from the study. This percentage subsequently followed a fluctuating pattern, rising to 59% (235/400) at 6 months and then dropping to 43% (173/400) and 41% (165/400) at 9 and 12 months, respectively. By the time of the 24-month interview, the study cohort had reduced by 67% (132/400). The characteristics of the mothers and infants of the sub-cohort that completed the timing questionnaire are described in Table 1. No statistically significant differences were observed between the cohort (400) and the sub-cohort (148), as already reported [16,17]. In brief, 89% of mothers (mean age 33.7 years; Standard Deviation 4.4) had a medium-to-high level of education, 95% declared they were employed before birth and 80% were in employment at six months after birth. Most infants (90%) were born between 38 and 42 weeks of gestation and 82% by vaginal delivery. The majority (91%) weighed between 2500 g and 4199 g at birth, and 79% were between 46 and 52 cm long. The infants' mean BMI was calculated at three and six months: 70% and 75% of infants had a BMI that fell within the normal range (between the 15th and the 85th WHO percentile), 15% and 3% were below the 15th percentile, while 15% and 21% were over the 85th percentile, respectively.

Table 1. Characteristics of mothers at enrolment and children at birth.

	Cohort	Sub-Cohort	
Mothers	***n* (%)**	***n* (%)**	*p* *
Age (years)	(n = 399)	(n = 148)	0.713
≤29	90 (23)	29 (20)	
30–34	160 (40)	59 (40)	
≥35	149 (37)	60 (40)	
Born in Italy	(n = 400)	(n = 148)	0.451
Yes	351 (88)	134 (91)	
No	49 (12)	14 (9)	
Education	(n = 348)	(n = 147)	0.158
≤Secondary school	59 (17)	16 (11)	
Completed high school or equivalent	154 (44)	64 (43)	
Bachelor degree or higher	135 (39)	67 (46)	
Employment before birth	(n = 323)	(n = 136)	1.000
Yes	306 (95)	129 (95)	
No	17 (5)	7 (5)	
Employment at 6 months after birth	(n = 218)	(n = 147)	0.790
Yes	176 (81)	117 (80)	
No	42 (19)	30 (20)	
Allergy of mother or of other family member	(n = 263)	(n = 148)	0.812
Yes	64 (24)	38 (26)	
No	199 (76)	110 (74)	
Children	***n* (%)**	***n* (%)**	*p*
Gestational age (weeks)	(n = 339)	(n = 147)	0.730
36–37	29 (9)	14 (9)	
38–42	310 (91)	133 (91)	
Infant gender	(n = 345)	(n = 148)	0.142
male	173 (50)	85 (57)	
female	172 (50)	63 (43)	
Birth weight (g)	(n = 344)	(n = 148)	0.552
<2500	3 (1)	2 (1)	
2500–4199	324 (94)	136 (92)	
≥4200	17 (5)	10 (7)	
Birth length (cm)	(n = 342)	(n = 148)	0.563
<46	5 (1)	2 (1)	
46–52.9	283 (83)	117 (79)	
≥53	54 (16)	29 (20)	

* *p*-Value is calculated using a two-tailed Fisher Exact test.

3.2. Timing of Complementary Feeding

At six months of age, 73% of infants were still receiving breast milk but, in contrast with WHO recommendations, only 7% were exclusively breastfed; 40% received formula and breast milk, 27% only formula and 26% breast milk and complementary food. One infant was given food other than milk before the age of three months, 7% at three months, 32% at four, 47% at five months. Only 14% of infants were given their first complementary food at six months or more

The median age of introduction of solid foods was 5.2 months (min 2.8; max 7.2). The interval between the first tasting and the complete introduction of the different food categories ranged from 6 to 32 days. The range was narrower for food groups such as dairy products, vegetables, and cereals (6, 6, and 7 days, respectively) and wider for honey, sugar, and cow milk (32, 29, and 22 days, respectively). The timetable of the complete introduction of each food category is reported in Figure 2.

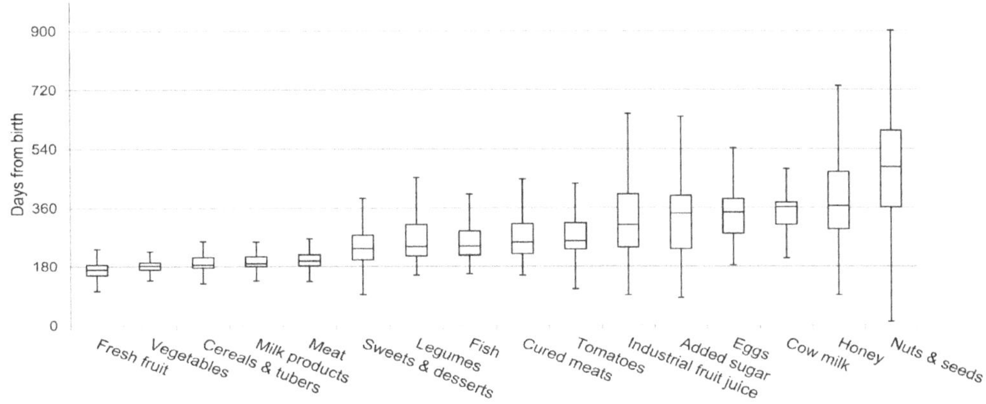

Figure 2. Timing of introduction of the single food groups in days from birth. The ends of the whiskers are set at 1.5*IQR above the third quartile (Q3) and 1.5*IQR below the first quartile (Q1). If the Minimum or Maximum values are outside this range, then they are shown as outliers. IQR = Inter Quartile Range.

In the figure, the cereals/tubers categories and the sweets/desserts categories, which include sweets and creamy porridge, have been merged for representational purposes. The first food group to be introduced was fresh fruit (at a median age of 170 days); followed by vegetables (182 days); cereals, including bread, pasta with gluten, and rice (193 days); milk products (189 days); and meat (197 days). The last food groups to be introduced were cow milk (362 days), honey (365 days), and nuts and seeds (484 days). In 80% of the cases, the first type of food to be offered was the apple, followed by vegetable soup (41%), and baby cereals (41%). The use of gluten-free products (bread, pasta, and desserts) was low (17% of infants) and the timing of their introduction was similar to that of the products with gluten. The introduction of pasta with gluten occurred at a median of 234 days, as opposed to 224 days for gluten-free pasta. The most frequently used commercial baby food types were: milk products (67%), fish (62%), sweets and desserts (61%), cured meat (52%), cereals (52%), meat (49%), fruit (27%), and vegetables (3%).

3.3. Compliance with WHO Recommendations

Table 2 shows the percentage of mothers who complied with the WHO recommendations on complementary feeding. The recommendations to which most mothers adhered were the minimum diversity diet (96%) and the introduction of honey after 12 months of age (80%), while 62% of the mothers complied with the recommendation to limit the use of commercial baby foods. However, the analysis of the "maximum diversity diet" indicated that, by the age 12 months, only 45% of children had introduced all seven food groups and, in particular, eggs and legumes had been introduced by 53% and 74% of infants, respectively.

Table 2. Percentage of mothers who followed the WHO recommendations (n = 148).

Items Included in the Score	(n)
Introduction of solid foods ≥6 months	14% (21)
Reduced use of commercial baby foods	62% (92)
Introduction of cow's milk ≥12 months	63% (94)
Introduction of honey ≥12 months	80% (118)
Minimum dietary diversity	96% (142)

As shown in Figure 3, eight mothers (5%) complied with all five recommendations and eight (5%) complied with only one, while 34% complied with at least three recommendations. Within this subgroup, the least frequently adhered to recommendation was the introduction of complementary feeding after the age of six months (19%).

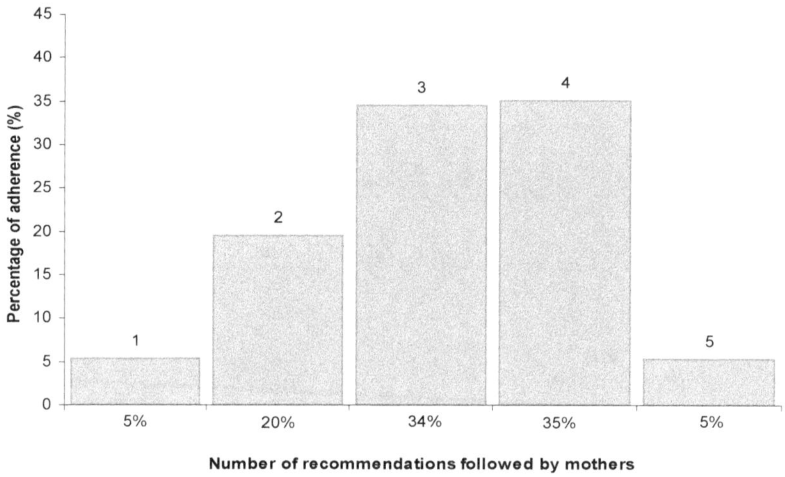

Figure 3. Number of recommendations (0, 1, 2, 3, 4 and 5) followed by mothers and percentage of compliance.

3.4. Regression Analyses

The stratified analyses showed that only few of the outcomes considered were significantly associated with selected mothers' characteristics. The introduction of cow milk after 12 months was significantly associated with the introduction of the first foods at 21 weeks of age or more if mothers were not breastfeeding their infants at six months (66%, $p = 0.03$), did not have a family history of allergy (80%, $p < 0.01$), had a BMI (kg/m^2) of less than 25 (72%, $p = 0.02$), and were younger than 35 years old (76%, $p = 0.02$). The test of homogeneity showed significant differences only between mothers with or without a history of allergy ($p = 0.03$).

Compliance with at least three out of five recommendations was significantly associated with the introduction of the first food at 21 weeks of age or more, if mothers where not breastfeeding their infants at six months (63%, $p = 0.05$), did not have a family history of allergy (74%, $p = 0.01$), had a BMI (kg/m^2) of less than 25 (71%, $p = 0.02$), and if they had received information on infant feeding from a midwife (68%, $p = 0.03$).

The multivariate logistic regression analyses showed no significant associations between the outcomes and maternal characteristics, probably due to the small size of the sample. The results are reported in the Supplementary Materials section (Tables S2–S6).

4. Discussion

As already observed in other studies [20,22,29], the timing of the introduction of complementary foods tends to follow a standard pattern: the infant's diet includes only few categories of food and differs substantially from that of the family, with commercial baby foods taking up a considerable share. Our study shows that the feeding practices of this cohort follow the same pattern and fall short of the WHO recommendations on breast and complementary feeding. Seventy five percent of mothers adhered to three or more out of five WHO recommendations on adequate complementary feeding, but only 5% complied with all five. The lowest rate of compliance related to the recommendation to introduce complementary foods at six months or more, with 86% of infants receiving complementary foods before the age of six months. This percentage is higher than the one reported in a recent study in the Netherlands [14], but close to the data reported in a nutrition survey from the UK [30] and in a WHO multicenter study of comparable sample size conducted in different countries [31]. However, comparisons with other studies are difficult because most of them adopt a cut-off of 17 weeks of age for early introduction, as recommended by ESPGHAN [12].

Despite the evidence that, in terms of prevention of allergies, there is no benefit in delaying the introduction of potentially allergenic foods [15] and that, in fact, early contact with food can induce tolerance and desensitization [32], the mothers in our cohort deferred the introduction of tomatoes, eggs, fish, and nuts and seeds, to between 8 (fish) and 16 months of age (nuts and seeds), as shown in Figure 2. This may have contributed to the lack of "maximum dietary diversity" by 12 months observed in more than half of the infants in our cohort. Indeed, as noted in a recent national survey [33,34], in a developed country such as Italy, without nutritional deficiencies and with high availability of nutrients, the "maximum dietary diversity" index could, and should, be higher.

It has been shown that the process of food learning starts very early and that there is a period in which new foods are relatively easily accepted [35,36]. Because food preferences developed at an early age may have long-lasting influence [37], it would be desirable to expose infants to as many tastes as possible in the first year of life. In her study [38], Cashdan showed that infants introduced to solids unusually late maintain a reduced diet and food range throughout childhood, perhaps as a result of the contraction of the sensitive period.

The partial compliance with WHO recommendations observed in our cohort, has already been reported by others [22,29,39]. Considering that 98% of the mothers in our study declared they received information on complementary feeding from their paediatrician and that in 62% of the cases, this advice was followed, the role of health professionals seems to be crucial, despite the lack of a statistically significant association in our regression analyses.

One of the possible reasons for the lack of correct and consistent information on the timing and type of complementary feeding is that in Italy there are no specific national Ministry of Health guidelines incorporating the WHO recommendations. These are therefore unevenly acquired by health professionals and poorly transferred to parents.

To our knowledge, this is the first study to explore in detail timing of complementary feeding and compliance with WHO recommendations, and associated factors, in Italy. The study does, however, have a number of limitations. The main problem is the loss to follow up of enrolled mother-infant pairs between birth and 36 months of age (37%), which greatly reduced the availability of complete data and thus the power to detect significant associations by multivariate analyses. The second major limitation is the complexity of the food timetable which required regular updating over a long period of time with detailed information regarding newly introduced food types. Although this tool is designed to provide high quality data, in our case this was at the expense of the sample size, making it difficult to compare our results with those of other national surveys.

5. Conclusions

Our paper describes the partial compliance with WHO recommendations on complementary feeding, in northeast Italy. Most of the infants in our cohort were started on complementary foods before the age of six months. They shared a very similar diet, which was very different from the family diet and characterized by the delayed introduction of certain food types. Further research will be needed to clarify the association between compliance with recommendations and socio-economic variables, in order to identify vulnerable groups in the population, including migrant families.

Taken together, our results suggest that Italy would greatly benefit from national evidence-based guidelines on infant feeding to support the development of solid public health strategies. These guidelines should be free from commercial interests, consistently adhered to, and promoted by all health professionals, especially in the light of the considerable influence their advice seems to have on parental practices.

Supplementary Materials:
Table S1: Association between introduction of first foods after 21 weeks and compliance with WHO recommendations

both as stand-alone variables and as overall compliance with any three out of five and selected variables by bivariate logistic regression analysis ($n = 148$), Table S2: Association between introduction of first foods after 21 weeks and introduction of honey after 12 months adjusted by selected variables by multivariate logistic regression analysis ($n = 130$), Table S3: Association between introduction of first foods after 21 weeks and introduction of cow milk after 12 months adjusted by selected variables by multivariate logistic regression analysis ($n = 130$), Table S4: Association between introduction of first foods after 21 weeks and less consumption of baby food adjusted by selected variables by multivariate logistic regression analysis ($n = 130$), Table S5: Association between introduction of first foods after 21 weeks and minimum dietary diversity recommendation adjusted by selected variables by multivariate logistic regression analysis ($n = 130$), Table S6: Association between introduction of first foods after 21 weeks and compliance with three out of five WHO recommendations adjusted by selected variables by multivariate logistic regression analysis ($n = 130$).

Acknowledgments: The authors wish to thank the mothers who participated in the study. The study was funded by the Institute for Maternal and Child Health IRCCS Burlo Garofolo, Trieste, Italy, and was approved by its Ethics Committee (RC 32/06).

Author Contributions: A.C. designed and supervised the study, helped analyze and interpret the results, and revised the manuscript. P.P., C.C. and A.K. conducted the study, collected the data, constructed the database, helped analyze and interpret the results, and wrote the manuscript. L.M. was in charge of the statistical analysis and revised the manuscript. All authors read and approved the final manuscript.

References

1. World Health Organization. *Complementay Feeding: Report of the Global Consultation, and Summary of Guiding Principles for Complementary Feeding of the Breastfed Child*; WHO: Geneva, Switzerland, 2002.
2. Monteiro, P.O.A.; Victora, C.G. Rapid growth in infancy and childhood and obesity in later life—A systematic review. *Obes. Rev.* **2005**, *6*, 143–154. [CrossRef] [PubMed]
3. Reynolds, C.M.; Gray, C.; Li, M.; Segovia, S.A.; Vickers, M.H. Early Life Nutrition and Energy Balance Disorders in Offspring in Later Life. *Nutrients* **2015**, *7*, 8090–8111. [CrossRef] [PubMed]
4. Ersino, G.; Henry, C.J.; Zello, G.A. Suboptimal Feeding Practices and High Levels of Undernutrition Among Infants and Young Children in the Rural Communities of Halaba and Zeway, Ethiopia. *Food Nutr. Bull.* **2016**, *37*, 409–424. [CrossRef] [PubMed]
5. Saaka, M.; Wemakor, A.; Abizari, A.R.; Aryee, P. How well do WHO complementary feeding indicators relate to nutritional status of children aged 6–23 months in rural Northern Ghana? *BMC Public Health* **2015**, *15*, 1157. [CrossRef] [PubMed]
6. World Health Organization; The United Nations Children's Fund. *Global Strategy for Infant and Young Child Feeding*; WHO: Geneva, Switzerland, 2002.
7. Arenz, S.; Ruckerl, R.; Koletzko, B.; von Kries, R. Breast-feeding and childhood obesity—A systematic review. *Int. J. Obes. Relat. Metab. Disord.* **2004**, *28*, 1247–1256. [CrossRef] [PubMed]
8. Huh, S.Y.; Rifas-Shiman, S.L.; Taveras, E.M.; Oken, E.; Gillman, M.W. Timing of solid food introduction and risk of obesity in preschool-aged children. *Pediatrics* **2011**, *127*, 544–551. [CrossRef] [PubMed]
9. Pearce, J.; Taylor, M.A.; Langley-Evans, S.C. Timing of the introduction of complementary feeding and risk of childhood obesity: A systematic review. *Int. J. Obes. (Lond.)* **2013**, *37*, 1295–1306. [CrossRef] [PubMed]
10. De Beer, M.; Vrijkotte, T.G.; Fall, C.H.; van Eijsden, M.; Osmond, C.; Gemke, R.J. Associations of infant feeding and timing of linear growth and relative weight gain during early life with childhood body composition. *Int. J. Obes. (Lond.)* **2015**, *39*, 586–592. [CrossRef] [PubMed]
11. Della Salute, M. *Linee di Indirizzo Nazionali Sulla Protezione, la Promozione ed il Sostegno Dell'allattamento al Seno*; Gazzetta Ufficiale: Roma, Italy, 2008.
12. Agostoni, C.; Decsi, T.; Fewtrell, M.; Goulet, O.; Kolacek, S.; Koletzko, B.; Michaelsen, K.F.; Moreno, L.; Puntis, J.; Rigo, J.; et al. Complementary feeding: A commentary by the ESPGHAN Committee on Nutrition. *J. Pediatr. Gastroenterol. Nutr.* **2008**, *46*, 99–110. [CrossRef] [PubMed]
13. Cattaneo, A.; Williams, C.; Pallas-Alonso, C.R.; Hernandez-Aguilar, M.T.; Lasarte-Velillas, J.J.; Landa-Rivera, L.; Rouw, E.; Pina, M.; Volta, A.; Oudesluys-Murphy, A.M. ESPGHAN's 2008 recommendation for early introduction of complementary foods: How good is the evidence? *Matern. Child Nutr.* **2011**, *7*, 335–343. [CrossRef] [PubMed]
14. World Health Organization. *Exclusive Breastfeeding for Six Months Best for Babies Everywhere*; WHO: Geneva, Switzerland, 2011.

15. Michaelsen, K.F.; Weaver, L.; Branca, F.; Robertson, A. *Feeding and Nutrition of Infants and Young Children*, 87th ed.; WHO Regional Publications, European Series; WHO Regional Office for Europe: Copenhagen, Denmark, 2000.
16. World Health Organization. *Complementary Feeding: Family Foods for Breasfed Infants*; WHO: Geneva, Switzerland, 2000.
17. Scott, J.A.; Binns, C.W.; Graham, K.I.; Oddy, W.H. Predictors of the early introduction of solid foods in infants: Results of a cohort study. *BMC Pediatr.* **2009**, *9*, 60. [CrossRef] [PubMed]
18. Tromp, I.I.M.; Briede, S.; Kiefte-de Jong, J.C.; Renders, C.M.; Jaddoe, V.W.; Franco, O.H.; Hofman, A.; Raat, H.; Moll, H.A. Factors associated with the timing of introduction of complementary feeding: The Generation R Study. *Eur. J. Clin. Nutr.* **2013**, *67*, 625–630. [CrossRef] [PubMed]
19. Giovannini, M.; Riva, E.; Banderali, G.; Scaglioni, S.; Veehof, S.H.; Sala, M.; Radaelli, G.; Agostoni, C. Feeding practices of infants through the first year of life in Italy. *Acta Paediatr.* **2004**, *93*, 492–497. [PubMed]
20. Pani, P.; Carletti, C.; Knowles, A.; Parpinel, M.; Concina, F.; Montico, M.; Cattaneo, A. Patterns of nutrients' intake at six months in the northeast of Italy: A cohort study. *BMC Pediatr.* **2014**, *14*, 127. [CrossRef] [PubMed]
21. Carletti, C.; Pani, P.; Knowles, A.; Monasta, L.; Montico, M.; Cattaneo, A. Breastfeeding to 24 months of age in the northeast of Italy: A cohort study. *Breastfeed. Med.* **2011**, *6*, 177–182. [CrossRef] [PubMed]
22. Schiess, S.; Grote, V.; Scaglioni, S.; Luque, V.; Martin, F.; Stolarczyk, A.; Vecchi, F.; Koletzko, B.; European Childhood Obesity Project. Introduction of complementary feeding in 5 European countries. *J. Pediatr. Gastroenterol. Nutr.* **2010**, *50*, 92–98. [CrossRef] [PubMed]
23. Biro, G.; Hulshof, K.F.; Ovesen, L.; Amorim Cruz, J.A.; EFCOSUM Group. Selection of methodology to assess food intake. *Eur. J. Clin. Nutr.* **2002**, *56*, S25–S32. [CrossRef] [PubMed]
24. Buzzard, M. 24-Hour dietary recall and food record methods. In *Nutritional Epidemiology*, 2nd ed.; Willett, W., Ed.; Oxford University Press: Oxford, UK, 1998; pp. 50–73.
25. World Health Organization; The United Nations Children's Fund. Indicators for assessing infant and young child feeding practices. In Proceedings of the Conclusions of a Consensus Meeting, Washington, DC, USA, 6–8 November 2007; WHO: Geneva, Switzerland, 2008.
26. World Health Organization. *Guideline: Vitamin A Supplementation in Infants and Children 6–59 Months of Age*; WHO: Geneva, Switzerland, 2011.
27. Clayton, H.B.; Li, R.; Perrine, C.G.; Scanlon, K.S. Prevalence and reasons for introducing infants early to solid foods: Variations by milk feeding type. *Pediatrics* **2013**, *131*, 1108–1114. [CrossRef] [PubMed]
28. Baker, J.L.; Michaelsen, K.F.; Rasmussen, K.M.; Sørensen, T.I. Maternal prepregnant body mass index, duration of breastfeeding, and timing of complementary food introduction are associated with infant weight gain. *Am. J. Clin. Nutr.* **2004**, *80*, 1579–1588. [PubMed]
29. Dratva, J.; Merten, S.; Ackermann-Liebrich, U. The timing of complementary feeding of infants in Switzerland: Compliance with the Swiss and the WHO guidelines. *Acta Paediatr.* **2006**, *95*, 818–825. [CrossRef] [PubMed]
30. Lennox, A.; Sommerville, J.; Ong, K.; Handerson, H.; Allen, R. *Diet and Nutrition Survey of Infants and Young Children, 2011*; Department of Health and Food Standards Agency: London, UK, 2013.
31. WHO Multicenter Growth Reference Study Group. Complementary feeding in the WHO Multicenter Growth Reference Study. *Acta Paediatr.* **2006**, *450*, 27–37.
32. Longo, G.; Berti, I.; Burks, A.W.; Krauss, B.; Barbi, E. IgE-mediated food allergy in children. *Lancet* **2013**, *382*, 1656–1664. [CrossRef]
33. Leclercq, C.; Arcella, D.; Piccinelli, R.; Sette, S.; Le Donne, C.; Turrini, A.; INRAN-SCAI 2005-06 Study Group. The Italian National Food Consumption Survey INRAN-SCAI 2005-06: Main results in terms of food consumption. *Public Health Nutr.* **2009**, *12*, 2504–2532. [CrossRef] [PubMed]
34. Sette, S.; Le Donne, C.; Piccinelli, R.; Arcella, D.; Turrini, A.; Leclercq, C.; INRAN-SCAI 2005-6 Study Group. The third Italian National Food Consumption Survey, INRAN-SCAI 2005-06—Part 1: Nutrient intakes in Italy. *Nutr. Metab. Cardiovasc. Dis.* **2011**, *21*, 922–932. [CrossRef] [PubMed]
35. Lange, C.; Visalli, M.; Jacob, S.; Chabanet, C.; Schlich, P.; Nicklaus, S. Maternal feeding practices during the first year and their impact on infants' acceptance of complementary food. *Food Qual. Prefer.* **2013**, *29*, 89–98. [CrossRef]
36. Schwartz, C.; Scholtens, P.A.; Lalanne, A.; Weenen, H.; Nicklaus, S. Development of healthy eating habits early in life. Review of recent evidence and selected guidelines. *Appetite* **2011**, *57*, 796–807. [PubMed]

37. Nicklaus, S.; Remy, E. Early origins of overeating: Tracking between early food habits and later eating patterns. *Curr. Obes. Rep.* **2013**, *2*, 179–184. [CrossRef]
38. Cashdan, E. A sensitive period for learning about food. *Hum. Nat.* **1994**, *5*, 279–291. [CrossRef] [PubMed]
39. O'Donovan, S.M.; Murray, D.M.; Hourihane, J.O.; Kenny, L.C.; Irvine, A.D.; Kiely, M. Adherence with early infant feeding and complementary feeding guidelines in the Cork BASELINE Birth Cohort Study. *Public Health Nutr.* **2015**, *18*, 2864–2873. [CrossRef] [PubMed]

13

The Effect of Gestational and Lactational Age on the Human Milk Metabolome

Ulrik K. Sundekilde [1,*], Eimear Downey [2], James A. O'Mahony [2], Carol-Anne O'Shea [3], C. Anthony Ryan [3], Alan L. Kelly [2] and Hanne C. Bertram [1]

1 Department of Food Science, Aarhus University, Årslev 5792, Denmark; hannec.bertram@food.au.dk
2 School of Food and Nutritional Sciences, University College Cork, Cork T12 YN60, Ireland; eimeardowney@gmail.com (E.D.); sa.omahony@ucc.ie (J.A.M.); a.kelly@ucc.ie (A.L.K.)
3 Department of Paediatrics and Child Health, University College Cork, Cork T12 YN60, Ireland; Ca.OShea@ucc.ie (C.A.S.); tony.ryan@ucc.ie (C.A.R.)
* Correspondence: uksundekilde@food.au.dk

Abstract: Human milk is the ideal nutrition source for healthy infants during the first six months of life and a detailed characterisation of the composition of milk from mothers that deliver prematurely (<37 weeks gestation), and of how human milk changes during lactation, would benefit our understanding of the nutritional requirements of premature infants. Individual milk samples from mothers delivering prematurely and at term were collected. The human milk metabolome, established by nuclear magnetic resonance (NMR) spectroscopy, was influenced by gestational and lactation age. Metabolite profiling identified that levels of valine, leucine, betaine, and creatinine were increased in colostrum from term mothers compared with mature milk, while those of glutamate, caprylate, and caprate were increased in mature term milk compared with colostrum. Levels of oligosaccharides, citrate, and creatinine were increased in pre-term colostrum, while those of caprylate, caprate, valine, leucine, glutamate, and pantothenate increased with time postpartum. There were differences between pre-term and full-term milk in the levels of carnitine, caprylate, caprate, pantothenate, urea, lactose, oligosaccharides, citrate, phosphocholine, choline, and formate. These findings suggest that the metabolome of pre-term milk changes within 5–7 weeks postpartum to resemble that of term milk, independent of time of gestation at pre-mature delivery.

Keywords: pre-term; infant; nutrition; human milk; metabolites; NMR; metabolomics

---

1. Introduction

Human milk (HM) is the recognised gold standard for feeding new-born full-term healthy infants. HM is a unique food source that contains all the exacting amounts of required nutrients to support the growth and development of term infants during the first six months of life. The health benefits of HM have been well documented [1]. Current data suggest that the quantity of HM consumed by healthy term infants is on average 0.778 kg human milk/day, with males consuming 0.056 kg/day more than females. Human milk consumption rises rapidly during the first month postpartum to ~0.6 kg/day and increases to ~0.82 kg/day in 3–4 month old infants [2].

Human milk is also regarded as particularly important for feeding pre-mature infants. There are many health benefits related to providing a pre-term infant with HM, including improvements in digestion, nutrient absorption, gastrointestinal function, and neurodevelopment of the infant [3,4]. In addition, an exclusive HM diet has been associated with lower rates of necrotizing enterocolitis, a potentially fatal gastrointestinal complication, in premature infants [5]. Human milk oligosaccharides (HMO) are known to affect the gut microbiota and it has been speculated that HMOs could account for the lower observed incidences of necrotizing enterocolitis [6].

Mother's milk is inadequate for rapidly growing pre-term neonates, which can be ascribed to a higher protein and energy requirement of pre-term neonates, particularly those of low birth weight and <28 weeks gestation, leading to insufficient weight gain and nutrition deficits [7,8]. For extremely pre-term and very low birth weight infants, the fortification of HM using commercial fortifiers is often recommended in order to supply the neonate with the nutrients required to support its rapid rate of growth. Studies have shown that the addition of HM fortifier can improve weight, length, and head circumference growth, in addition to bone mineralization and neurological outcomes [9–13].

It is known that the composition of pre-term milk differs from that of milk of full-term mothers, with higher reported levels of total protein, fat, carbohydrate and energy in pre-term milk [14]. Differences in the proteome of the two types of milk have also been reported [15]. Generally, studies have focused on the macronutrient content of pre-term and term HM without consideration of micronutrients such as biologically significant metabolites [14].

Previous work on milk metabolomes has predominantly considered bovine milk [16–20] and human milk [21–28]. Recently, a multi-analytical platform study identified 710 metabolites in human milk by using a combination of MS- and NMR-based analytical techniques [21]. Moreover, a recent study identified subtle differences between some milk metabolites during the first month of lactation [27]. However, the changes in pre-term and full-term human milk metabolomes over a full lactation time course have not yet been reported in detail.

In this study, we report how gestational age affects the low-molecular-weight metabolome of HM from mothers of pre-term and term infants over range of stages of lactation. The milk metabolomes were compared using proton nuclear magnetic resonance spectroscopy (^{1}H NMR)-based metabolomics from milk samples from mothers at different gestational ages. Longitudinal samples were also examined to analyse how pre-term milk develops with time postpartum compared with term milk.

2. Materials and Methods

2.1. Ethical Approval

Ethical approval for this study was granted by The Clinical Research Ethics Committee of the Cork Teaching Hospitals, Cork, Ireland (clinical number reference ECM 4(s) 06/08/13).

2.2. Samples and Sample Collection

2.2.1. Pre-term Samples

Multiple frozen (−20 °C) longitudinal pre-term HM samples were collected from 15 individual mothers of pre-term infants (Table 1). The HM samples were collected from the freezers of the neonatal intensive care unit of Cork University Maternity Hospital (Wilton, Co. Cork, Ireland). Each bottle of HM was dated allowing for an accurate calculation of the gestational age of the infant when the milk was expressed. The HM samples from each individual mother were pooled according to 'day postpartum' up to 14 days and according to 'week postpartum' after this, creating n = 62 pre-term HM samples. For one donor (Pre-1), information on number of days postpartum was unavailable and accordingly samples from this donor were removed from multivariate models using gestational age or days postpartum for modelling or visualization purposes.

2.2.2. Full-term Samples

Frozen (−20 °C) HM samples (n = 30) were obtained from The Western Trust Milk Bank, Irvinestown, Co. Fermanagh, Ireland (Table 2). The HM samples were from 30 individual mothers of healthy full-term infants who donated milk with consent for use for research purposes. The mothers expressed milk in a domestic setting and stored milk at −20 °C before shipping to The Western Trust Milk Bank, Ireland. HM was pasteurised and microbiologically screened before being frozen and shipped to University College Cork where it was stored at −20 °C. Milk samples were categorized according to the length of time postpartum; colostrum (<5 days postpartum; n = 5), transitional (6 days–2 weeks postpartum; n = 4), mature (>2 weeks, n = 21).

Table 1. Sample information from mothers of pre-term infants.

Sample Id	Secretor Status	Gestation	Infant Weight, Grams	Age of Mother, Years	Gravida [1]	Para [2]	Number of Samples	Postpartum Span [3]
Pre 01	Se^+	–	–	–	–	–	4	–
Pre 02	Se^+	38 weeks	3210	35	2	2	4	7–11 weeks
Pre 03	Se^+	28 weeks	1190	33	1	1	9	4–12 days
Pre 04	Se^+	31 weeks	1830	36	3	3	5	1–5 weeks
Pre 05	Se^+	30 weeks	1340	29	1	1	7	4 days–7 weeks
Pre 06	Se^+	32 weeks + 2 days	2340	42	2	2	1	8 days
Pre 07	Se^-	24 weeks + 4 days	540	33	1	1	4	1–4 days
Pre 08	Se^-	31 weeks	1680	35	2	2	2	5–14 weeks
Pre 09	Se^+	35 weeks + 6 days	2410	33	1	1	3	2–5 weeks
Pre 10	Se^+	35 weeks + 2 days	3100	26	1	1	2	4–5 days
Pre 11	Se^+	33 weeks + 4 days	1800	29	6	5	2	4–6 days
Pre 12	Se^+	35 weeks + 4 days	3260	45	4	3 + 2 [4]	2	9–10 days
Pre 13	Se^+	26 weeks	650	40	–	–	15	6 days–8 weeks
Pre 14	Se^-	28 weeks + 3 days	–	–	–	–	1	13 weeks
Pre 15	Se^+	32 weeks	–	–	–	–	1	9 weeks

[1] Number of pregnancies, including the current pregnancy; [2] number of times the mother has given birth; [3] time range indicates days postpartum of first and last samples from that donor; [4] indicates twin pregnancy.

2.3. NMR Spectroscopy

NMR spectroscopy was essentially performed as described earlier [29]. Briefly, the samples skimmed by centrifugation at 4000 g for 15 min and removal of the top fat layer before filtering to remove residual lipids and protein using Amicon Ultra 0.5 mL 10 kDa (Millipore, Billerica, MA, USA) spin filters at 10,000 g for 30 min at 4 °C. A filtered sample (500 μL) was mixed with 100 μL D_2O containing 0.025% 3-(trimethylsilyl) propionic-2,2,3,3-d_4 acid, sodium salt (TSP; Sigma-Aldrich, St. Louis, MO, USA) as an internal chemical shift reference. ^{1}H NMR spectroscopy was performed at 298 K on a Bruker Avance III 600 spectrometer, operating at a ^{1}H frequency of 600.13 MHz, and equipped with a 5-mm ^{1}H TXI probe (Bruker BioSpin, Rheinstetten, Germany). The sample sequence was randomized prior to acquisition and standard one-dimensional spectra were acquired using a single 90° pulse experiment with a relaxation delay of 5 s. Water suppression was achieved by irradiating the water peak during the relaxation delay, and a total of 64 scans were collected into 32,768 data points spanning a spectral width of 12.15 ppm. All ^{1}H spectra were initially referenced to the TSP signal at 0 ppm. Prior to Fourier transformation, the data were multiplied by a 0.3 Hz line-broadening function. The proton NMR spectra were phase and baseline corrected manually using Topspin 3.2 (Bruker Biospin, Rheinstetten, Germany). NMR signals were assigned in accordance with existing literature [20,21,25,29], 2D NMR spectroscopy, Chenomx NMR Suite 8.1.2 (Chenomx Inc, Edmonton, AB, Canada) and the Human Metabolome Database [30].

Table 2. Sample information from mothers of term infants.

Sample ID	Secretor status	Time postpartum	Group
Term 01	Se^+	<5 days	Colostrum
Term 02	Se^+	<5 days	Colostrum
Term 03	Se^+	<5 days	Colostrum
Term 04	Se^+	<5 days	Colostrum
Term 05	Se^+	<5 days	Colostrum
Term 06	Se^+	2 weeks	Transitional
Term 07	Se^+	2 weeks	Transitional
Term 08	Se^-	6 days	Transitional
Term 09	Se^-	2 weeks	Transitional
Term 10	Se^-	15 weeks	Mature
Term 11	Se^-	9 weeks	Mature
Term 12	Se^+	15 weeks	Mature
Term 13	Se^-	11 weeks	Mature
Term 14	Se^-	15 weeks	Mature
Term 15	Se^-	11 weeks	Mature
Term 16	Se^+	16 weeks	Mature
Term 17	Se^-	9 weeks	Mature
Term 18	Se^+	19 weeks	Mature
Term 19	Se^+	24 weeks	Mature
Term 20	Se^+	11 weeks	Mature
Term 21	Se^+	7–10 weeks	Mature
Term 22	Se^+	13 weeks	Mature
Term 23	Se^+	13 weeks	Mature
Term 24	Se^+	14 weeks	Mature
Term 25	Se^+	5 weeks	Mature
Term 26	Se^+	27 weeks	Mature
Term 27	Se^-	33 weeks	Mature
Term 28	Se^-	27 weeks	Mature
Term 29	Se^+	29 weeks	Mature
Term 30	Se^+	33 weeks	Mature

2.4. Secretor Status

Maternal secretor status was determined as previously described [25]. In brief the absence or presence of 2-FL was used to determine secretor status quantified by NMR spectroscopy (2-FL corresponds to NMR signal at δ 5.32 ppm). Milk from mothers classified as non-secretors did not have any detectable levels of 2-FL, whereas milk from mothers classified as secretors did contain 2-FL.

2.5. Multivariate Data and Statistical Analyses

NMR spectra of milk samples were aligned using Icoshift by co-shifting of the whole spectra according to the anomeric lactose proton at 5.23 ppm [31]. The proton NMR spectra were subdivided into 0.01 ppm bins, reducing each spectrum into 957 separate variables in the regions 10.00–5.00 and 4.72–0.5 ppm. Principal component analysis (PCA) and orthogonal partial least squares discriminant analysis (OPLS-DA) were performed in order to identify differences in the metabolite profiles. The data was mean-centred and Pareto-scaled prior to analysis. The OPLS-DA model was cross-validated using segmentation with seven splits. Covariance was investigated by analysis of OPLS-DA regression coefficients back-transformed to original data and colour coded by the loading weights [32]. The multivariate data analysis was performed using SIMCA-P + 13 (Umetrics AB, Umeå, Sweden). Alignment by Icoshift, binning, and analysis of OPLS-DA plots were performed in MATLAB 7.13 using in-house developed scripts (MathWorks Inc., Natick, MA, USA). Univariate statistical significance was evaluated by Student's *t*-test using the Statistics Toolbox in MATLAB 7.13 (MathWorks Inc., Natick, MA, USA).

3. Results

HM samples ($n = 92$) were collected from 45 individual mothers with different gestational ages at delivery, ranging from 24.6–35.8 weeks in the case of pre-term samples and more than 37 weeks for full-term samples (Tables 1 and 2). For pre-mature deliveries, infant birth weight ranged from 540 g to 3260 g. Age of the mothers of pre-term infants ranged from 26–45 years, and all had at least one previous pregnancy longer than 24 weeks gestation (Table 1).

The median spectrum of all 92 milk samples is shown in Figure 1. Each signal corresponds to proton resonances in milk metabolites according to assignments in Table 3. Differences in fucosylated human milk oligosaccharides (HMO) have previously been described to depend on maternal secretor status [33]. Accordingly, secretor status of the mothers was determined by examining the specific patterns of fucosylated oligosaccharides (Figure 1B) [25]. Thirteen mothers were found to be non-secretors, accounting for 28.9% of the mothers included in the study (Tables 1 and 2).

The collected milk samples were analysed for changes during lactation following both full-term (Figure 2) and pre-term (Figure 3) delivery. Figure 2 shows a scores plot of principal component (PC) 2 and PC3 from a principal component analysis (PCA) model of full-term milk samples. The samples are grouped into colostrum, transitional, and mature groups and coloured according to days postpartum. The scores plot shows the distinct groupings of the milk samples, and indicates a gradual change in the milk metabolome as the milk develops from colostrum towards mature milk (Figure 2). In addition, no detectable differences were observed between mature milk samples in the intervals before 26 weeks and after 26 weeks (Figure 2). There was an apparent difference in milk metabolites depending on secretor status in term milk samples, as the milk samples were separated into secretor or non-secretor groups along PC2 (Figure 2).

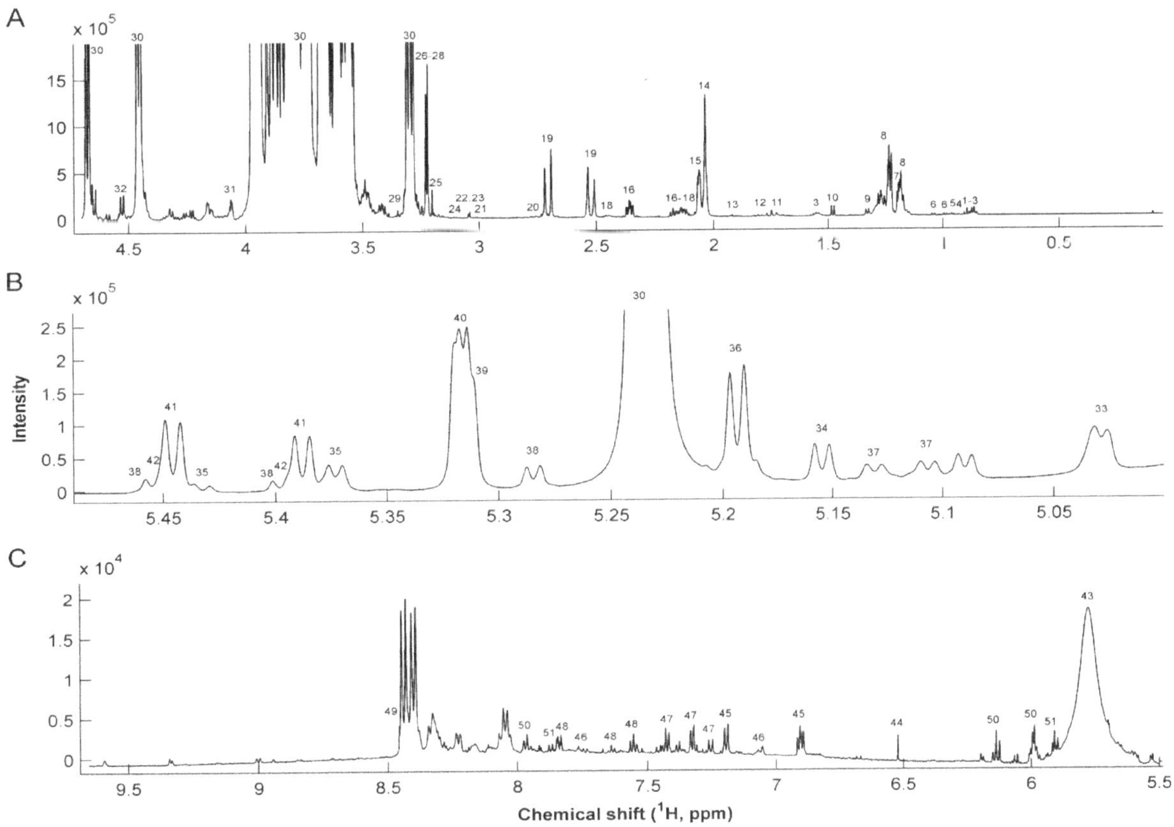

Figure 1. Median ^{1}H NMR spectrum of 92 human milk samples. (**A**) Aliphatic region 4.6–0 ppm (**B**) Human milk oligosaccharides in 5.45–5.00 ppm region; and (**C**) aromatic region 9.7–5.5 ppm region. For peak assignments refer to Table 3.

Table 3. List of metabolites in human milk with chemical shifts in ppm from internal TSP standard and assignment of resonances.

#	Metabolite	¹H Chemical shift (ppm)	Assignment	#	Metabolite	¹H Chemical shift (ppm)	Assignment
1	Caprylate	0.85	CH_3	29	Methanol	3.37	CH_3
		1.53	CH_2	30	Lactose	3.23, 3.5–4.0	Multiple
2	Caprate	0.85	CH_3	31	Gluconate	4.05	CH
		1.53	CH_2	32	Galactose	4.57	CH
3	Butyrate	0.88	CH_3	33	Fuc α1,4 GlcNAc	5.03	CH-1
		1.55	β-CH_2	34	Fuc α1,3 GlcNAc	5.19	CH-1
		2.16	α-CH_2	35	LNDFH II	5.03	Fuc (α1-4) CH-1
4	Pantothenate	0.91	CH_3			5.38	Fuc (α1-3) αGlc CH-1
5	Leucine	0.94	CH_3			5.43	Fuc (α1-3) βGlc CH-1
6	Valine	0.98	γ-CH_3	36	LNDFH I	5.16	Fuc (α1-2) CH-1
		1.03	γ′-CH_3			5.03	Fuc (α1-4) CH-1
7	3-BHBA	1.18	CH_3	37	LNFP III	5.11	Fuc (α1-3) GlcNAc CH-1
		2.39	CH_2			5.13	Fuc (α1-3) GlcNAc CH-1
8	Fucosyl moieties	1.19	CH_3-6	38	LDFT	5.29	Fuc (α1-2) CH-1
		1.23–1.29	CH_3-6			5.4	Fuc (α1-3) αGlc CH-1
9	Lactate	1.32	CH_3			5.46	Fuc (α1-3) βGlc CH-1
10	Alanine	1.47	CH_3	39	LNFP I	5.32	Fuc (α1-2) CH-1
11	6′-SL	1.73	CH_3	40	2′FL	5.32	Fuc (α1-2) CH-1
12	3′-SL	1.78	CH_3	41	3′FL	5.39	Fuc (α1-3) αGlc CH-1
13	Acetate	1.91	CH_3			5.44	Fuc (α1-3) βGlc CH-1
14	GlcNAc	2.04	CH_3	42	LNFP V	5.39	Fuc(α1-3)αGlc CH-1
15	Sialic acid	2.06	CH_3			5.44	Fuc (α1-3) βGlc CH-1
16	Glutamate	2.12	β-CH_2	43	Urea	5.76	NH_2
		2.33	γ-CH_2	44	Fumarate	6.51	CH = CH
17	Methionine	2.13	CH_3	45	Tyrosine	6.9	CH-3,5
18	Glutamine	2.11	β-CH_2			7.2	CH-2,6
		2.46	γ-CH_2	46	Methylhistidine	7.06	CH-4
19	Citrate	2.51	α-CH_2			7.8	CH-2
		2.69	α′-CH_2	47	Phenylalanine	7.32	CH-2,6
20	Dimethylamine	2.72	2 CH_3			7.37	CH-4
21	2-oxogluturate	2.99	CH_2			7.42	CH-3,5
22	Creatinine	3.02	CH_3	48	Hippurate	7.54	CH-2,6
23	Creatine	3.03	CH_3			7.63	CH-4
24	Malonate	3.12	CH_2			7.82	CH-3,5
25	Choline	3.19	3 CH_3	49	Formate	8.44	CH
26	O-Phosphocholine	3.21	3 CH_3	50	Cytidine triphosphate	5.99	CH-2
		4.16	CH_2			6.13	CH-10
27	Carnitine	2.42	CH_2			7.97	CH-11
		3.21	3 CH_3	51	Uridine	5.89	CH-2
28	Betaine	3.24	3 CH_3			5.91	CH-10
						7.87	CH-11

Abbreviations: 3-BHBA, 3-betahydroxybutyrate; FL, fucosyllactose; Fuc, Fucose; GlcNAc, *N*-acetylglucosamine; LDFT, lactodifucotetraose; LNDFH, lacto-*N*-difucohexaose, LNFP, lacto-*N*-fucopentaose; SL, sialyllactose.

Several milk metabolites were found to be present in significantly different concentration in colostrum, transitional, and mature milk. Fucosylated oligosaccharides, and also components of oligosaccharides (Fucose, *N*-acetylneuraminic acid, *N*-acetylglucosamine), were found at the highest levels in colostrum, and levels decreased in mature milk samples (Figure 2B). Moreover, levels of valine, leucine, pantothenate, citric acid, lactic acid, betaine, and creatinine were higher in colostrum and transitional milk compared with mature HM, and levels of glutamate, butyrate, caprylate, and caprate were higher in mature HM compared with colostrum and transitional milk. The level of β-hydroxybutyrate was found to be independent of milk maturity in full-term HM (Figure 2B). Milk from non-secretor mothers did not contain oligosaccharides with α1-2 fucosylated structures (Figure 2B); however, the level of 3′ fucosyllactose (3′-FL) was increased in non-secretor mothers compared with secretor mothers.

Similarly, the pre-term milk samples were also examined for an effect of stage of lactation on the milk metabolome. The scores plot of a two component PCA model of milk samples from pre-term mothers is shown in Figure 3, in which samples are coloured according to number of days postpartum. The scores and loadings plots clearly show the changes in milk metabolome occurring over time in pre-term milk. Levels of fucosyl moieties, *N*-acetylneuraminic acid, *N*-acetylglucosamine, 3′-sialyllactose, 6′-sialyllactose, 2′-fucosyllactose, citric acid, choline, and creatinine decreased with time postpartum (Figure 3B), while levels of 3-FL, lacto-*N*-difucohexaose I (LNDFH I), butyrate, caprylate, caprate, lactic acid, valine, leucine, alanine, glutamate, and pantothenate increased with time postpartum (Figure 3B). Only two mothers, who donated seven milk samples in total, were identified as non-secretors (Table 1). Thus, it was not possible to identify differences in the PCA model for pre-term samples on the basis of secretor status.

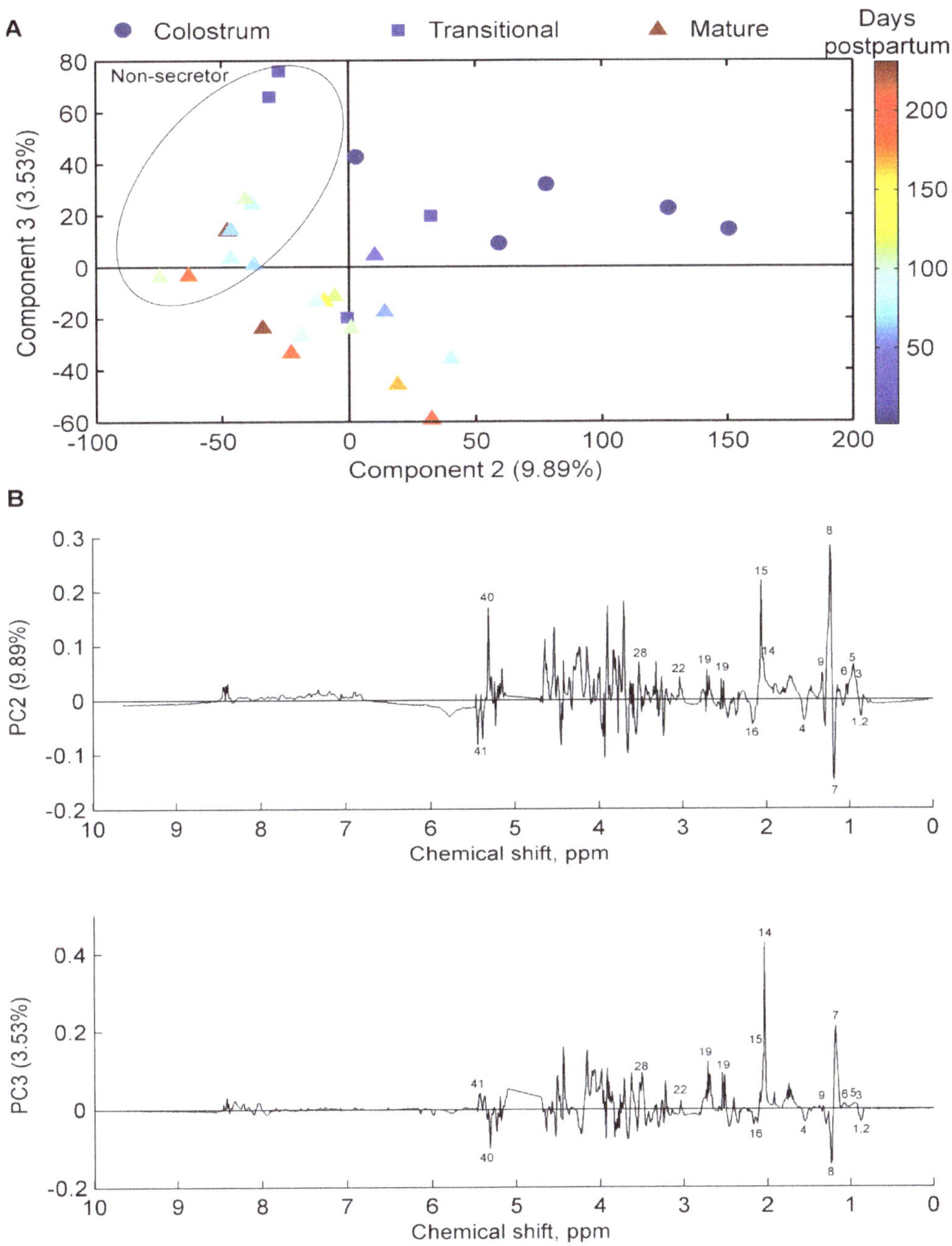

Figure 2. (**A**) Principal component analysis scores plot of full-term milk samples from 30 mothers (n = 30)); samples are coloured according to days postpartum; Colostrum (dots), transitional (squares), and mature (triangles); the circle denotes samples from non-secretor mothers, while remaining samples are from secretor mothers; and (**B**) corresponding loading line plots. For peak assignments refer to Table 3.

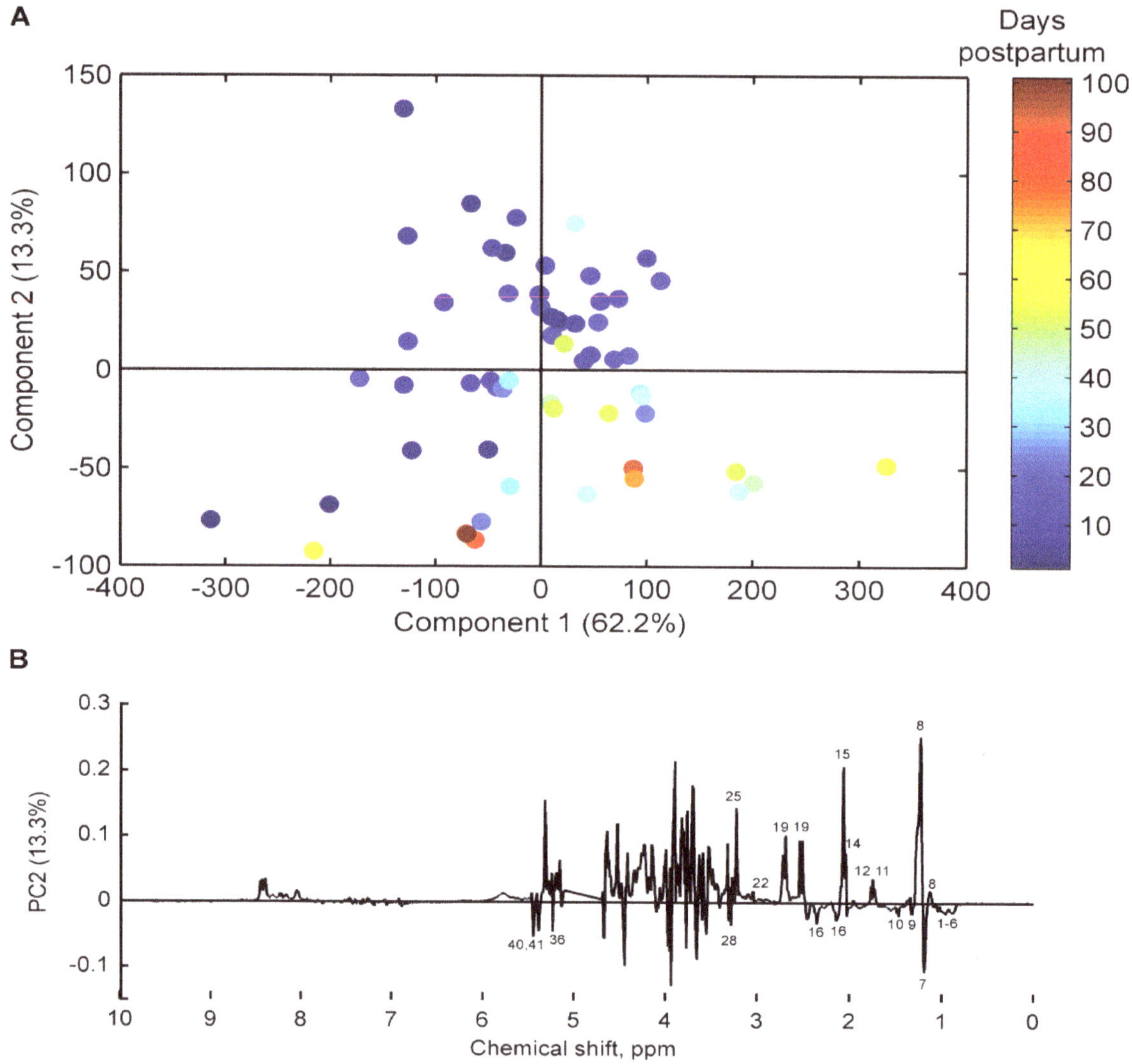

Figure 3. (**A**) Principal component analysis scores plot of pre-term milk samples from 15 mothers (n = 58), coloured according to number of days postpartum; and (**B**) corresponding loading line plot. For peak assignments refer to Table 3.

As some of the same time-related changes were apparent in both pre-term and full-term milk samples, the difference between the pre-term and full-term milk metabolomes of similar days postpartum was investigated. Citrate (P = 0.00057), lactose (P = 0.0039), and phosphocholine (P = 0.049 were found to be present in significantly higher levels in pre-term milk samples compared with full-term milk samples (Figure 4). Citrate level is known to decrease with time postpartum [28], while lactose is the major milk metabolite identified by NMR spectroscopy [20].

Thus, in the following analysis, NMR resonances originating from lactose were removed in order to increase the weight of other metabolites in the multivariate models. A PCA of pre-term and full-term milk samples (n = 88) was generated using two principal components which, together, explained 80.8% of the total variance described by the PCA model (Figure 5). From the PCA model, it is apparent that the milk metabolite profile from mothers of pre-term infants older than 5–7 weeks resembles that of full-term milk, as they are positioned in close proximity to the full-term milk samples, independent of time of gestation at delivery (Figure 5).

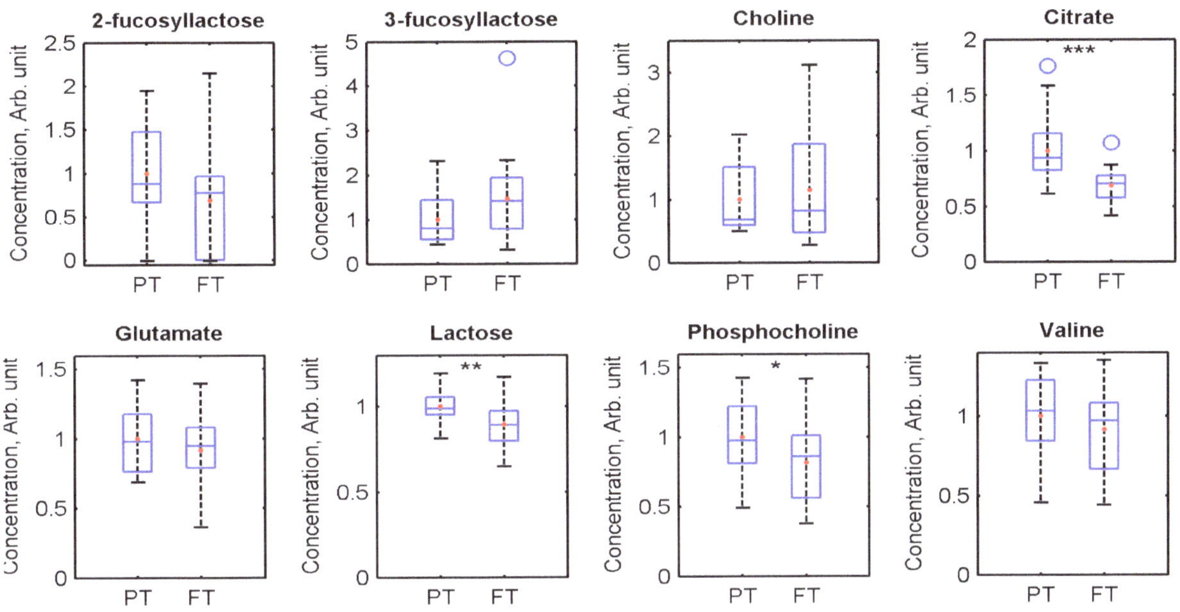

Figure 4. Box plots showing the distributions of 2-fucosyllactose, 3-fucosyllactose, choline, citrate, glutamate, lactose, phosphocholine, and valine concentrations in pre-term (PT) and full-term (FT) milk. Pre-term milk samples <14 days postpartum and full-term colostrum, transitional, and mature >26 weeks were excluded from the analysis in order to compare milk with a similar range of days postpartum. Horizontal lines indicate medians; coloured boxes specify interquartile ranges and dashed lines the ranges without outliers. The open circles indicate outliers (falls in-between 1.5× and 3× the interquartile range). *** = $P < 0.001$, ** = $P < 0.01$, * = $P < 0.05$; the comparisons were made using two-tailed Student's t-test.

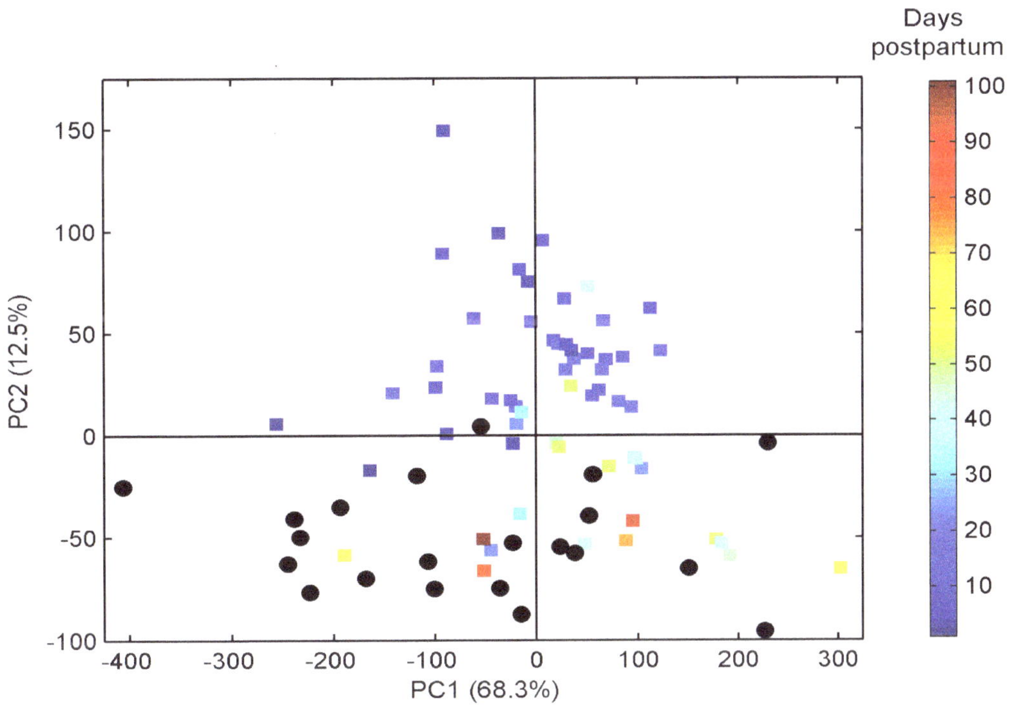

Figure 5. Principal component analysis scores plot of mature milk samples from pre-term (squares, $n = 58$) and full-term (circles, $n = 30$) mothers. Pre-term milk samples are coloured according to days postpartum.

OPLS-DA was also performed on the pre-term and full-term milk samples (Figure 6). Full-term and pre-term colostrum and transitional milk were excluded from the analysis, due to there being too few samples of these, and to be able to compare milk samples with similar days postpartum. The OPLS-DA model shows that significant differences exist between the metabolite profiles of pre-term and full-term milk (Figure 6B). In full-term milk, carnitine, caprylate, caprate, pantothenate, beta-hydroxybutyrate, and urea were found to be present in higher levels compared with pre-term milk, while lactose (Figure 4), Fucosyl moieties, *N*-acetylneuraminic acid, *N*-acetylglucosamine, 3′-sialyllactose, 6′-sialyllactose, lacto-*N*-difucohexaose I (LNDFH I), glutamate, citric acid, phosphocholine, choline, and formic acid were found in higher levels in pre-term milk (Figure 6).

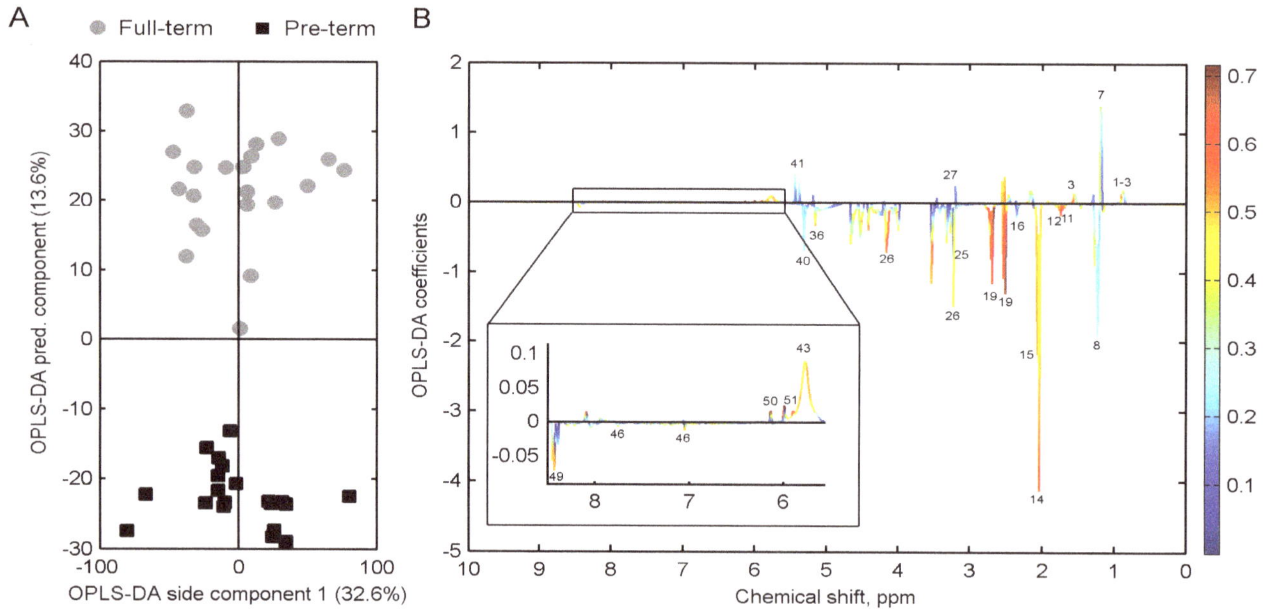

Figure 6. (**A**) Orthogonal partial least squares discriminant analysis of pre-term (n = 20, days postpartum range 3–14 weeks) and full-term (n = 21, days postpartum range 3–26 weeks) milk. Full-term colostrum, transitional, and pre-term milk <2 weeks postpartum have been excluded. Cross-validation, Q2: 0.70; (**B**) corresponding OPLS-DA coefficients plot. Each variable has been coloured according to the OPLS-DA loadings (correlation between NMR variables and pre-term/ full-term classes); for peak assignments refer to Table 3.

4. Discussion

Pre-mature birth is considered to have long-lasting adverse effects on health, and it has been proposed that the introduction of metabolomics technologies may facilitate better understanding of these effects [34]. The exact causes of preterm delivery are not clear, but often associated with inflammation [35]. In the present study, causes of the preterm delivery were not known. In this study, differences in metabolomic profiles of HM were associated with gestational age. Previous studies have shown many health benefits of breast-feeding pre-term infants. However, mother's milk may not always be adequate for pre-term infants with high nutrition density requirements, which can lead to insufficient weight gain and nutrition deficits. To date, only a few metabolomics studies have been performed on pre-term human milk in the first few weeks of lactation [27]. To our knowledge, this is the first study to comprehensively characterize and compare the pre-term and full-term human milk metabolome over a lactation time-course (up to 14 weeks postpartum). Milk metabolomics may be used in a clinical setting [23], in order to establish the milk metabolome for infant nutrition in cases where the optimal nutrition is a key advantage as in pre-term infants. Milk metabolomics studies in cows' milk have previously shown an ability to yield information about the health status of the cow [29,36]. It can likewise be hypothesized that the milk metabolome of lactating mothers can give information that can be used in a clinical setting.

Previous studies have shown that several factors influence the variability in the milk metabolome. The epithelial cells in the mammary gland are accountable for the milk production, and these cells are ultimately responsible for converting most precursors into milk components, but many other cell types are also involved in milk production [37]. Development of the mammary epithelial cells during pregnancy has been shown to influence transport pathways in the mammary gland responsible for different protein profiles of milk [38]. Moreover, insulin has been shown to be actively transported into milk and maternal diabetes affect milk insulin levels [39]. Maternal factors such as diet, lifestyle and phenotype have been shown to influence the milk composition [26]. Moreover, secretor status is also important for the biosynthesis of milk oligosaccharides [26]. The presence of α1,2 fucosyltransferase gene (FUT2) is important for the milk oligosaccharides since non-secretors, which lack the FUT2 gene, are unable to biosynthesize HMOs with a fucose bound to a *N*-acetylglucosamine via a glycosidic α1,2 linkage. Non-secretor status occurs in approximately 20% of most human populations [40,41]. In the present study, non-secretor status, identified by increased level of 3-FL, was found in 28.9 % of milk donors. Gestational age and the stage of lactation are also known to influence the milk proteins [14], lipids [42], and lactose [43]. Preliminary HM metabolomic studies have shown a difference between the metabolite profiles of pre-term and full-term HM [22,24]. Additionally, the metabolite extraction procedure in sample preparation prior to NMR spectroscopy has shown to influence the milk metabolite levels. In a recent paper, a sample preparation method using ultrafiltration as employed in the present study, was found to be superior compared with methanol/chloroform extraction in terms of separating small molecules from proteins and lipids [28]. Levels of HMO and its components are known to decrease with time [44]. A specific HMO, lacto-*N*-tetraose, has also been shown to be elevated in pre-term milk [45]. Interestingly, specific HMOs, LNDFH I, 3′-sialyllactose, and 6′-sialyllactose, and common components of HMO, including fucose, *N*-acetylglucosamine, and *N*-acetylneuraminic acid were identified to be present in higher concentrations in pre-term milk. HMOs have previously been shown to prevent necrotizing enterocolitis in neonatal rats [6], which may be linked to alterations in the microbiota of the infant's gut [46]. Thus, the elevated amounts of HMOs in pre-term milk may be a factor in the observed association of lower rates of necrotizing enterocolitis in premature infants fed HM [5].

Most of the free amino acids in HM steadily decrease in level as the milk matures [42]. However, the pre-term milk amino acid composition has not been well characterized throughout the course of lactation [47–49]. Glutamate is known to increase with lactation time [47] and this was also found in both pre-term and full-term milk in the present study. Valine and leucine, two essential amino acids, were found at the highest concentration in full-term colostrum and decreased with time postpartum, in agreement with other human milk metabolomics studies [27]. In contrast, increases in valine and leucine levels were observed in pre-term milk with time post-partum, which is in contrast to the pattern observed in full-term milk and that previously reported for pre-term milk [48,49].

Short- and medium-chain fatty acids (SMCFA; butyrate, caprylate, and caprate) were found in higher concentrations in full-term milk compared with pre-term milk. Moreover, the levels of SMCFA increased with time postpartum, as previously reported [50]. Choline is of high nutritional value, as it is abundant in cell membranes and acts as a precursor for the important messenger acetylcholine, and infants require high amounts of choline in order to sustain their rapid growth. Phosphocholine was found in higher levels in pre-term milk than in full-term milk, which is in agreement with previous reports on phosphocholine [51]. In contrast, pre-term milk has previously been shown to contain lesser amounts of choline [51], which is contradictory to findings in the present study.

In this study, it was shown that, after 5–7 weeks the metabolite profiles of pre-term milk resembled that of full-term milk, independently of gestational age. For extremely early pre-term infants born at a gestational age of, e.g., 24 weeks, these findings suggest that mother's milk becomes equivalent to mature milk for term infants by the time the infant reaches ~29 weeks post-menstrual age. This is a significant finding concerning a period in which the infant still requires advanced nutritional support to maintain its growth and long-term developmental requirements. Clinical metabolomics could potentially be advantageous to determine when milk metabolites levels become inadequate due to maturation of milk, if causal relationships between milk metabolites and infant growth parameters can be established. Previous studies have shown that protein concentration remains at higher levels in pre-term human milk even after 8 weeks of lactation [13]; however, we believe this to be the first study to document the changes in the metabolomics profile of pre-term human milk as it evolves to resemble that of full-term milk, and to show that this occurs independent of gestational age at delivery.

In conclusion, specific differences in milk metabolites exist between milk from mothers delivering pre-maturely and at term. Moreover, milk metabolite composition is associated with gestational age and the metabolome of pre-term milk changes within 5–7 weeks postpartum to resemble that of full-term milk, independent of time of gestation at delivery. However, as this study did not systematically collect samples from a cohort of mothers in a longitudinal design, further studies of this kind are recommended to more fully understand the significance of the changes reported herein.

Acknowledgments: The authors would like to acknowledge the Western Trust Milk Bank, Irvinestown, Co. Fermanagh, Ireland, the staff of the neonatal intensive care unit of Cork University Maternity Hospital and all of the mother and infants that kindly donated their milk. The authors are grateful for financial support from the Danish Research Council FTP through the project "Advances in Food quality and Nutrition Research through implementation of metabolomic strategies".

Author Contributions: All authors participated in the conception, design and writing of the manuscript. All authors read and approved the final manuscript.

Abbreviations

The following abbreviations are used in this manuscript:

HM	Human milk
HMO	Human milk oligosaccharide
NMR	Nuclear magnetic resonance

1. Wu, T.C.; Chen, P.H. Health consequences of nutrition in childhood and early infancy. *Pediatr. Neonatol.* **2009**, *50*, 135–142. [CrossRef]
2. Da Costa, T.H.M.; Haisma, H.; Wells, J.C.K.; Mander, A.P.; Whitehead, R.G.; Bluck, L.J.C. How much human milk do infants consume? Data from 12 countries using a standardized stable isotope methodology. *J. Nutr.* **2010**, *140*, 2227–2232. [PubMed]
3. Isaacs, E.B.; Morley, R.; Lucas, A. Early diet and general cognitive outcome at adolescence in children born at or below 30 weeks gestation. *J. Pediatr.* **2009**, *155*, 229–234. [CrossRef] [PubMed]
4. Lawrence, R.M. Breastfeeding, Host-resistance factors and immunologic significance of human milk. In *Breastfeeding. A guide for the medical profession*; Lawrence, R.A., Lawrence, R.M., Eds.; Elsevier: Philadelphia, PA, USA, 2006; pp. 171–214.
5. Sullivan, S.; Schanler, R.J.; Kim, J.H.; Patel, A.L.; Trawöger, R.; Kiechl-Kohlendorfer, U.; Chan, G.M.; Blanco, C.L.; Abrams, S.; Cotten, C.M.; *et al.* An exclusively human milk-based diet is associated with a lower rate of necrotizing enterocolitis than a diet of human milk and bovine milk-based products. *J. Pediatr.* **2010**, *156*, 562–567. [CrossRef] [PubMed]
6. Jantscher-Krenn, E.; Zherebtsov, M.; Nissan, C.; Goth, K.; Guner, Y.S.; Naidu, N.; Choudhury, B.; Grishin, A.V.; Ford, H.R.; Bode, L. The human milk oligosaccharide disialyllacto-*N*-tetraose prevents necrotising enterocolitis in neonatal rats. *Gut* **2012**, *61*, 1417–1425. [CrossRef] [PubMed]
7. Mikkola, K.; Ritari, N.; Tommiska, V.; Salokorpi, T.; Lehtonen, L.; Tammela, O.; Pääkkönen, L.; Olsen, P.; Korkman, M.; Fellman, V. Neurodevelopmental outcome at 5 years of age of a national cohort of extremely low birth weight infants who were born in 1996–1997. *Pediatrics* **2005**, *116*, 1391–1400. [CrossRef] [PubMed]

8. Sauer, P.J. Can extrauterine growth approximate intrauterine growth? Should it? *Am. J. Clin. Nutr.* **2007**, *85*, 608S–613S. [PubMed]
9. Faerk, J.; Petersen, S.; Peitersen, B.; Michaelsen, K.F. Diet and bone mineral content at term in premature infants. *Pediatr. Res.* **2000**, *47*, 148–156. [CrossRef] [PubMed]
10. Gross, S.J. Bone mineralization in preterm infants fed human milk with and without mineral supplementation. *J. Pediatr.* **1987**, *111*, 450–458. [CrossRef]
11. Martins, E.C.; Krebs, V.L.J. Effects of the use of fortified raw maternal milk on very low birth weight infants. *J. Pediatr.* **2009**, *85*, 157–162. [CrossRef]
12. Nicholl, R.M.; Gamsu, H.R. Changes in growth and metabolism in very low birthweight infants fed with fortified breast milk. *Acta. Paediatr.* **1999**, *88*, 1056–1061. [CrossRef] [PubMed]
13. Pettifor, J.M.; Rajah, R.; Venter, A.; Moodley, G.P.; Opperman, L.; Cavaleros, M.; Ross, F.P. Bone mineralization and mineral homeostasis in very low-birth-weight infants fed either human milk or fortified human milk. *J. Pediatr. Gastroenterol. Nutr.* **1989**, *8*, 217–224. [CrossRef] [PubMed]
14. Bauer, J.; Gerss, J. Longitudinal analysis of macronutrients and minerals in human milk produced by mothers of preterm infants. *Clin. Nutr.* **2011**, *30*, 215–220. [CrossRef] [PubMed]
15. Armaforte, E.; Curran, E.; Huppertz, T.; Ryan, C.A.; Caboni, M.F.; O'Connor, P.M.; Ross, R.P.; Hirtz, C.; Sommerer, N.; Chevalier, F.; *et al.* Proteins and proteolysis in pre-term and term human milk and possible implications for infant formulae. *Int. Dairy J.* **2010**, *20*, 715–723. [CrossRef]
16. Boudonck, K.J.; Mitchell, M.W.; Wulff, J.; Ryals, J.A. Characterization of the biochemical variability of bovine milk using metabolomics. *Metabolomics* **2009**, *5*, 375–386. [CrossRef]
17. Buitenhuis, A.J.; Sundekilde, U.K.; Poulsen, N.A.; Bertram, H.C.; Larsen, L.B.; Sørensen, P. Estimation of genetic parameters and detection of quantitative trait loci for metabolites in Danish Holstein milk. *J. Dairy Sci.* **2013**, *96*, 3285–3295. [CrossRef] [PubMed]
18. Klein, M.S.; Almstetter, M.F.; Schlamberger, G.; Nurnberger, N.; Dettmer, K.; Oefner, P.J.; Meyer, H.H.D.; Wiedemann, S.; Gronwald, W. Nuclear magnetic resonance and mass spectrometry-based milk metabolomics in dairy cows during early and late lactation. *J. Dairy Sci.* **2010**, *93*, 1539–1550. [CrossRef] [PubMed]
19. Maher, A.D.; Hayes, B.; Cocks, B.; Marett, L.; Wales, W.J.; Rochfort, S. Latent biochemical relationships in the blood-milk metabolic axis of dairy cows revealed by statistical integration of ^{1}H NMR spectroscopic data. *J. Proteome Res.* **2013**, *12*, 1428–1435. [CrossRef] [PubMed]
20. Sundekilde, U.K.; Larsen, L.B.; Bertram, H.C. NMR-Based Milk Metabolomics. *Metabolites* **2013**, *3*, 204–222. [PubMed]
21. Andreas, N.J.; Hyde, M.J.; Gomez-Romero, M.; Lopez-Gonzalvez, M.A.; Villaseñor, A.; Wijeyesekera, A.; Barbas, C.; Modi, N.; Holmes, E.; Garcia-Perez, I. Multiplatform characterization of dynamic changes in breast milk during lactation. *Electrophoresis* **2015**, *36*, 2269–2285. [CrossRef] [PubMed]
22. Longini, M.; Tataranno, M.L.; Proietti, F.; Tortoriello, M.; Belvisi, E.; Vivi, A.; Tassini, M.; Perrone, S.; Buonocore, G. A metabolomic study of preterm and term human and formula milk by proton MRS analysis: Preliminary results. *J. Matern. Neonatal Med.* **2014**, *27*, 27–33. [CrossRef] [PubMed]
23. Marincola, F.C.; Dessì, A.; Corbu, S.; Reali, A.; Fanos, V. Clinical impact of human breast milk metabolomics. *Clin. Chim. Acta.* **2015**, *451*, 103–106. [CrossRef] [PubMed]
24. Marincola, F.C.; Noto, A.; Caboni, P.; Reali, A.; Barberini, L.; Lussu, M.; Murgia, F.; Santoru, M.L.; Atzori, L.; Fanos, V. A metabolomic study of preterm human and formula milk by high resolution NMR and GC/MS analysis: Preliminary results. *J. Matern. Neonatal Med.* **2012**, *25*, 62–67. [CrossRef] [PubMed]
25. Praticò, G.; Capuani, G.; Tomassini, A.; Baldassarre, M.E.; Delfini, M.; Miccheli, A. Exploring human breast milk composition by NMR-based metabolomics. *Nat. Prod. Res.* **2014**, *28*, 95–101. [CrossRef] [PubMed]
26. Smilowitz, J.T.; O'Sullivan, A.; Barile, D.; German, J.B.; Lönnerdal, B.; Slupsky, C.M. The human milk metabolome reveals diverse oligosaccharide profiles. *J. Nutr.* **2013**, *143*, 1709–1718. [CrossRef] [PubMed]
27. Spevacek, A.R.; Smilowitz, J.T.; Chin, E.L.; Underwood, M.A.; German, J.B.; Slupsky, C.M. Infant maturity at birth reveals minor differences in the maternal milk metabolome in the first month of lactation. *J. Nutr.* **2015**, *145*, 1698–1708. [CrossRef] [PubMed]
28. Wu, J.; Domellöf, M.; Zivkovic, A.M.; Larsson, G.; Öhman, A.; Nording, M.L. NMR-based metabolite profiling of human milk: A pilot study of methods for investigating compositional changes during lactation. *Biochem. Biophys. Res. Commun.* **2015**, *469*, 626–632. [CrossRef] [PubMed]

29. Sundekilde, U.K.; Poulsen, N.A.; Larsen, L.B.; Bertram, H.C. Nuclear magnetic resonance metabonomics reveals strong association between milk metabolites and somatic cell count in bovine milk. *J. Dairy Sci.* **2013**, *96*, 290–299. [CrossRef] [PubMed]
30. Wishart, D.S.; Knox, C.; Guo, A.C.; Eisner, R.; Young, N.; Gautam, B.; Hau, D.D.; Psychogios, N.; Dong, E.; Bouatra, S.; *et al.* HMDB: A knowledgebase for the human metabolome. *Nucleic Acids Res.* **2009**, *37*, D603–D610. [CrossRef] [PubMed]
31. Savorani, F.; Tomasi, G.; Engelsen, S.B. icoshift: A versatile tool for the rapid alignment of 1D NMR spectra. *J. Magn. Reson.* **2010**, *202*, 190–202. [CrossRef] [PubMed]
32. Cloarec, O.; Dumas, M.E.; Trygg, J.; Craig, A.; Barton, R.H.; Lindon, J.C.; Nicholson, J.K.; Holmes, E. Evaluation of the orthogonal projection on latent structure model limitations caused by chemical shift variability and improved visualization of biomarker changes in ^{1}H NMR spectroscopic metabonomic studies. *Anal. Chem.* **2005**, *77*, 517–526. [CrossRef] [PubMed]
33. Thurl, S.; Munzert, M.; Henker, J.; Boehm, G.; Müller-Werner, B.; Jelinek, J.; Stahl, B. Variation of human milk oligosaccharides in relation to milk groups and lactational periods. *Br. J. Nutr.* **2010**, *104*, 1261–1271. [CrossRef] [PubMed]
34. Dessì, A.; Ottonello, G.; Fanos, V. Physiopathology of intrauterine growth retardation: From classic data to metabolomics. *J. Matern. Neonatal Med.* **2012**, *25* (Suppl. 5), 13–18. [CrossRef] [PubMed]
35. Palmas, F.; Fattuoni, C.; Noto, A.; Barberini, L.; Dessì, A.; Fanos, V. The choice of amniotic fluid in metabolomics for the monitoring of fetus health. *Expert Rev. Mol. Diagn.* **2016**, *7159*, 1–14. [CrossRef] [PubMed]
36. Klein, M.S.; Buttchereit, N.; Miemczyk, S.P.; Immervoll, A.K.; Louis, C.; Wiedemann, S.; Junge, W.; Thaller, G.; Oefner, P.J.; Gronwald, W. NMR metabolomic analysis of dairy cows reveals milk glycerophosphocholine to phosphocholine ratio as prognostic biomarker for risk of ketosis. *J. Proteome Res.* **2012**, *11*, 1373–1381. [CrossRef] [PubMed]
37. McManaman, J.L.; Neville, M.C. Mammary physiology and milk secretion. *Adv. Drug Deliv. Rev.* **2003**, *55*, 629–641. [CrossRef]
38. Molinari, C.E.; Casadio, Y.S.; Hartmann, B.T.; Livk, A.; Bringans, S.; Arthur, P.G.; Hartmann, P.E. Proteome mapping of human skim milk proteins in term and preterm milk. *J. Proteome Res.* **2012**, *11*, 1696–1714. [CrossRef] [PubMed]
39. Whitmore, T.J.; Trengove, N.J.; Graham, D.F.; Hartmann, P.E. Analysis of insulin in human breast milk in mothers with type 1 and type 2 diabetes mellitus. *Int. J. Endocrinol.* **2012**, *2012*, 296368. [CrossRef] [PubMed]
40. Kelly, R.J.; Rouquier, S.; Giorgi, D.; Lennon, G.G.; Lowe, J.B. Sequence and Expression of a Candidate for the Human Secretor Blood Group (1,2) Fucosyltransferase Gene (FUT2): Homozygosity for an enzyme-inactivating nonsense mutation commonly correlates with the non-secretor phenotype. *J. Biol. Chem.* **1995**, *270*, 4640–4649. [CrossRef] [PubMed]
41. Totten, S.M.; Zivkovic, A.M.; Wu, S.; Ngyuen, U.; Freeman, S.L.; Ruhaak, L.R.; Darboe, M.K.; German, J.B.; Prentice, A.M.; Lebrilla, C.B. Comprehensive profiles of human milk oligosaccharides yield highly sensitive and specific markers for determining secretor status in lactating mothers. *J. Proteome Res.* **2012**, *11*, 6124–6133. [CrossRef] [PubMed]
42. Beijers, R.J.W.; Schaafsma, A. Long-chain polyunsaturated fatty acid content in Dutch preterm breast milk; differences in the concentrations of docosahexaenoic acid and arachidonic acid due to length of gestation. *Early Hum. Dev.* **1996**, *44*, 215–223. [CrossRef]
43. Coppa, G.V.; Gabrielli, O.; Pierani, P.; Catassi, C.; Carlucci, A.; Giorgi, P.L. Changes in carbohydrate composition in human milk over 4 months of lactation. *Pediatrics* **1993**, *91*, 637–641. [PubMed]
44. Villaseñor, A.; Garcia-Perez, I.; Garcia, A.; Posma, J.M.; Fernández-López, M.; Nicholas, A.J.; Modi, N.; Holmes, E.; Barbas, C. Breast milk metabolome characterization in a single-phase extraction, multiplatform analytical approach. *Anal. Chem.* **2014**, *86*, 8245–8252. [CrossRef] [PubMed]
45. De Leoz, M.L.A.; Gaerlan, S.C.; Strum, J.S.; Dimapasoc, L.M.; Mirmiran, M.; Tancredi, D.J.; Smilowitz, J.T.; Kalanetra, K.M.; Mills, D.A.; German, J.B.; *et al.* Lacto-*N*-tetraose, fucosylation, and secretor status are highly variable in human milk oligosaccharides from women delivering preterm. *J. Proteome Res.* **2012**, *11*, 4662–4672. [CrossRef] [PubMed]
46. Torrazza, R.M.; Neu, J. The altered gut microbiome and necrotizing enterocolitis. *Clin. Perinatol.* **2013**, *40*, 93–108. [CrossRef] [PubMed]

47. Zhang, Z.; Adelman, A.S.; Rai, D.; Boettcher, J.; Lőnnerdal, B. Amino acid profiles in term and preterm human milk through lactation: A systematic review. *Nutr.* **2013**, *5*, 4800–4821. [CrossRef] [PubMed]
48. Atkinson, S.; Anderson, G.; Bryan, M. Human milk: Comparison of the nitrogen composition in milk from mothers of premature and full-term infants. *Am. J. Clin. Nutr.* **1980**, *33*, 811–815. [PubMed]
49. Chuang, C.K.; Lin, S.P.; Lee, H.C.; Wang, T.J.; Shih, Y.S.; Huang, F.Y.; Yeung, C.Y. Free amino acids in full-term and pre-term human milk and infant formula. *J. Pediatr. Gastroenterol. Nutr.* **2005**, *40*, 496–500. [CrossRef] [PubMed]
50. Moltó-Puigmartí, C.; Castellote, A.I.; Carbonell-Estrany, X.; López-Sabater, M.C. Differences in fat content and fatty acid proportions among colostrum, transitional, and mature milk from women delivering very preterm, preterm, and term infants. *Clin. Nutr.* **2011**, *30*, 116–123. [CrossRef] [PubMed]
51. Holmes-McNary, M.Q.; Cheng, W.L.; Mar, M.H.; Fussell, S.; Zeisel, S.H. Choline and choline esters in human and rat milk and in infant formulas. *Am. J. Clin. Nutr.* **1996**, *64*, 572–576. [PubMed]

14

The Effects of Mild Gestational Hyperglycemia on Exclusive Breastfeeding Cessation

Sergio Verd [1,2,*], Diego de Sotto [3], Consuelo Fernández [2] and Antonio Gutiérrez [4,5]

1 Department of Primary Care, Balearic Health Authority, Health Sciences Research Institute IUNICS, 10 Alexandre Rosselló Ave, 07002 Palma de Mallorca, Spain
2 Department of Primary Care, Balearic Health Authority, 07003 Palma de Mallorca, Spain; consuelofernandez@ibsalut.caib.es
3 Endocrinology Unit, Department of Paediatrics, Hospital Son Espases, Valldemossa Road, 79, 07010 Palma de Mallorca, Spain; diego.desotto@ssib.es
4 Molecular Biology Unit, Division of Hematology, Son Espases University Hospital, Valldemossa Road, 79, 07010 Palma de Mallorca, Spain; antoniom.gutierrez@ssib.es
5 Palma de Mallorca Institute of Health Research (IdISPa), Valldemossa Road, 79, 07010 Palma de Mallorca, Spain
* Correspondence: drsverd@gmail.com

Abstract: Gestational diabetes increases the risk of a range of adverse perinatal outcomes, including breastfeeding failure, but the best cut-off point for gestational diabetes is unknown. The purpose of this study was to evaluate the association between mild gestational glucose tolerance impairment and the early cessation of exclusive breastfeeding (EBF). This is an observational study of 768 women with full term pregnancies that were screened for gestational diabetes at 24–28 weeks gestation. Subjects were divided into two groups: those with a normal 1-h glucose challenge test and those with an elevated 1-h glucose challenge test but still did not qualify for gestational diabetes. We constructed multivariable logistic regression models using data from 616 women with normal gestational glucose tolerance and 152 women with an isolated positive 1-h glucose challenge test. The risk of early exclusive breastfeeding cessation was found to increase in women with mildly impaired glucose tolerance during pregnancy (adjusted OR, 1.65; 95% CI: 1.11, 2.45). Risks of early EBF cessation were also independently associated with the amount of neonatal weight loss and admission to the neonatal ward. Instead, parity was associated with a decreased risk for shorter EBF duration. Insulin resistance—even in the absence of gestational diabetes mellitus—may be an impeding factor for EBF.

Keywords: breastfeeding; gestational diabetes; neonate; glucose tolerance test; prediabetes; insulin resistance; pregnancy outcomes

---

1. Introduction

The role of maternal metabolic health on early lactation success is only recently gaining recognition. A wide range of entangled factors may contribute to reduced milk supply. We know that gestational diabetes predisposes women to both perinatal depression and undesired weaning [1–3]. Several authors have reported that glucose homeostasis during pregnancy may affect breast development [4] and could correlate with breastfeeding outcomes [5,6]. Insulin resistance may act at the lactocyte level [7]. Pregnant women at risk of metabolic syndrome are prone to delayed onset of lactogenesis stage II (DLII) [8]—a risk factor for early breastfeeding cessation [9]. In recent years, it has been shown that most of the time, variation in onset of lactogenesis stage II (LII) is predicted by 1-h post-glucose challenge (1-hOGTT) at 26 weeks of gestation [8]. This finding is in line with current data suggesting that the correlation between any degree of glucose tolerance impairment and adverse offspring outcome follows a continuous pattern, and that even mild degrees of hyperglycemia may be associated with complications [10].

Taken together, these data suggest that suboptimal maternal glucose tolerance may be a key factor in the establishment of breastfeeding. Despite the rising prevalence of gestational prediabetes, studies on neonatal outcomes of this condition are still scarce. To shed some light on this issue, we conducted a secondary analysis and evaluated the following research question: is there an association between mild gestational hyperglycemia and the early cessation of exclusive breastfeeding (EBF)?

2. Experimental Section

2.1. Enrollment

We enrolled a population-based sample of mother–infant dyads attending a general care pediatric clinic in a middle-class neighborhood in Majorca, Spain. The enrollment phase lasted from January 2007 to December 2012. We invited all mothers who attempted breastfeeding to participate in "a study on infant feeding" upon their first well-child visit. The study was approved by the Institutional Review Boards of the Health Authority of the Balearic Islands, and participants consent was obtained prior to their inclusion in the study.

2.2. Selection Criteria and Data Collection

This analysis was conducted in the context of an ongoing observational study of breastfeeding natural history. The study protocol has previously been described in detail [11,12]. In brief, the study was conducted as a review of medical records from a Pediatric Office where approximately 120 babies are enrolled every year. Prenatal inclusion criteria were: (1) the routinely administered 24 to 28-week gestation 1-hOGTT, and (2) mothers had to be free of gestational diabetes (GDM). Post-birth inclusion criteria were (3) delivery at term (37 weeks of gestation), and (4) the mother initiated breastfeeding as planned. We extracted additional data on patient characteristics and on infant feeding from the prenatal and pediatric medical records. From the pediatric record, information on infant feeding was collected at discharge from the hospital and at the scheduled well-baby visits. Information about the duration of EBF was obtained from pediatric records, information previously collected from mother's report of how the baby was being fed at the time of well-baby visits at 2 weeks, and at 2, 4, 6, and 9 months of age. Duration of EBF was defined as the last notation in the record when the infant was fed only breast milk. According to the WHO, exclusive breastfeeding means that the infant receives only breast milk. No other solids are given, with the exception of vitamins, minerals, or medicines. Of the eligible mother–infant dyads, 768 had information available for all key variables, and were therefore included in the analyses presented here.

2.3. Glucose Challenge Test

According to the recommendations of the American College of Obstetrics and Gynecology (ACOG) [13], standard practice in our setting involves universal screening for GDM in all pregnant women at 24–28 weeks' gestation by a nonfasting 1-h 50 g glucose challenge test. Patients testing positive for the 1-hOGTT (1-h plasma glucose 7.8 mmol/L) were asked to return for a 3-h 100 g oral glucose tolerance test (3-hOGTT).

Categorization. Based on 1-hOGTT and 3-hOGTT, subjects were stratified into the following three glucose tolerance groups:

(i) Normal glucose tolerance (NGT), defined by normal 1-hOGTT results (1-h plasma glucose < 7.8 mmol/L);
(ii) Mild impairment of glucose tolerance (MIGT), defined by a single abnormal value greater than or equal to 7.8 mmol/L, but less than 10.6 mmol/L;

(iii) GDM, requires at least two of the following on the 3-hOGTT: fasting glucose 5.8 mmol/L, 1-h glucose 10.6 mmol/L, 2-h glucose 9.2 mmol/L, or 3-h glucose 8.1 mmol/L.

2.4. Data Analysis

Our outcome measure was discontinuation of EBF. Dichotomization: this variable has been split at the median to form short and normal breastfeeding duration groups. Our primary predictor was MIGT in pregnancy. Patients were allocated to the NGT group or to the MIGT group. Data were analyzed using the IBM-SPSS (V22.0) Package (IBM Corp., Armonk, NY, USA). First, we examined distributions and summary measures for each variable. Table 1 shows, for each study group, continuous variables as median followed by range, while categorical variables are presented as proportions. Univariate differences across the groups were assessed using Mann–Whitney test for continuous variables, and either chi square or Fisher's exact test for categorical variables. Multiple regression analysis was used to identify perinatal factors that independently predicted a short duration of EBF. Covariates considered included parity, glucose tolerance status in pregnancy, delivery type, birth weight, admission to the neonatal ward, and neonatal weight loss at discharge. A series of models were constructed using these covariates. The final models included main effects significant at $p < 0.05$.

Table 1. Patient characteristics.

Variable	NGT: 1-h Plasma Glucose < 7.8 mmol/L (N = 616)	MIGT: 10.6 mmol/L > 1-hOGTT Results $\geq$ 7.8 mmol/L (N = 152)	p
Gender:			
Male	51%	53%	0.72
Female	49%	47%	
Parity:			
1	64%	65%	1
>1	36%	35%	
Mother's age (years)	33 (20–45)	33 (25–42)	0.064
Gestational weight gain	12 (1–39)	12 (4–27)	0.84
Weeks of gestation	40 (37–42)	40 (37–42)	0.79
Delivery type:			
Eutocic	82%	18%	0.67
Instrumental	80%	20%	
C-section	79%	21%	
Birth weight	3272 (1995–4800)	3395 (2050–4390)	0.018
Birth height	49.5 (33–54)	50 (45.5–53.5)	0.13
Birth head circumference	34.5 (31–37)	34.5 (31–37.5)	0.74
Percent of loss of birth weight to discharge	6 (−0.32–0.21)	7 (−7–13)	0.41

Abbreviations: 1-h post-glucose challenge (1-hOGTT); mild impairment of glucose tolerance (MIGT); normal glucose tolerance (NGT).

3. Results

3.1. Patient Characteristics

Table 1 shows the demographic and perinatal characteristics of the 768 study participants stratified into our two predefined glucose tolerance categories in pregnancy: NGT (n = 616) and MIGT (n = 152). Around eighty percent (80.2%) of subjects tested in the normal range for glucose tolerance. This was a predominantly middle-class cohort from a general pediatric clinic where most participants had private health insurance. There were no significant differences between the groups with respect to most baseline characteristics, but birth weight was lowest in the NGT group (p = 0.018), and birth height was lower in the NGT group than in the MIGT group—though this difference did not reach statistical significance (p = 0.13).

3.2. EBF Outcome: Univariate Analysis

Table 2 shows that, upon univariate analysis, the rate of EBF adverse outcomes was significantly higher in the MIGT than in the NGT group (58% vs. 48%; $p = 0.03$). In fact, in the MIGT cohort, median duration of EBF was 56 days (1–300), while in the NGT cohort, it was significantly longer: 100 days (1–360) ($p = 0.045$). Other significant findings for decreased EBF duration included parity, gender of the newborn infant, neonatal weight loss at discharge, and admission to the neonatal ward.

Table 2. Results for univariate analysis of exclusive breastfeeding (EBF) duration.

EBF Discontinuation	Before Day 100 ($N = 384$)	Equal or Later than Day 100 ($N = 384$)	p
MIGT	58%	42%	0.03 *
NGT	48%	52%	
Gender:			
Male	214 (54%)	169 (43%)	0.001 **
Female	179 (45%)	225 (57%)	
Parity:			
1	271(72%)	214 (57%)	<0.001 ***
>1	107 (28%)	159 (28%)	
Mother's age (years)	33 (18–42)	33 (21–45)	0.92
Gestational weight gain	12 (1–30)	12 (4–39)	0.05
Weeks of gestation	40 (37–42)	40 (37–42)	0.27
Delivery type:			
Eutocic	184 (50%)	207 (57%)	0.38
Instrumental	61 (17%)	55 (15%)	
C-section	119 (33%)	110 (30%)	
Birth weight	3252 (1995–4390)	3330 (2310–4800)	0.02 *
Birth height	49.5 (33–54)	50 (45.5–54)	0.32
Birth head circumference	34.5 (31–37)	34.5 (31–37.5)	0.36
Percent of loss of birth weight to discharge	7 (−7–21)	6 (−32–20)	<0.001 ***

Abbreviations: mild impairment of glucose tolerance (MIGT); normal glucose tolerance (NGT). * $p < 0.05$; ** $p < 0.01$; *** $p < 0.001$.

3.3. EBF Outcome: Multivariate Analysis

We reanalyzed the association between MIGT and EBF outcome after adjustment for significant univariate variables (Table 3). EBF duration—as a dichotomous variable (<100 days)—was independently associated with the MIGT group (OR: 1.65; CI: 1.11–2.45). In addition, neonatal weight loss at discharge and admission to the neonatal ward were identified as significant risk factors for short EBF duration in the multivariable model. Instead, parity was associated with a decreased risk for shorter EBF duration.

Table 3. Multivariate analysis of factors independently associated with reduction in exclusive breastfeeding duration.

	AOR (95% CI)	p
Mildly impaired glucose tolerance	1.65 (1.11–2.45)	0.01
Early neonatal weight loss	1.73 (1.26–2.36)	0.001
Admission to neonatal ward	3.32 (1.04–10.60)	0.04
Parity	0.57 (0.41–0.79)	0.001

Abbreviations: AOR, adjusted odds ratio.

4. Discussion

In this report, we aimed to determine whether an abnormal 1-hOGTT is independently associated with adverse EBF outcomes despite a normal subsequent 3-hOGTT. We have shown that MIGT during pregnancy predicts a shortened breastfeeding duration. To our knowledge, there is only one other study on the lactational implications of mild gestational hyperglycemia. Interestingly, it shows that testing positive in the 1-hOGTT is the main contributing factor to a delay or failure in the onset of LII [9], and specifically, that DLII is a clinical indicator of women at risk of early postpartum breastfeeding cessation. Three groups have evaluated the effect of DLII on breastfeeding outcomes. Chapman et al. showed that among women planning to breastfeed $\geq$6 months, women without DLII were more likely to continue breastfeeding [14]. In the analyses by Hruschka and colleagues, immediate postpartum supplementation was associated with DLII [15]. Finally, data from over 2400 mothers showed that DLII was associated with the cessation of any and exclusive breastfeeding at 4-weeks postpartum [9].

Since O'Sullivan first described gestational glucose intolerance, progressively lower thresholds have been proposed for the diagnosis and treatment of GDM. New data have demonstrated that the risk of adverse outcomes increases, even among women with sub-threshold results in fasting and post-load glucose screening [16]. Furthermore, it was recently reported that pregnant women with an isolated abnormal glucose value at 1-hOGTT carry a severe metabolic perturbation, characterized by markedly reduced beta-cell function; their metabolic phenotype resembles that of GDM, and may be associated with the same adverse outcomes as GDM [17]. The Hyperglycemia and Adverse Pregnancy Outcome (HAPO) study showed associations between increasing levels of fasting, 1-h, and 2-h plasma glucose obtained on oral glucose-tolerance testing and each of the adverse perinatal outcomes examined: birth weight above the 90th percentile and cordblood serum C-peptide level above the 90th percentile, premature delivery, shoulder dystocia or birth injury, intensive neonatal care, hyperbilirubinemia, and preeclampsia [18]. The effects of GDM on short-term breastfeeding outcomes have been clearly documented, unlike the effects of MIGT. Yet, women with a history of GDM face challenges with EBF in the critical period for setting up breastfeeding success. A recent systematic review of ten original papers from 1989 to 2013 on the effect of GDM on LII onset shows that all studies consistently identified that LII occurred later among gestationally diabetic mothers than in non-diabetic mothers [19]. LII is characterized by changes in breastmilk components—in particular, a decrease in breastmilk sodium. Conversely, the presence of GDM increases the risk of an elevated breastmilk sodium level on day three postpartum [20]. A case–control study revealed that women diagnosed with low milk supply were significantly more likely to have had GDM compared with women with other lactation outcomes [21]. Poorer sucking patterns have been found among newborn infants of mothers with GDM [22]. A cross-sectional analysis including 2038 women found that the adjusted odds of EBF at hospital discharge were lower among women with GDM compared to women without GDM [23].

Overt GDM is associated with significantly increased risks of adverse breastfeeding outcomes. Whereas, until recently, women with an abnormal 1-hOGTT (with normal 3h-OGTT) were regarded as a false positive result, emerging data suggest that current diagnostic criteria for GDM are too restrictive, and that lesser degrees of hyperglycemia also increase offspring risks [10]. Despite the associated adverse pregnancy outcomes, no international consensus exists that identifies a cut-off value for the definition of GDM. Current criteria of the International Association of Diabetes and Pregnancy Study Groups (IADPSG) are lower than the ACOG 2013 thresholds (fasting glucose 5.1 versus 5.8 mmol/L, or 1-h glucose 10.0 versus 10.6 mmol/L). It has been reported that applying the IADPSG criteria to the population would increase the rate of GDM from 7.3% to 10.3% [24]. A 2013 National Institutes of Health (NIH) panel states that there are clear benefits to the standardization of international diagnostic criteria. Nevertheless, the panel is concerned with the adoption of new criteria that would increase the prevalence of GDM (and the corresponding costs and interventions), without clear demonstration of improvements in health outcomes [25]. Therefore, new tools—such as Capula's index—continue to be developed to improve the accuracy and cost-effectiveness of this screening [26].

A brief literature review shows that it is well established that insulin resistance is a strong predictor of short breastfeeding duration, but the underlying causal contributors remained unclear until very recently. Over the last years, insulin-sensitive gene expression has been shown to be upregulated during the lactation cycle, and insulin is now considered to play a direct role in lactation [27].

The established dogma has been that women are never physiologically unable to lactate, but rather that low milk supply is a mistaken belief on their part. Thus, most interventions have focused on improving breastfeeding education. However, emerging clinical research suggests an important association between suboptimal glucose tolerance and lactation difficulty. Our findings add to the evidence that a woman's metabolic complications adversely affect her lactation outcomes. 1-hOGTT may be a useful clinical indicator to identify women at risk of early postpartum breastfeeding cessation. These results have clinical implications, underlining that breastfeeding support of women with abnormal glucose tolerance should be individualized. Given the current insulin resistance epidemic, caregivers face the challenge of meeting the growing need for clinical guidance of women with both metabolic disturbances and low milk supply. Further translational research is needed to successfully implement interventions that will enable more women to avoid undesired breastfeeding cessation.

These analyses have several limitations. First, this is a secondary analysis. Second, the nature of these data did not allow for evaluation of the contribution of interactions between conditions previously reported (e.g., gestational weight gain and maternal obesity, neonatal weight loss and DLII). Third, our significant findings may be inauthentic due to unmeasured confounding. A factor that influences a woman's ability to breastfeed is the presence of personal or professional support. Other mother-centered factors include social barriers, work-related barriers, or a dislike of breastfeeding. We do not have data on all maternal factors that may affect milk production and composition. Finally, our assessment of metabolic dysregulation was done prenatally. We do not know to what extent maternal metabolic status in the early postpartum is affected.

Strengths of this study include the consistency with existing literature and the prospective design to collect breastfeeding duration and exclusivity data. The study does not rely on later recall of breastfeeding outcomes. Although the study populations and availability of pertinent confounders differed, the current study confirms that 1-hOGTT represents an important metabolic perturbation in pregnancy, characterized not only by increased risk for adverse pregnancy outcomes, but also by early breastfeeding dysfunction. It is becoming clear that long glucose challenge tests are not superior to short glucose challenge tests in the assessment of prenatal glucose tolerance.

Finally, we clearly identified several additional independent risk factors for early breastfeeding cessation (e.g., neonatal weight loss, admission to the neonatal ward, and parity).

5. Conclusions

In summary, women who test positive for 1-hOGTT may be less able to sustain EBF at 100 days. These findings suggest that 1-hOGTT may already identify a high-risk population of mothers in need of interventions to increase breast milk production.

Acknowledgments: We want to thank all mothers who participated in this study. We also acknowledge Silvia Celorio, SHO, for her cooperation in participant recruitment. This project would not have been possible without editorial assistance assistance from Berta Verd.

Author Contributions: All authors contributed extensively to the work presented in this paper. S.V. and D.d.S. conceived the study; C.F. and A.G. developed the methdology; D.d.S. and C.F. monitored data collection; A.G. analyzed the data; S.V. wrote the paper.

Abbreviations

The following abbreviations are used in this manuscript:

1-hOGTT	1-h post-glucose challenge
3-hOGTT	3-h glucose tolerance test
ACOG	American College of Obstetricians and Gynecologists
DLII	delayed onset of lactogenesis stage II
EBF	exclusive breastfeeding
GDM	gestational diabetes
IADPSG	International Association of Diabetes and Pregnancy Study Groups
LII	lactogenesis stage II
MIGT	mild impairment of glucose tolerance
NGT	normal glucose tolerance

References

1. Herring, S.J.; Rich-Edwards, J.W.; Oken, E.; Rifas-Shiman, S.L.; Kleinman, K.P.; Gillman, M.W. Association of postpartum depression with weight retention 1 year after childbirth. *Obesity* **2008**, *16*, 1296–1301. [CrossRef] [PubMed]
2. Dennis, C.L.; McQueen, K. Does maternal postpartum depressive symptomatology influence infant feeding outcomes? *Acta Paediatr.* **2007**, *96*, 590–594. [CrossRef] [PubMed]
3. Matias, S.L.; Dewey, K.G.; Quesenberry, C.P., Jr.; Gunderson, E.P. Maternal prepregnancy obesity and insulin treatment during pregnancy are independently associated with delayed lactogenesis in women with recent gestational diabetes mellitus. *Am. J. Clin. Nutr.* **2014**, *99*, 115–121. [CrossRef] [PubMed]
4. Vanky, E.; Nordskar, J.J.; Leithe, H.; Hjorth-Hansen, A.K.; Martinussen, M.; Carlsen, S.M. Breast size increment during pregnancy and breastfeeding in mothers with polycystic ovary syndrome: A follow-up study of a randomised controlled trial on metformin versus placebo. *BJOG* **2012**, *119*, 1403–1409. [CrossRef] [PubMed]
5. Nommsen-Rivers, L.A.; Chantry, C.J.; Peerson, J.M.; Cohen, R.J.; Dewey, K.G. Delayed onset of lactogenesis among first-time mothers is related to maternal obesity and factors associated with ineffective breastfeeding. *Am. J. Clin. Nutr.* **2010**, *92*, 574–584. [CrossRef] [PubMed]
6. Stuebe, A.M.; Horton, B.J.; Chetwynd, E.; Watkins, S.; Grewen, K.; Meltzer-Brody, S. Prevalence and Risk Factors for Early, Undesired Weaning Attributed to Lactation Dysfunction. *J. Women's Health* **2014**, *23*, 404–412. [CrossRef] [PubMed]
7. Lemay, D.G.; Ballard, O.A.; Hughes, M.A.; Morrow, A.L.; Horseman, N.D.; Nommsen-Rivers, L.A. RNA sequencing of the human milk fat layer transcriptome reveals distinct gene expression profiles at three stages of lactation. *PLoS ONE* **2013**, *8*, e67531. [CrossRef] [PubMed]
8. Nommsen-Rivers, L.A.; Dolan, L.M.; Huang, B. Timing of stage II lactogenesis is predicted by antenatal metabolic health in a cohort of primiparas. *Breastfeed. Med.* **2012**, *7*, 43–49. [CrossRef] [PubMed]
9. Brownell, E.; Howard, C.R.; Lawrence, R.A.; Dozier, A.M. Delayed onset lactogenesis II predicts the cessation of any or exclusive breastfeeding. *J. Pediatr.* **2012**, *161*, 608–614. [CrossRef] [PubMed]
10. Melamed, N.; Hiersch, L.; Hod, M.; Chen, R.; Wiznitzer, A.; Yogev, Y. Is abnormal 50-g glucose-challenge testing an independent predictor of adverse pregnancy outcome? *J. Matern. Fetal Neonatal Med.* **2012**, *25*, 2583–2587. [CrossRef] [PubMed]
11. Verd, S.; Nadal-Amat, J.; Gich, I.; Leshem, M. Salt preference of nursing mothers is associated with earlier cessation of exclusive breastfeeding. *Appetite* **2010**, *54*, 233–236. [CrossRef] [PubMed]
12. Verd, S.; Barriuso, L.; Gich, I.; Gutiérrez, A.; Nadal-Amat, J.; Carreras, E. Risk of early breastfeeding cessation among symmetrical, small for gestational age infants. *Ann. Hum. Biol.* **2013**, *40*, 146–151. [CrossRef] [PubMed]
13. American College of Obstetricians and Gynecologists. Practice Bulletin No. 137: Gestational diabetes mellitus. *Obstet. Gynecol.* **2013**, *122*, 406–416.
14. Chapman, D.J.; Perez-Escamilla, R. Does delayed perception of the onset of lactation shorten breastfeeding duration? *J. Hum. Lact.* **1999**, *5*, 107–111. [CrossRef]

15. Hruschka, D.J.; Sellen, D.W.; Stein, A.D.; Martorell, R. Delayed onset of lactation and risk of ending full breast-feeding early in rural Guatemala. *J. Nutr.* **2003**, *133*, 2592–2599. [PubMed]
16. Stuebe, A.M.; Landon, M.B.; Lai, Y.; Klebanoff, M.; Ramin, S.M.; Wapner, R.J.; Varner, M.W.; Rouse, D.J.; Sciscione, A.; Catalano, P.; et al. Is There a Threshold Oral Glucose Tolerance Test Value for Predicting Adverse Pregnancy Outcome? *Am. J. Perinatol.* **2015**, *32*, 833–838. [PubMed]
17. Retnakaran, R.; Qi, Y.; Sermer, M.; Connelly, P.W.; Zinman, B.; Hanley, A.J. Isolated hyperglycemia at 1 h on oral glucose tolerance test in pregnancy resembles gestational diabetes mellitus in predicting postpartum metabolic dysfunction. *Diabetes Care* **2008**, *31*, 1275–1281. [CrossRef] [PubMed]
18. HAPO Study Cooperative Research Group; Metzger, B.E.; Lowe, L.P.; Dyer, A.R.; Trimble, E.R.; Chaovarindr, U.; Coustan, D.R.; Hadden, D.R.; McCance, D.R.; Hod, M. Hyperlycemia and adverse pregnancy outcomes. *N. Engl. J. Med.* **2008**, *358*, 1991–2002. [PubMed]
19. De Bortoli, J.; Amir, L.H. Is onset of lactation delayed in women with diabetes in pregnancy? A systematic review. *Diabet. Med.* **2016**, *33*, 17–24. [CrossRef] [PubMed]
20. Galipeau, R.; Goulet, C.; Cgagnon, M. Infant and maternal factors influencing breastmilk sodium among primiparous mothers. *Breastfeed. Med.* **2012**, *7*, 290–294. [CrossRef] [PubMed]
21. Riddle, S.W.; Nommsen-Rivers, L.A. A case control study of diabetes during pregnancy and low milk supply. *Breastfeed. Med.* **2016**, *11*, 80–85. [CrossRef] [PubMed]
22. Bromiker, R.; Rachamim, A.; Hammerman, C.; Schimmel, M.; Kaplan, M.; Medoff-Cooper, B. Immature suckling patterns in infants of mothers with diabetes. *J. Pediatr.* **2006**, *49*, 640–643. [CrossRef] [PubMed]
23. Haile, Z.T.; Oza-Frank, R.; Azulay Chertok, I.R.; Passen, N. Association between history of gestational diabetes and exclusive breastfeeding at hospital discharge. *J. Hum. Lact.* **2015**. [CrossRef] [PubMed]
24. Mayo, K.; Melamed, N.; Vandenbergh, H.; Berger, H. The impact of adoption of the international association of diabetes in pregnancy study group criteria for the screening and diagnosis of gestational diabetes. *Am. J. Obstet. Gynecol.* **2015**, *212*, e1–e9. [CrossRef] [PubMed]
25. Vandorten, J.P.; Dodson, W.C.; Espeland, M.A.; Grobman, W.A.; Guise, J.M.; Mercer, B.M.; Minkoff, H.L.; Poindexter, B.; Prosser, L.A.; Sawaya, G.F.; et al. NIH consensus development conference: Diagnosing gestational diabetes mellitus. *NIH Consens. State Sci. Statements* **2013**, *29*, 1–31.
26. Capula, C.; Chiefari, E.; Borelli, M.; Oliverio, R.; Vero, A.; Foti, D.; Puccio, L.; Vero, R.; Brunetti, A. A new predictive tool for the early risk assessment of gestational diabetes mellitus. *Prim Care Diabetes* **2016**, *10*, 315–323. [CrossRef] [PubMed]
27. Nommsen-Rivers, L.A. Does insulin explain the relationship between maternal obesity and poor lactation outcomes? An overview of the literature. *Adv. Nutr.* **2016**, *7*, 407–414. [CrossRef] [PubMed]

Food and Nutrient Intake among 12-Month-Old Norwegian-Somali and Norwegian-Iraqi Infants

Navnit Kaur Grewal [1,*], Lene Frost Andersen [2], Cathrine Solheim Kolve [1], Ingrid Kverndalen [1] and Liv Elin Torheim [1]

1 Department of Nursing and Health Promotion, Faculty of Health Sciences, Oslo and Akershus University College of Applied Sciences, P.O. Box 4 St. Olavs Plass, 0130 Oslo, Norway; cathrinekolve@gmail.com (C.S.K.); ingrid.kverndalen@hotmail.com (I.K.); liv.elin.torheim@hioa.no (L.E.T.)
2 Department of Nutrition, Institute of Basic Medical Sciences, University of Oslo, P.O. Box 1046 Blindern, 0317 Oslo, Norway; l.f.andersen@medisin.uio.no
* Correspondence: navnit-kaur.grewal@hioa.no

Abstract: The aim of the present paper was to describe food and nutrient intake among 12-month-old Norwegian-Somali and Norwegian-Iraqi infants, with a focus on iron and vitamin D intake. A cross-sectional survey was conducted from August 2013 through September 2014. Eighty-nine mothers/infants of Somali origin and 77 mothers/infants of Iraqi origin residing in Eastern Norway participated in the study. Data were collected using two 24-h multiple-pass recalls. Forty percent of the Norwegian-Somali infants and 47% of the Norwegian-Iraqi infants were breastfed at 12 months of age ($p = 0.414$). Median energy percentages (E%) from protein, fat and carbohydrates were within the recommended intake ranges, except the level of saturated fats (12–13 E%). Median intakes of almost all micronutrients were above the recommended daily intakes. Most of the infants consumed iron-enriched products (81%) and received vitamin D supplements (84%). The median intakes of iron and vitamin D were significantly higher among infants receiving iron-enriched products and vitamin D supplements compared to infants not receiving such products ($p < 0.001$). The findings indicate that the food and nutrient intake of this group of infants in general seems to be in accordance with Norwegian dietary recommendations. Foods rich in iron and vitamin D supplements were important sources of the infants' intake of iron and vitamin D and should continue to be promoted.

Keywords: food; nutrient intake; infants; immigrants; Norway

---

1. Introduction

The first two years of a child's life are particularly important as this is a period of rapid growth when nutritional needs are high [1,2]. Knowledge about infants' and toddlers' food and nutrient intake is therefore important to evaluate their diet and identify potential challenges. In Norway, national dietary surveys of infants and toddlers have been performed at the ages of 6, 12 and 24 months [3–5]. Due to methodological issues, infants and toddlers of immigrant mothers were excluded from these surveys, and separate surveys for these children have been called for by the Norwegian Directorate of Health [6].

Consequently, compared to infants of Norwegian-born parents, less is known about the food and nutrient intake of infants of immigrant parents in Norway. However, some previous smaller studies of Norwegian immigrant children have shown some potential nutrition challenges, such as high prevalence of iron and vitamin D deficiencies and a relatively high added sugar intake [7–9]. It has further been suggested that immigrant children may be introduced to cow's milk at a younger age than ethnic Norwegian children, although inconsistent trends have been observed [9]. As cow's milk contains very little iron, consumption >500 mL/day has been associated with reduced iron stores in young children [10,11]. However, intake of fortified foods seems to improve iron status in late infancy [12].

To address the paucity of data on food and nutrient intake and infant feeding practices among Norwegian children with immigrant backgrounds, the InnBaKost study was initiated in 2012. Information on breastfeeding and complementary feeding practices among 6-month-old Norwegian-Somali and Norwegian-Iraqi infants was recently published [13]. The present paper aimed to describe and compare food and nutrient intake among 12-month-old Norwegian-Somali and Norwegian-Iraqi infants, with a focus on iron and vitamin D intake.

2. Materials and Methods

2.1. Subjects and Design

A cross-sectional survey was carried out from August 2013–September 2014. Mothers born in Somalia or Iraq and living in Oslo, Akershus or Buskerud were eligible for inclusion. These two immigrant groups were chosen, as they are the two non-Western immigrant groups in Norway with the highest number of births per year [14]. Children on a special diet due to serious illness were excluded. If the mother had twins or triplets, only one child was included by random selection.

Mothers who participated in the InnBaKost survey of 6-month-old infants [13] were contacted again when their children turned 12 months old. These mothers had not received any information about the results in the 6-months survey or dietary counselling which could influence dietary habits at the infants' 12 months of age. In the 6-month survey, 107 Norwegian-Somali mothers and infants and 80 Norwegian-Iraqi mothers and infants participated [13]. Of these, 70 Norwegian-Somali infants and 61 Norwegian-Iraqi infants participated in the 12-month follow-up survey. Seven of the Somali-born mothers and eight of the Iraqi-born mothers declined to participate further, while 30 Somali-born mothers and 11 Iraqi-born mothers could not be reached. Along with the mothers/infants participating in the 6-month survey, 19 additional Somali-born mothers and 16 additional Iraqi-born mothers were recruited. The additional mothers were recruited through lists obtained from the National Population Register. Mothers who were not reached from these lists in the 6-month survey were approached again when the infants were 12 months. A total sample of 89 Norwegian-Somali infants and 77 Norwegian-Iraqi infants were included for the present analysis.

To collect data on the food intake of the 12-month-old infants, two 24-h multiple-pass recalls were conducted face-to-face as closely as possible to the child's 12-month birthday. Eight trained female fieldworkers speaking the relevant language performed the interviews in Somali, Arabic, Kurdish or Norwegian. A total of 8% ($n = 13$) only completed one single 24-h recall. For mothers who were unable to meet in person, the interview was conducted over the telephone. Of all the participants, 3% ($n = 5$) had both interviews conducted over the telephone, while 4% ($n = 7$) had one of the two interviews conducted over the telephone. The interviews were conducted at a time and place chosen by individual mothers. The average time between the two 24-h recalls was 2 weeks. For 7% of the participants, there were more than 4 weeks between the two interviews. Approximately 78% of all the dietary recalls were collected for intakes on weekdays and 22% were collected for intakes on weekends among Norwegian-Somali infants, and the numbers were 83% and 17%, respectively, for Norwegian-Iraqi infants. In both groups, over 85% of the recall days were reported as representative of the usual daily dietary intake of the child. Each mother who completed the two 24-h recalls received a voucher for a baby shop worth approximately US $25.

The Regional Committees for Medical and Health Research Ethics (2012/957) approved the study, and informed consent was obtained from all the participating mothers.

2.2. 24-h Multiple-Pass Recall Method

The 24-h multiple-pass recall method was used to collect data on the 12-month-old Norwegian-Somali and Norwegian-Iraqi infants. The method was first developed and pilot tested on 12 Somali-born and Iraqi-born mothers from January to June 2013 [15].

Briefly, in this dietary recall method, the mothers were to be interviewed twice about the exact food and beverage intake of their children during the preceding 24 h. A 24-h period was defined as from the time the child woke up the previous day until the time the child woke up the day of the interview.

The dietary recall was divided into three passes. In the first pass, the mothers were asked to report everything that their children had consumed the previous day, including during the night. Each breastfeeding occurrence was also to be reported. In the second pass, mothers were asked to provide additional detailed information about each item of food and drink consumed by the children. This included type of product, brand names, cooking methods, amounts and leftovers. For homemade dishes, the mothers were asked for the recipes, and the list of ingredients was recorded. The third pass was a review of the recall, and the mothers were given the opportunity to provide any additional information regarding the children's food and drink consumption. During the last pass, the field workers were also instructed to prompt for information about foods and drinks not mentioned that were considered to be easy to forget, such as snacks, fruits, water, juices and supplements, which the field workers read from a list.

Two photographic booklets previously used in Norwegian national dietary surveys, were utilized during the interviews as an aid to estimate portion sizes. The *Spedkost* booklet [4] containing 17 colour photograph series of infant portion sizes of selected foods and drinks was mostly employed. The *Norkost* booklet [16] containing a series of adult portion sizes was mainly used to estimate portion sizes of different kinds of bread.

A picture library containing 405 pictures divided into 19 folders on an iPad was used to help identify the types of foods/drinks/products given to the children. The development of the picture library has been described in more detail elsewhere [15].

2.3. Questionnaire and Background Characteristics

A questionnaire with 19 questions on five topics was used to collect additional information about the infants. The questions related to breastfeeding (whether the infant was breastfed, and if so, the frequency of breastfeeding), the age of introduction to various foods and drinks, whether the infant had any allergies/intolerances, the use of dietary supplements and arenas for receiving infant nutrition information.

In Norway, healthcare personnel routinely measure the length and weight of children during regular check-ups at children's health clinics, including at 12 months of age. Participating mothers were asked to bring their infant's health cards to the interview in order to record these data. Other background characteristics, such as infants' gender, mothers' age, mothers' age when they immigrated to Norway, number of children, parental education levels and fathers' origins, were already provided from the 6-month survey. The same questions were asked of newly recruited mothers. All mothers were also asked to provide information on current work status and person/place in charge of day-care for the infants. When possible, other persons in charge of the day-care of the infant during the recall days were consulted on the infants' dietary intake during those hours.

2.4. Food Intake and Nutrient Calculations

Information from the 24-h recalls was manually coded by nutritionists. All foods and beverages consumed by each child were converted into grams of edible portions. For recipes, a modified version of the summing method was applied to calculate the intake of each ingredient [17]. A breast milk intake of 124 mL per feed or an intake of 497 mL for children whose mothers reported to have breastfed their children four times or more was used, as described by Grewal et al. [15]. The daily nutrient intakes (averaged over the two days) were computed using a food database and a dietary calculation system (KBS, version 7.2, database AE-10) developed at the Department of Nutrition, University of Oslo, Oslo, Norway. The food database used is mainly based on the official Norwegian food composition table but is also continuously supplemented with data on new food items and nutrient content. Relevant food products missing from KBS were added, and the nutrient content was based on the nutrient content listed on the products' nutritional label. Nutrients from dietary supplements and from fortified foods consumed during the recall days were included in the calculated nutrient intake. The calculated average daily nutrient intake from the two recalls was compared to the recommended intake ranges for macronutrients and recommended daily intakes (RI) for micronutrients [18].

2.5. Statistical Analysis

Data from the questionnaire and background characteristics were manually entered into the statistical software package IBM SPSS Statistics version 22.0. Data about the food and nutrient intakes estimated from KBS were transferred to SPSS. All data were further processed and analysed in SPSS. Energy intake information acquired during the telephone interviews ($n = 12$) did not differ from those who completed two face-to-face 24-h recalls and were therefore included in the analyses. Mothers who only completed one 24-h recall were also included.

The weight and length of the children were converted into Z-scores for weight-for-age, height-for-age and weight-for-height according to 2006 WHO child growth standards [19] using WHO Anthro (version 3.2.2, January 2011, Geneva, Switzerland) and macros. Cow's milk and yoghurt were categorized as 'dairy products' in the analysis. Infant formula and infant cereals were categorized as 'iron-enriched products'.

Iron intake was compared between infants receiving and not receiving dairy products and between infants receiving and not receiving iron-enriched products. The intake of dairy products and the intake of iron-enriched products were tested by different background characteristics. The intake of vitamin D was compared between infants receiving and not receiving vitamin D supplements. The intake of vitamin D supplements was tested by different background characteristics. The data did not adhere to a normal distribution, and continuous variables are presented as median and 25th and 75th percentiles (P_{25}–P_{75}) and were tested using a Mann-Whitney U test. Categorical variables were tested using a Chi-square test.

3. Results

Selected characteristics of the infants and their parents are presented in Table 1. The Norwegian-Somali infants had significantly higher Z-scores for height-for-age (1.4 vs. 0.6, $p = 0.001$) but not for weight-for-height (0.7 vs. 0.2, $p = 0.087$) compared to the Norwegian-Iraqi infants. The Somali-born mothers were younger (29 years vs. 32 years, $p = 0.026$), had lived in Norway for a longer period of time (10 years vs. 7 years, $p = 0.012$) and a higher percentage were working at the time of interviewing (27% vs. 13%, $p = 0.026$) compared to the Iraqi-born mothers. A higher proportion of the Iraqi-born mothers had higher education compared to the Somali-born mothers (64% vs. 38%, $p = 0.001$).

3.1. Breastfeeding

At 12 months of age, 40% of the Norwegian-Somali infants and 47% of the Norwegian-Iraqi infants were breastfed ($p = 0.414$). The median breastfeeding frequency among those breastfeeding was 4.5 times a day in both groups.

Table 1. Characteristics of the infants and parents sampled (n = 166).

Characteristics	Total (n = 166) †		Somali Origin (n = 89) †		Iraqi Origin (n = 77) †		p-Value *
Infants							
Boys/girls ‡	55/45		60/40		49/51		0.154
Weight at 12 months (g) ‡	10,000	(9286–11,100)	10,270	(9779–11,811)	9708	(9093–10,575)	0.001
Boys	10,120	(9470–11,293)	10,350	(9824–11,800)	9940	(8600–10,885)	0.034
Girls	9815	(9175–10,960)	10,185	(9481–12,104)	9460	(9100–10,500)	0.012
Length at 12 months (cm) ‡	77.5	(75.0–79.9)	78.9	(77.0–81.5)	76.5	(74.4–78.3)	<0.001
Boys	78.0	(75.6–80.5)	78.3	(76.8–81.0)	77.8	(74.4–79.3)	0.110
Girls	77.0	(75.0–79.0)	79.5	(76.5–82.8)	76.0	(74.1–77.4)	<0.001
Z-score							
Weight-for-age	0.5	(0.0–1.5)	0.9	(0.2–1.9)	0.4	(0.0–1.1)	0.020
Height-for-age	0.8	(0.8–1.7)	1.4	(0.4–2.4)	0.6	(0.0–1.1)	0.001
Weight-for-height	0.3	(−0.4–1.2)	0.7	(−0.4–1.5)	0.2	(−0.4–0.9)	0.087
Mothers							
Age (years) ‡	30.0	(27.0–34.0)	29.0	(27.0–33.0)	32.0	(27.0–36.5)	0.026
Age when immigrated to Norway ‡	22.0	(15.0–26.3)	20.0	(12.0–24.0)	23.0	(19.0–29.0)	0.001
Number of years lived in Norway ‡	10.0	(5.0–14.0)	10.0	(5.0–15.0)	7.0	(3.0–13.0)	0.012
Education ‡							
No/basic education	50		62		36		0.001
High school/higher education	50		38		64		
Current employment status ‡							
Not working	79		73		87		0.026
Working (full-time/part-time)	21		27		13		
Primiparous ‡	28		28		27		0.891
Fathers							
Origin ‡							
Somalia/Iraq	92		95		88		0.102
Other	8		5		12		
Education ‡							
No/basic education	28		29		27		0.285
High school/higher education	63		59		68		
Do not know	9		12		5		
Responsible for child during daytime ‡							0.021
Mother	58		48		68		
Others (e.g., partner, day-care, etc.)	19		21		17		
Mother and others	23		31		15		

* Comparison of parents and infants of Somali and Iraqi origin. † Percentages for categorical variables, and medians (25th and 75th percentiles) for continuous variables; ‡ Data on gender are missing for three infants from Somalia. The lengths of 44 infants are missing (37 from Somalia and 7 from Iraq). The weights of 42 infants are missing (33 from Somalia and 9 from Iraq). Among male infants, data on length are missing for 26 infants and data on weight are missing for 26 infants. Among female infants, data on length are missing for 16 infants and data on weight are missing for 15 infants. The ages of four Somali-born mothers are missing. The ages when immigrated to Norway are missing for six Somali-born mothers and two Iraqi-born mothers. Mothers' and fathers' highest completed education is missing for four mothers and five fathers from Somalia. Current work status is missing for one Somali-born mother and one Iraqi-born mother. Primiparous data and father's origin is missing for four Somali-born mothers. Who is responsible for the child during daytime is missing for one Norwegian-Iraqi infant. These are not included in the analysis.

3.2. Food Intake

Data from the 24-h recalls on daily intakes of various types of foods and drinks among all infants are presented in Table 2. Percentages of and intake among consumers are presented in Table 3. Norwegian-Somali infants had significantly higher median daily intakes of commercial infant cereals, commercial fruit purees, fish/fish products, yoghurt and cow's milk compared to the Norwegian-Iraqi infants (Table 2). Norwegian-Iraqi infants, on the other hand, had significantly higher daily intakes of refined flour bread, cake, meat and meat products, eggs, fruits and berries, added sugar, tea and water than Norwegian-Somali infants (Table 2).

Commercial infant cereals and fruit purees, potatoes and fish/fish products were consumed by a significantly higher proportion of Norwegian-Somali infants compared to Norwegian-Iraqi infants, while bread, grain products, cake, meat, eggs, fruit/berries and tea were more commonly consumed by Norwegian-Iraqi infants (Table 3).

3.3. Energy and Nutrient Intake

The average energy and nutrient intake from the 24-h recalls are shown in Table 4. The median energy intake among Norwegian-Somali infants was 3791 kJ compared to 4122 kJ among Norwegian-Iraqi infants ($p = 0.059$). The median energy percentages (E%) from protein, fat and carbohydrates were within the recommended intake ranges in both groups; however, the intake of saturated fats was above the recommended upper level of 10 E%. The intake of added sugar, on the other hand, was below 5 E% in both groups.

The main sources of saturated fat intake in the total diet of the Norwegian-Somali infants were cow's milk (which contributed with 22%), breast milk (22%), commercial infant cereals (9%) and cheese (8%) (data not shown). The main sources of saturated fats among the Norwegian-Iraqi infants were breast milk (23%), meat and meat products (11%), cow's milk (9%) and cheese (9%). Yoghurt was the main source of the added sugar intake among both the Norwegian-Somali and Norwegian-Iraqi infants (38% vs. 23%).

The median intake of all micronutrients, except iron and niacin in both groups and zinc among Norwegian-Somali infants were above the RI.

3.4. Factors Associated with Iron Intake

The main sources of dietary iron were commercial infant cereals (which contributed with 51% among Norwegian-Somali vs. 34% among Norwegian-Iraqi infants), iron supplements (13% vs. 9%), infant formula (10% vs. 19%) and bread and other grain products (10% vs. 8%). During the recall days, 6% of the Norwegian-Somali infants and 8% of the Norwegian-Iraqi infants received supplements containing iron ($p = 0.574$, data not shown). Table 5 shows the percentage of the infants receiving dairy products and iron-enriched products and also median intakes of iron among infants receiving dairy products and iron-enriched products. There were no significant differences between the two groups regarding the proportion who had received dairy products, whether it concerned any dairy products or more than 500 g dairy products per day. A higher proportion of Norwegian-Somali infants had received iron-enriched products compared to Norwegian-Iraqi infants (88% vs. 73%, respectively; $p = 0.015$). Intakes of iron did not differ significantly between infants receiving dairy products compared to infants not receiving dairy products. However, the median intake of iron was significantly higher among infants receiving iron-enriched products (8.1 mg/day) compared to infants not receiving iron-enriched products (3.7 mg/day; $p < 0.001$). Neither intake of dairy products nor intake of iron-enriched products differed significantly between genders, according to mothers' ages, number of years lived in Norway, education level, current work status or number of children.

Table 2. Median intake of foods and drinks (g/day) among all infants at 12 months of age.

	Total (n = 166)		Somali Origin (n = 89)		Iraqi Origin (n = 77)		p-Value *
	Median	(P_{25}, P_{75})	Median	(P_{25}, P_{75})	Median	(P_{25}, P_{75})	
Infant foods							
Breastmilk	0	(0, 372)	0	(0, 310)	0	(0, 454)	0.139
Infant formula	0	(0, 190)	0	(0, 103)	0	(0, 275)	0.092
Commercial infant cereal †	125	(0, 275)	200	(102, 300)	58	(0, 150)	<0.001
Commercial infant dinners	0	(0, 0)	0	(0, 0)	0	(0, 0)	0.762
Commercial fruit puree	0	(0, 3)	0	(0, 45)	0	(0, 0)	0.004
Commercial baby drinks	0	(0, 0)	0	(0, 0)	0	(0, 0)	0.884
Bread	17	(4, 31)	18	(0, 31)	16	(6, 31)	0.281
100% sifted flour	0	(0, 0)	0	(0, 0)	0	(0, 4)	0.001
<50% wholemeal flour	0	(0, 0)	0	(0, 0)	0	(0, 8)	<0.001
>50% wholemeal flour	4	(0, 21)	9	(0, 30)	0	(0, 16)	0.055
Grain products	13	(4, 30)	11	(2, 30)	14	(6, 29)	0.268
Cake	0	(0, 7)	0	(0, 0)	6	(0, 15)	<0.001
Potatoes	13	(0, 26)	16	(6, 26)	10	(0, 27)	0.090
Vegetables	37	(22, 66)	41	(26, 67)	33	(16, 64)	0.239
Meat/meat products	17	(0, 35)	5	(0, 23)	24	(11, 49)	<0.001
Fish/fish products	0	(0, 17)	9	(0, 21)	0	(0, 0)	<0.001
Eggs	0	(0, 0)	0	(0, 0)	0	(0, 22)	<0.001
Fruit and berries	43	(7, 90)	36	(0, 58)	58	(22, 121)	<0.001
Yoghurt	41	(0, 94)	57	(0, 110)	25	(0, 63)	0.009
Cheese	2	(0, 12)	1	(0, 11)	3	(0, 13)	0.512
Margarine, butter and oils	4	(2, 8)	4	(2, 8)	4	(2, 8)	0.602
Added sugar	0	(0, 0)	0	(0, 0)	0	(0, 2)	0.045
Drinks							
Cow's milk	60	(0, 320)	188	(0, 344)	26	(0, 245)	0.025
Whole milk	0	(0, 0)	0	(0, 0)	0	(0, 0)	0.623
Partly skimmed milk	31	(0, 250)	110	(0, 313)	3	(0, 185)	0.013
Skimmed milk	0	(0, 0)	0	(0, 0)	0	(0, 0)	0.127
Nido	0	(0, 0)	0	(0, 0)	0	(0, 0)	0.127
Juice	0	(0, 30)	0	(0, 30)	0	(0, 30)	0.187
Soda/squash with sugar	0	(0, 0)	0	(0, 0)	0	(0, 0)	0.872
Soda/squash, light	0	(0, 0)	0	(0, 0)	0	(0, 0)	0.397
Tea	0	(0, 0)	0	(0, 0)	0	(0, 0)	0.028
Water	180	(120, 270)	160	(98, 248)	187	(126, 299)	0.041

* Comparison of the intake of foods and drinks among infants of Somali and Iraqi origin, Mann–Whitney U test; † Prepared with water, infant formula, Nido and/or cow's milk.

Table 3. Percentage of consumers and median intake of foods and drinks (g/day) among consumers at 12 months of age.

	Total (n = 166)			Somali Origin (n = 89)			Iraqi Origin (n = 77)			p-Value
	% Consumers	Median	(P_{25}–P_{75})	% Consumers	Median	(P_{25}–P_{75})	% Consumers	Median	(P_{25}–P_{75})	*
Infant foods										
Breastmilk	43	434	(310–497)	40	372	(248–455)	47	474	(326–497)	0.414
Infant formula	31	330	(217–540)	26	291	(192–492)	36	385	(240–649)	0.143
Commercial infant cereal †	74	200	(109–300)	88	214	(125–305)	57	140	(75–298)	<0.001
Commercial infant dinners	13	95	(44–148)	14	95	(42–134)	12	98	(45–173)	0.729
Commercial fruit puree	25	50	(45–98)	34	50	(45–100)	14	45	(45–90)	0.004
Commercial baby drinks	2	40	(26–88)	2	40	(-)	3	63	(-)	0.883
Bread	79	23	(11–35)	70	25	(16–36)	90	17	(8–33)	0.002
100% sifted flour	18	12	(5–17)	8	25	(13–38)	30	10	(4–15)	<0.001
<50% wholemeal flour	24	16	(6–23)	12	19	(8–23)	36	13	(5–25)	<0.001
>50% wholemeal flour	52	21	(11–33)	57	25	(15–33)	46	17	(8–33)	0.128
Grain products	84	18	(9–32)	75	18	(9–39)	91	17	(8–31)	0.020
Cake	37	17	(6–19)	16	11	(5–14)	62	14	(6–19)	<0.001
Potatoes	71	20	(12–34)	82	18	(11–28)	58	22	(13–37)	0.001
Vegetables	95	38	(25–68)	94	43	(27–69)	96	34	(18–67)	0.605
Meat/meat products	72	24	(13–46)	60	21	(8–31)	86	32	(16–51)	<0.001
Fish/fish products	46	18	(11–37)	65	16	(10–31)	23	29	(16–43)	<0.001
Eggs	21	28	(13–45)	11	10	(4–34)	33	28	(22–45)	0.001
Fruit and berries	80	55	(31–101)	64	54	(38–88)	99	59	(25–123)	<0.001
Yoghurt	70	63	(36–107)	70	95	(50–112)	70	46	(20–75)	0.948
Cheese	53	10	(4–20)	52	10	(4–18)	55	11	(4–21)	0.713
Margarine, butter and oils	95	4	(2–8)	94	4	(2–8)	96	5	(2–8)	0.605
Added sugar	22	4	(1–8)	17	2	(1–9)	29	4	(2–7)	0.070
Drinks										
Cow's milk	68	248	(60–420)	71	286	(152–440)	64	121	(29–404)	0.327
Whole milk	17	173	(23–250)	15	245	(179–392)	20	28	(15–170)	0.403
Partly skimmed milk	58	215	(60–368)	65	239	(117–365)	51	180	(32–375)	0.058
Skimmed milk	1	11	(-)	0	-	(-)	3	11	(-)	0.126
Nido	3	156	(68–537)	1	156	(-)	5	169	(49–689)	0.126
Juice	45	31	(19–93)	38	53	(29–105)	52	30	(13–91)	0.076
Soda/squash with sugar	16	31	(15–100)	16	45	(16–100)	17	31	(14–105)	0.841
Soda/squash, light	2	43	(31–58)	3	35	(-)	1	60	(-)	0.385
Tea	8	15	(5–30)	3	63	(-)	13	13	(4–23)	0.021
Water	100	180	(120–270)	100	160	(98–248)	100	187	(126–299)	-

* Comparison of the percentage of consumers among infants of Somali and Iraqi origin, Chi-square test; † Prepared with water, infant formula, Nido and/or cow's milk.

Table 4. Average energy and nutrient intake among infants of Somali and Iraqi origin at 12 months of age.

	RI † (1–2 Years)	Total (n = 166)		Somali Origin (n = 89)		Iraqi Origin (n = 77)		p-Value *
		Median	(P_{25}–P_{75})	Median	(P_{25}–P_{75})	Median	(P_{25}–P_{75})	
Energy intake (kJ)		3945	(3235–4562)	3791	(2989–4544)	4122	(3454–4751)	0.059
Protein (E%)	10–15	14.5	(12.3–17.0)	14.8	(12.8–17.6)	13.8	(11.7–16.2)	0.074
Total fat (E%)	30–40	35.0	(30.0–39.3)	33.8	(29.9–37.6)	36.5	(32.5–40.9)	0.004
Saturated fat	<10	12.1	(10.1–14.7)	11.7	(9.7–13.7)	12.7	(11.1–15.6)	0.001
Monounsaturated fatty acids		12.6	(10.3–14.5)	11.8	(9.4–13.9)	13.4	(11.3–15.0)	0.002
Polyunsaturated fatty acids		5.7	(4.8–6.8)	5.3	(4.4–6.5)	6.1	(5.3–7.3)	0.003
Total carbohydrates (E%)	45–60	48.5	(44.8–51.9)	49.5	(46.8–51.9)	47.2	(42.9–52.1)	0.048
Added sugars	<10	3.2	(1.3–5.9)	4.0	(1.5–6.1)	2.5	(1.3–5.0)	0.063
Fibre (g)		7.4	(5.4–10.3)	7.4	(5.3–10.2)	7.4	(5.5–10.9)	0.753
Vitamin A (µg)	300 (RAE)	666	(483–878)	717	(574–933)	561	(400–874)	0.011
Vitamin D (µg)	10	12.6	(8.6–17.4)	13.9	(10.2–17.7)	11.7	(7.2–17.0)	0.029
Vitamin E (mg)	4 (µ-TE) ‡	10.5	(5.3–14.6)	12.1	(8.5–15.4)	7.3	(4.6–12.3)	<0.001
Thiamine (mg)	0.5	0.61	(0.42–0.80)	0.62	(0.42–0.80)	0.60	(0.41–0.80)	0.864
Riboflavin (mg)	0.6	0.72	(0.44–1.00)	0.77	(0.48–1.08)	0.66	(0.44–0.86)	0.039
Niacin (mg)	7 (NE) ‡	6.3	(4.4–8.6)	6.1	(4.5–8.3)	6.5	(4.4–8.7)	0.593
B6 (mg)	0.5	0.56	(0.39–0.75)	0.50	(0.37–0.73)	0.60	(0.44–0.82)	0.033
Folate (µg)	60	95	(72–135)	85	(66–121)	108	(80–151)	0.002
B12 (µg)	0.6	1.8	(0.8–2.9)	2.1	(1.1–3.0)	1.3	(0.6–2.6)	0.022
Vitamin C (mg)	25	72	(46–113)	74	(45–110)	69	(48–121)	0.755
Calcium (mg)	600	727	(519–954)	777	(587–984)	633	(480–938)	0.017
Iron (mg)	8	7.1	(4.6–10.3)	7.3	(4.9–10.3)	6.7	(4.5–11.4)	0.523
Zinc (mg)	5	5.1	(3.9–6.4)	4.8	(3.9–6.0)	5.3	(4.0–6.9)	0.117

* Comparison of infants of Somali and Iraqi origin, Mann–Whitney U test; † RI = Recommended intake ranges for macronutrients and recommended daily intakes for micronutrients. ‡ TE = tocopherol equivalent, NE = niacin equivalent.

Table 5. Percentage of Norwegian-Somali and Norwegian-Iraqi infants receiving dairy products and iron-enriched products and median iron intake (mg/day) among infants receiving dairy products and iron-enriched products.

	Total	Somali Origin	Iraqi Origin	*p*-Value [†]	Iron mg/Day		*p*-Value [‡]
	(n = 166)	(n = 89)	(n= 77)		Median	(P_{25}–P_{75})	
Dairy products							
No (n = 21)	13	9	16	0.199	9.4	(5.2–11.1)	0.327
Yes (n = 145)	87	91	84		7.0	(4.5–10.2)	
Dairy products							
≤500 g/day (n = 140)	84	80	90	0.082	7.2	(4.8–10.7)	0.170
>500 g/day (n = 26)	16	20	10		6.4	(4.2–8.9)	
Iron–enriched products *							
No (n = 32)	19	12	27	0.015	3.7	(2.6–5.5)	<0.001
Yes (n = 145)	81	88	73		8.1	(5.7–11.2)	

* Include infant formula and infant cereals; [†] Tested by Chi-square test; [‡] Tested by Mann–Whitney U test.

3.5. Factors Associated with Vitamin D Intake

Vitamin D supplements comprised more than half of the vitamin D intake in both groups (61% among Norwegian-Somali infants vs. 52% among Norwegian-Iraqi infants). Other sources of vitamin D were commercial infant cereals (19% in both groups), infant formula (7% vs. 17%) and fish and fish products (6% vs. 3%) among Norwegian-Somali and Norwegian-Iraqi infants, respectively. During the recall days, a total of 84% of the infants had received vitamin D supplements. Significantly more among the Norwegian-Somali infants compared to the Norwegian-Iraqi infants had received vitamin D supplements during the recall days (94% vs. 71%, respectively; $p < 0.001$) The median (P_{25}–P_{75}) intake of vitamin D among those receiving vitamin D supplements was 14.5 (10.8–18.1) µg/day compared to 4.1 (1.5–7.6) µg/day among those not receiving vitamin D supplements ($p < 0.001$). The intake of vitamin D supplements did not differ significantly between genders, according to mothers' ages, number of years lived in Norway, education level, current work status or number of children.

4. Discussion

The present paper describes the food and nutrient intake in a group of 12-month-old Norwegian infants of mothers who immigrated to Norway from Somalia and Iraq. The findings indicate that the nutrient intake in this group of infants in general seems to be in accordance with Norwegian dietary recommendations, with the possible exception of certain micronutrients. The intake of added sugar was low, whereas the median intake of saturated fats exceeded the recommendations.

4.1. Breastfeeding

In this group of infants with immigrant backgrounds, 40% of the Norwegian-Somali infants and 47% of the Norwegian-Iraqi infants were breastfed at 12 months of age, with a median frequency of 4.5 times a day. This is quite similar to the 46% found to be breastfed in the Norwegian national dietary survey of infants at 12 months of age who had an average breastfeeding frequency of 3.5 times a day [4]. Breastfeeding patterns have been shown to vary between ethnic subgroups in a society, but also to depend on country of residence [20–22]. Data from a nationally representative population based cohort study from Ireland [21] and the National Survey of Children's Health in the US [22] reported higher breastfeeding initiation and longer duration among immigrant mothers compared to the native mothers. However, the breastfeeding prevalence in Ireland and the US were in general lower than what is common in Norway and other Scandinavian countries [23]. This may explain the opposite findings and the greater differences between immigrant and native mothers compared to our findings.

4.2. Food Intake

Commercial infant cereals, bread, potatoes and vegetables, fruit and berries, meat/meat products and fish/fish products were the most commonly consumed foods among the Norwegian-Somali and Norwegian-Iraqi infants. These foods were also consumed by a high proportion of infants in the Norwegian national dietary survey [4]. Commercial infant dinners were consumed by a higher proportion of infants in the national dietary survey compared to infants in the present survey [4]. Homemade dinners were also more common than commercial infant dinners at 6 months of age among Norwegian-Somali and Norwegian-Iraqi infants [13]. The lower use of commercial infant dinners among the children with immigrant background may be due, as reported in a study of Somali mothers in the US, to concerns about the lack of freshness of commercially produced baby foods and also the practice of feeding children the same foods as adults [24].

One important consideration when comparing these results is that the Norwegian national dietary survey used a semi-quantitative food frequency questionnaire (FFQ) to assess the infants' dietary intake at 12 months of age [4], while the present study used repeated 24-h recalls due to limited knowledge about Norwegian-Somali and Norwegian-Iraqi infants' diets. Thus, any comparison between the two studies should be undertaken with caution because the results from the national dietary survey represent the infants' intake over a longer period of time.

4.3. Energy and Nutrient Intake

The energy intake among both Norwegian-Somali and Norwegian-Iraqi infants was lower than the mean intake of 5100 kJ reported in the national dietary survey, which only reported the energy and nutrient intake of non-breastfed infants [4]. The average daily energy requirement for boys and girls at 12 months of age is 337 kJ/kg and 333 kJ/kg, respectively, according to Nordic nutrition recommendations [25]. Based on the median weights of the infants in the sample, Norwegian-Somali infants would have an average daily energy requirement of 3440 kJ and Norwegian-Iraqi infants would have an average daily energy requirement of 3252 kJ, which is lower than the average energy intake found in this study. However, the quality of the data on weight and height may have some limitations as each child health clinic may differ in terms of accuracy in reporting the measurements and the measurements may have been taken a few weeks before or after the 24-h recalls were performed. In addition, the weights of several infants were not registered, which may also have affected the median weights reported in this study. Furthermore, breast milk amounts were only estimated and this, along with possible misreporting of dietary intakes, may give inaccurate energy intake data.

The median E% of protein, total fat and carbohydrates were all within the recommended intake ranges [18]. Saturated fat was above the recommended 10 E%. However, one of the major sources of saturated fats in the diet was breast milk, which is recommended to give to infants until 12 months of age and beyond [18]. Other main sources of saturated fats was cow's milk and meat and meat products. Parents could reduce the infants' intake of saturated fats by changing high-fat dairy products with low-fat products as well as using lean cuts of meat. The intake of added sugar was appreciably lower than the recommended upper level of 10 E%, which is a positive finding. These results are quite similar to those reported in the national dietary survey, where saturated fats accounted for 12 E% and added sugar only accounted for 4 E%. Previous studies of young children with immigrant backgrounds in Norway and other countries have suggested that high sugar and sweetened beverage intake could be prevalent in this group [9,26–28]. However, the studies from Norway were conducted several years ago, and it could be that the trend of reducing the intake of added sugar, which has been reflected in the national dietary surveys, is also the case for this group of children. In the national dietary surveys, the intake of added sugar decreased from 10 E% in 1999 to 4 E% in 2007 due to the reduced intake of sugary drinks among Norwegian infants and the reduced levels of added sugar in commercial infant products [4,29]. In addition, a qualitative survey among Somali-born mothers in Norway revealed that most mothers thought that their infants at 12 months were too young to be given sugar [30]. However, the older siblings were usually eating candy and the majority of mothers had sweets available at home at all times, which may indicate that sweets and sugary drinks may be introduced at a later stage in the child's life.

4.4. Factors Associated with Iron Intake

Iron deficiency has been reported to be prevalent among both immigrant and non-immigrant children in Europe [7,31,32], however, some studies have suggested a higher prevalence among immigrant children [7,32]. The consumption of milk with low iron content and the excessive consumption of cow's milk have been reported in the literature to be factors that may cause iron deficiency [32,33]. On the other hand, iron-enriched products may be a protective factor against inadequate iron intake [32].

In the present study, we found no significant differences in iron intake among infants who consumed dairy products compared to those who did not consume dairy products. There were no significant differences among those who consumed more than 500 g/day of dairy products compared to those who consumed less. Still, high consumption of cow's milk is not recommended as it may inhibit the iron absorption [34]. Higher iron intakes were observed among infants who received iron-enriched products compared to those who did not receive these products. This has also been found among one-year-old children in other studies [12,35]. The majority of infants in the present study received iron-enriched products; however, the median intake of iron was lower than the RI [18] and the intake reported in the national dietary survey (12.8 mg/day) [4] for both Norwegian-Somali and Norwegian-Iraqi infants. The higher intakes of iron among the infants in the national dietary survey may be explained by a lower consumption of cow's milk (92 g/day), with only 51% consumers, and a higher consumption of commercial infant cereals (293 g/day) and infant formula (144 g/day), with 82% and 40% consumers, respectively [4]. Commercial infant cereals and infant formula were the two major sources of iron in the diet of the infants in the national dietary survey, followed by bread and meat/meat products [4].

4.5. Factors Associated with Vitamin D Intake

The intake of vitamin D exceeded the recommended levels for both Norwegian-Somali and Norwegian-Iraqi infants. Severe vitamin D deficiency has been reported to be prevalent among 6-week-old infants of immigrant backgrounds in Norway who did not receive vitamin D supplements [8]. In the present study, vitamin D supplements were given to the majority of Norwegian-Somali and Norwegian-Iraqi infants, as was seen in the 6-month survey [13]. The proportion was lower among the Norwegian-Iraqi infants. Vitamin D supplements were more commonly given in this sample compared to the 67% reported in the national dietary survey; those infants also had lower average intake of vitamin D (6.8 μg/day) [4]. Those not receiving vitamin D supplements in the present survey were more likely to have much lower intakes of vitamin D than those receiving vitamin D supplements and also lower intakes than the RI of 10 μg/day [18]. Vitamin D supplementation has recently been reported by Moffat et al. [36] to be almost similar and high among both immigrants and Canadian-born mothers, although less so for refugee mothers. According to their findings, current public education on vitamin D supplementation delivered by nurses and other health educators seems to be similarly effective for Canadian and immigrant parents [36]. A study by Madar et al. showed significant improvement in vitamin D status among infants with immigrant backgrounds in Norway after receiving free vitamin D supply together with tailor-made information handouts [37]. Vitamin D supplements are provided for free to of non-Western immigrant backgrounds at child health centres in Norway due to concerns about inadequate vitamin D intakes in this group. [38]. The findings of this study suggest that this information may have reached the majority of the participating mothers.

4.6. Strengths and Limitations of the Study

Two very specific subgroups of the Norwegian population were chosen for the study, which is an important strength of the survey. According to lists from the National Population Register, the participating Norwegian-Somali and Norwegian-Iraqi infants accounted for approximately 19% and 27%, respectively, of all Norwegian-Somali and Norwegian-Iraqi infants who turned 12 months old during the recruitment period in the three Norwegian counties included. Recruitment challenges are widely reported in studies among immigrant populations [39], and was also observed in the present study. The advantage was the use of bilingual field workers, which enabled the recruitment of mothers with limited Norwegian language skills. A possible limitation is the relatively large number of mothers lost to follow-up at 12 months, although new mothers were recruited. However, a comparison of background characteristics from the 6-month survey [13] and a description of the two immigrant groups by Statistics Norway [40] suggest that the mothers are to some extent representative of Somali-born and Iraqi-born mothers in these three counties in Norway.

In general, the dietary assessment of infants can be complicated by the fact that dietary habits change rapidly in infancy. A review by Burrows et al. has indicated that weighed food records may provide the best dietary estimates for younger children from 0.5 to 4 years old [41]. However, the 24-h multiple-pass recall is less time consuming and is reportedly used more frequently among immigrant populations, along with FFQs [39,42]. The recalls were mainly performed face-to-face, which may be a benefit as potential misunderstandings can be easily clarified in a personal interview. On the other hand, the presence of a field worker may cause a perception of authority on the part of the mothers, which could lead to social desirability response bias [43].

Although the macronutrient composition may reflect the true dietary practices of the two immigrant groups, reporting errors such as underreporting or overreporting may contribute to apparently low or high intakes of certain foods [41]. For infants in particular, not all foods served are necessarily consumed as some is wasted. Furthermore, the mothers may share the responsibility for their children with other adults (e.g., partners, grandparents and day-care), and it may be more difficult for the mothers to assess children's intake during the hours they were not present [44].

In addition, biochemical indicators of iron and vitamin D status were not measured in the present study, which is necessary in order to assess the infants' iron and vitamin D status.

5. Conclusions

The findings of this study indicate that the food and nutrient intake of Norwegian-Somali and Norwegian-Iraqi infants in general seems to be in accordance with the Norwegian dietary recommendations. The intake of dairy products was generally higher among Norwegian-Somali infants compared to Norwegian-Iraqi infants, but dairy product intake did not seem to affect iron intake. Iron-enriched products and vitamin D supplements were important sources of the infants' iron and vitamin D intake. Vitamin D supplements and foods rich in iron should continue to be promoted. Infants with immigrant backgrounds are excluded from the Norwegian national dietary surveys, and the present study contributes with information about food and nutrient intake among two of these groups living in Norway. More research to investigate infant feeding practices among immigrant groups in Norway is needed.

Acknowledgments: The present study was financed and supported by the Norwegian Research Council (grant number 213460/H10). We would like to thank the field workers who assisted with the data collection and also the mothers/infants who participated in the study.

Author Contributions: N.K.G. designed the study and participated in the data collection, carried out the data analysis and wrote the manuscript. L.F.A. and L.E.T. designed the study, assisted in the data analysis and provided advice during all stages of the work. C.S.K. and I.K. coded the information from the 24-h recalls. All authors contributed to the development of the manuscript, including the drafting and editing of the manuscript. All authors read and approved the final manuscript.

References

1. Chomtho, S.; Wells, J.C.; Williams, J.E.; Davies, P.S.; Lucas, A.; Fewtrell, M.S. Infant growth and later body composition: Evidence from the 4-component model. *Am. J. Clin. Nutr.* **2008**, *87*, 1776–1784. [PubMed]
2. Victora, C.G. Nutrition in early life: A global priority. *Lancet* **2009**, *374*, 1123–1125. [CrossRef]
3. Øverby, N.C.; Kristiansen, A.L.; Andersen, L.F.; Lande, B. *Spedkost—6 Måneder. Landsomfattende Kostholdsundersøkelse Blant 6 Måneder Gamle Barn (Norwegian National Dietary Survey among 6-Month Old Infants)*; Norwegian Directorate of Health: Oslo, Norway, 2008.
4. Øverby, N.C.; Kristiansen, A.L.; Andersen, L.F.; Lande, B. *Spedkost—12 Måneder. Landsomfattende Kostholdsundersøkelse Blant 12 Måneder Gamle Barn (Norwegian National Dietary Survey among 12-Month Old Infants)*; Norwegian Directorate of Health: Oslo, Norway, 2009.
5. Kristiansen, A.L.; Andersen, L.F.; Lande, B. *Småbarnskost—2 år. Landsomfattende Kostholdesundersøkelse Blant 2 år Gamle Barn (Norwegian National Dietary Survey among 2-Year Old Children)*; Norwegian Directorate of Health: Oslo, Norway, 2009.
6. Lande, B.; Andersen, L.F.; Bærug, A.; Trygg, K.; Lund-Larsen, K.; Bjørneboe, G.E.A. Development of a method for use in a national representative dietary survey among norwegian infants and children—Spedkost/småbarnskost. *Nor. J. Epidemiol.* **2000**, *10*, 43–50.
7. Wandel, M.; Fagerli, R.A.; Olsen, P.T.; BorchIohnsen, B.; Ek, J. Iron status and weaning practices among norwegian and immigrant infants. *Nutr. Res.* **1996**, *16*, 251–265. [CrossRef]

8. Madar, A.A.; Stene, L.C.; Meyer, H.E. Vitamin d status among immigrant mothers from pakistan, turkey and somalia and their infants attending child health clinics in Norway. *Br. J. Nutr.* **2009**, *101*, 1052–1058. [CrossRef] [PubMed]
9. Kumar, B.; Wandel, M. Nutritional challenges among immigrant children and youth in Norway. In *Global Migration and Education*; Adams, L.D., Kirova, A., Eds.; Lawrence Erlbaum Associates: Mahwah, NJ, USA, 2007; pp. 67–81.
10. Maguire, J.L.; Lebovic, G.; Kandasamy, S.; Khovratovich, M.; Mamdani, M.; Birken, C.S.; Parkin, P.C.; Kids, T.A. The relationship between cow's milk and stores of vitamin d and iron in early childhood. *Pediatrics* **2013**, *131*, e144–e151. [CrossRef] [PubMed]
11. Soh, P.; Ferguson, E.L.; McKenzie, J.E.; Homs, M.Y.; Gibson, R.S. Iron deficiency and risk factors for lower iron stores in 6–24-month-old New Zealanders. *Eur. J. Clin. Nutr.* **2004**, *58*, 71–79. [CrossRef] [PubMed]
12. Thorisdottir, A.V.; Ramel, A.; Palsson, G.I.; Tomasson, H.; Thorsdottir, I. Iron status of one-year-olds and association with breast milk, cow's milk or formula in late infancy. *Eur. J. Nutr.* **2013**, *52*, 1661–1668. [CrossRef] [PubMed]
13. Grewal, N.K.; Andersen, L.F.; Sellen, D.; Mosdol, A.; Torheim, L.E. Breast-feeding and complementary feeding practices in the first 6 months of life among norwegian-somali and norwegian-iraqi infants: The innbakost survey. *Public Health Nutr.* **2016**, *19*, 703–715. [CrossRef] [PubMed]
14. Statistics Norway. Statbank Norway. Available online: http://www.ssb.no/statistikkbanken/SelectTable/hovedtabellHjem.asp?KortNavnWeb=innvbef&CMSSubjectArea=befolkning&StatVariant=&PLanguage=0&checked=true (accessed on 10 July 2015).
15. Grewal, N.K.; Mosdol, A.; Aunan, M.B.; Monsen, C.; Torheim, L.E. Development and pilot testing of 24-h multiple-pass recall to assess dietary intake of toddlers of somali- and iraqi-born mothers living in Norway. *Nutrients* **2014**, *6*, 2333–2347. [CrossRef] [PubMed]
16. Totland, T.H.; Melnæs, B.K.; Lundberg-Hallén, N.; Helland-Kigen, K.M.; Lund-Blix, N.A.; Myhre, J.B.; Johansen, A.M.W.; Løken, E.B.; Andersen, L.F. *Norkost 3—En Landsomfattende Kostholdsundersøkelse Blant Menn og Kvinner i Norge i Alderen 18–70 år, 2010–2011 (Norwegian National Dietary Survey among Adults 18–70 Years, 2010–2011)*; Norwegian Directorate of Health: Oslo, Norway, 2012.
17. Bergström, L. *Nutrient Losses and Gains in the Preparation of Foods*; National Food Administration: Uppsala, Sweden, 1994.
18. Norwegian Directorate for Health. *Recommendations for Diet, Nutrition and Physical Activity (Anbefalinger om Kosthold, Ernæring og Fysisk Aktivitet)*; Norwegian Directorate of Health: Oslo, Norway, 2014.
19. World Health Organization. The WHO Child Growth Standards. Available online: http://www.who.int/childgrowth/standards/en/ (accessed on 10 April 2015).
20. Van Rossem, L.; Vogel, I.; Steegers, E.A.P.; Moll, H.A.; Jaddoe, V.W.V.; Hofman, A.; Mackenbach, J.P.; Raat, H. Breastfeeding patterns among ethnic minorities: The generation r study. *J. Epidemiol. Community Health* **2010**, *64*, 1080–1085. [CrossRef] [PubMed]
21. Ladewig, E.L.; Hayes, C.; Browne, J.; Layte, R.; Reulbach, U. The influence of ethnicity on breastfeeding rates in Ireland: A cross-sectional study. *J. Epidemiol. Community Health* **2014**, *68*, 356–362. [CrossRef] [PubMed]
22. Singh, G.K.; Kogan, M.D.; Dee, D.L. Nativity/immigrant status, race/ethnicity, and socioeconomic determinants of breastfeeding initiation and duration in the United States, 2003. *Pediatrics* **2007**, *119* (Suppl. S1), S38–S46. [CrossRef] [PubMed]
23. Ibanez, G.; Martin, N.; Denantes, M.; Saurel-Cubizolles, M.J.; Ringa, V.; Magnier, A.M. Prevalence of breastfeeding in industrialized countries. *Rev. Epidemiol. Sante Publique* **2012**, *60*, 305–320. [CrossRef] [PubMed]
24. Steinman, L.; Doescher, M.; Keppel, G.A.; Pak-Gorstein, S.; Graham, E.; Haq, A.; Johnson, D.B.; Spicer, P. Understanding infant feeding beliefs, practices and preferred nutrition education and health provider approaches: An exploratory study with somali mothers in the USA. *Mater. Child Nutr.* **2010**, *6*, 67–88. [CrossRef] [PubMed]
25. Nordic Councel of Ministers. *Nordic Nutrition Recommendations 2012 Part 1: Summary, Principles and Use*; Nordic Council of Ministers: Copenhagen, Denmark, 2013.
26. Schneider, S.; Jerusalem, M.; Mente, J.; De Bock, F. Sweets consumption of preschool children—Extent, context, and consumption patterns. *Clin. Oral Investig.* **2013**, *17*, 1301–1309. [CrossRef] [PubMed]

27. De Hoog, M.L.; Kleinman, K.P.; Gillman, M.W.; Vrijkotte, T.G.; van Eijsden, M.; Taveras, E.M. Racial/ethnic and immigrant differences in early childhood diet quality. *Public Health Nutr.* **2014**, *17*, 1308–1317. [CrossRef] [PubMed]
28. Sahota, P.; Gatenby, L.A.; Greenwood, D.C.; Bryant, M.; Robinson, S.; Wright, J. Ethnic differences in dietary intake at age 12 and 18 months: The born in Bradford 1000 study. *Public Health Nutr.* **2015**, *19*, 1–9. [CrossRef] [PubMed]
29. Lande, B.; Andersen, L.F. *Spedkost 12 Måneder—Landsomfattende Kostholdsundersøkelse Blant Spedbarn i Norge (Norwegian National Dietary Survey among 12-Month Old Infants)*; Norwegian Directorate of Health: Oslo, Norway, 2005.
30. Lyngstad, J. Understanding Infant Feeding Practices, Relations to the Health Clinic and Experiences of Receiving Conflicting Advices: A Qualitative Study with Somali Mothers Living in Oslo. Master's Thesis, Faculty of Health Sciences, Department of Health, Nutrition and Management, Oslo and Akershus University College of Applied Sciences, Oslo, Norway, 2014.
31. Bramhagen, A.C.; Svahn, J.; Hallstrom, I.; Axelsson, I. Factors influencing iron nutrition among one-year-old healthy children in Sweden. *J. Clin. Nurs.* **2011**, *20*, 1887–1894. [CrossRef] [PubMed]
32. Verga, M.E.; Widmeier-Pasche, V.; Beck-Popovic, M.; Pauchard, J.Y.; Gehri, M. Iron deficiency in infancy: Is an immigrant more at risk? *Swiss Med. Wkly.* **2014**, *144*, w14065. [CrossRef] [PubMed]
33. Ziegler, E.E. Consumption of cow's milk as a cause of iron deficiency in infants and toddlers. *Nutr. Rev.* **2011**, *69* (Suppl. S1), S37–S42. [CrossRef] [PubMed]
34. Domellof, M.; Braegger, C.; Campoy, C.; Colomb, V.; Decsi, T.; Fewtrell, M.; Hojsak, I.; Mihatsch, W.; Molgaard, C.; Shamir, R.; et al. Iron requirements of infants and toddlers. *J. Pediatr. Gastroenterol. Nutr.* **2014**, *58*, 119–129. [CrossRef] [PubMed]
35. Virtanen, M.A.; Svahn, C.J.; Viinikka, L.U.; Raiha, N.C.; Siimes, M.A.; Axelsson, I.E. Iron-fortified and unfortified cow's milk: Effects on iron intakes and iron status in young children. *Acta Paediatr.* **2001**, *90*, 724–731. [CrossRef] [PubMed]
36. Moffat, T.; Sellen, D.; Wilson, W.; Anderson, L.; Chadwick, S.; Amarra, S. Comparison of infant vitamin d supplement use among Canadian-born, immigrant, and refugee mothers. *J. Transcult. Nurs.* **2015**, *26*, 261–269. [CrossRef] [PubMed]
37. Madar, A.A.; Klepp, K.I.; Meyer, H.E. Effect of free vitamin D (2) drops on serum 25-hydroxyvitamin d in infants with immigrant origin: A cluster randomized controlled trial. *Eur. J. Clin. Nutr.* **2009**, *63*, 478–484. [CrossRef] [PubMed]
38. Norwegian Directorate of Health. Gratis Vitamin D-tilskudd Til Spedbarn Med IKKE-Vestlig Innvandrerbakgrunn (Free Vitamin D Supplement to Infants with Non-Western Immigrant Backgrounds). Available online: http://www.matportalen.no/kosthold_og_helse/tema/kosttilskudd/gratis_vitamin_d-tilskudd_til_spedbarn_med_ikke-vestlig_innvandrerbakgrunn (accessed on 12 June 2015).
39. Ngo, J.; Gurinovic, M.; Frost-Andersen, L.; Serra-Majem, L. How dietary intake methodology is adapted for use in European immigrant population groups—A review. *Br. J. Nutr.* **2009**, *101* (Suppl. S2), S86–S94. [CrossRef] [PubMed]
40. Henriksen, K. *Levekår og Kjønnsforskjeller Blant Innvandrere Fra ti Land (Living Conditions and Gender Differences among Immigrants from Ten Countries)*; Statistics Norway: Oslo, Norway, 2010.
41. Burrows, T.L.; Martin, R.J.; Collins, C.E. A systematic review of the validity of dietary assessment methods in children when compared with the method of doubly labeled water. *J. Am. Diet. Assoc.* **2010**, *110*, 1501–1510. [CrossRef] [PubMed]
42. Garduno-Diaz, S.D.; Husain, W.; Ashkanani, F.; Khokhar, S. Meeting challenges related to the dietary assessment of ethnic minority populations. *J. Hum. Nutr. Diet.* **2014**, *27*, 358–366. [CrossRef] [PubMed]
43. Hebert, J.R.; Clemow, L.; Pbert, L.; Ockene, I.S.; Ockene, J.K. Social desirability bias in dietary self-report may compromise the validity of dietary intake measures. *Int. J. Epidemiol.* **1995**, *24*, 389–398. [CrossRef] [PubMed]
44. Livingstone, M.B.; Robson, P.J.; Wallace, J.M. Issues in dietary intake assessment of children and adolescents. *Br. J. Nutr.* **2004**, *92* (Suppl. S2), S213–S222. [CrossRef] [PubMed]

16

Food Consumption and Nutrient Intake by Children Aged 10 to 48 Months Attending Day Care in The Netherlands

R. Alexandra Goldbohm [1,*], Carina M. Rubingh [2], Caren I. Lanting [1,*] and Koen F. M. Joosten [3]

[1] Netherlands Organisation for Applied Scientific Research TNO, Schipholweg 77–89, Leiden 2316 ZL, The Netherlands

[2] Netherlands Organisation for Applied Scientific Research TNO, Utrechtseweg 48, Zeist 3700 AJ, The Netherlands; carina.dejong@tno.nl

[3] Erasmus University Medical Centre, Erasmus MC-Sophia Children's Hospital, Dr. Molewaterplein 60, Rotterdam 3015 GJ, The Netherlands; k.joosten@erasmusmc.nl

* Correspondence: ra.goldbohm@ziggo.nl (R.A.G.); caren.lanting@tno.nl (C.I.L.)

Abstract: The diet of young children is an important determinant of long-term health effects, such as overweight and obesity. We analyzed two-day food consumption records from 1526 young children (10–48 months old) attending 199 daycare centers across The Netherlands. Data were observed and recorded in diaries by caregivers at the day nursery and by parents at home on days that the children attended the daycare center. According to national and European reference values, the children had an adequate nutrient intake with exception of low intakes of total fat, *n*-3 fatty acids from fish and possibly iron. Intakes of energy and protein were substantially higher than recommended and part of the population exceeded the tolerable upper intake levels for sodium, zinc and retinol. Consumption of fruit, fats, fish, and fluids was substantially less than recommended. The children used mostly (semi-)skimmed milk products and non-refined bread and cereals, as recommended. Two thirds of the consumed beverages, however, contained sugar and contributed substantially to energy intake. In young children, low intakes of *n*-3 fatty acids and iron are a potential matter of concern, as are the high intakes of energy, protein, sugared beverages, and milk, since these may increase the risk of becoming overweight.

Keywords: young children; nutrition; dietary habits; childcare

---

1. Introduction

Proper nutrition of young children promotes optimal growth and development. The right amount of energy and nutrients also reduces the risk for developing overweight and obesity, dental caries, and gastrointestinal problems like constipation and diarrhea. In addition, there is some evidence that diet quality and especially breakfast consumption is related to cognitive functioning and academic performance of children [1,2]. Unfavorable dietary habits may have long-term implications, especially since childhood overweight tends to track into adulthood [3] and overweight and obesity are major risk factors for cardiovascular disease, type 2 diabetes mellitus, and cancer [4]. Early childhood is a critical period for prevention of diet-related disease later in life; dietary habits tend to be established at an early age and are maintained throughout later life [5].

In The Netherlands, about 40% of children until four years of age attend childcare [6]. Childcare providers are in a unique position to educate parents about healthy eating, to encourage children to eat healthy, and to provide a healthy environment for children to eat, grow and develop. In the current study, food consumption was registered in a large population of young children

(10–48 months old) attending day care across The Netherlands. Intakes of energy, macro- and micronutrients and on consumption of a complete set of food groups (e.g., bread, milk products, sweetened beverages) were established and compared with current recommendations. Some of the results have been published previously [7,8]; however, these were based on a smaller sample and only comprised a small selection of macronutrients and a few food groups.

2. Materials and Methods

2.1. Study Population

Details on the recruitment methods were previously published [7]. In brief, 199 childcare centers located across the Netherlands, were recruited between 2011 and 2014 to participate in the study, which was originally offered to all childcare centers in The Netherlands by Nutricia Nederland BV, Zoetermeer, The Netherlands, as a service to support their nutrition policy. Children between the age of 10 and 48 months who were attending the nursery for at least two days per week could participate in the study. The manager of the childcare center invited the children's parents to participate in the study and obtained written and signed informed consent from them. The study has been conducted in accordance with the Declaration of Helsinki and complied with national and EU data protection laws (Directive 95/46/EC). According to Dutch law, approval by a medical-ethical committee is exempted for this type of observational research.

2.2. Dietary Intake Assessment

Details on the assessment methods were previously published [7,8]. In brief, at the childcare center, food and beverage consumption was recorded on a structured poster by the carers for all children participating in the study during two days. Dutch children attending a childcare center usually eat breakfast and the main (hot) meal at home and lunch and a morning and afternoon snack at the childcare center. Few childcare centers serve a hot meal during lunchtime or in the evening. For the food and beverages consumed at home, a parent completed a structured diary at the same two days. Berdien van Wezel Dieticians (The Hague, The Netherlands), were responsible for data collection. Trained dieticians instructed carers and parents, supervised the recording and were responsible for coding and computer entry of the consumption data using the FoodFigures system [9].

2.3. Data Processing

A raw data set containing, for each child, records with food codes and a quantity (g or mL), eating occasion (e.g., breakfast), day and location (home or childcare center) per food code was exported from the FoodFigures system. Data checking and calculation of nutrient intake and food group consumption was performed using a software application in SAS [10,11] specifically developed for processing of dietary data [12]. The Dutch food composition database (NEVO), edition 2013, was used for calculation of nutrient intake [13]. In this edition of the NEVO database, dietary fiber is considered an energy-contributing nutrient (2 kcal/g fiber). A few food codes were derived from the NEVO database of 2011 or from an additional food composition database. Data were checked for inconsistencies and completeness of the records, i.e., two days, both at the childcare center and at home, should be present for each child. Potential outliers at the high and the low end of the quantity of consumed foods were listed and checked in the original diaries and posters. After correction of the database, a final check on potential outliers of the calculated nutrient intake was performed.

2.4. Data Analysis

Mean daily energy and nutrient intake was calculated for all children and for each age group (i.e., 10 and 11 months old and 1, 2 and 3 years old, which included children ⩾12–<24 months, ⩾24–<36 months, and ⩾36–<48 months, respectively). As (energy-adjusted) nutrient intake differed very little between boys and girls, their results are not separately presented. We used the "Statistical Program to

Assess Dietary Exposure" (SPADE) to transform the nutrient intake from the two days into a theoretical "usual" intake distribution of the population [14]. For all nutrients, we used the SPADE model for daily intakes, except for *n*-3 fish fatty acids and folic acid for which the module for episodical intakes was used and docosahexaenoic acid, for which no model was found that fitted the required criteria. We followed the European Food Safety Authority's (EFSA) guidance [15] to compare the usual intake distribution with dietary reference values (specifically, Adequate Intake and Tolerable Upper Intake Levels (TUIL)) as established by the Health Council of The Netherlands (HCN) [16–18] and, if relevant, more recent ones from the EFSA [19]. For this comparison, we assumed that the usual intake based on the two weekdays that the children attended the childcare center is representative for their true usual intake.

Furthermore, individual foods were divided into food groups to calculate the mean daily consumption of each food group. We defined several food group classifications. The first, a classic one, was based on type of food (e.g., meat, meat products, and poultry; bread; fruit). We used a second one, based on the food based dietary guidelines ("Schijf van Vijf") published by The Netherlands Nutrition Centre (NNC) [20], to compare mean daily consumption of the relevant food groups with the recommendations that apply to children from 1 to 3 years old. Finally, we subdivided the foods grouped according to the NNC classification in preferable or neutral foods and foods that should be eaten by exception only [21]. Preferable foods contribute positively to a diet preventive for chronic diseases, whereas "by exception" foods contribute negatively to such a diet. Classification of foods is based on their content of saturated fat, trans fat, sodium, dietary fiber and added sugar. For example, full-fat milk products (as opposed to skimmed milk) are classified as by-exception food, just as milk products and beverages with added sugar. The contribution of these food groups to the intake of selected nutrients was also calculated. Furthermore, we simulated the effect of replacing liquid cow's milk by formula among exclusive cow's milk users on usual iron and protein intake. In this simulation, liquid cow's milk was replaced by young children's formula (with a nutrient composition according to Nutrilon, Zoetermeer, The Netherlands, a brand from the Nutricia company).

3. Results

3.1. Study Population

Table 1 presents the characteristics of the study population (n = 1526). Body weight and height are not presented, as they were not considered sufficiently accurate and comprised a high proportion of missing values.

Table 1. Characteristics of the study population.

		n	%
Gender	Boy	759	49.7
	Girl	683	44.8
	Missing	84	5.5
Age	10–11 months old	31	2.0
	1 year old	411	26.9
	2 years old	497	32.6
	3 years old	410	26.9
	Missing	177	11.6
Zip-code based socioeconomic status of childcare centers	Low	381	25.0
	Medium	848	55.6
	High	218	14.3
	Missing	79	5.2
Number of days per week that the child attended childcare center	2 days	939	61.5
	3 days	348	22.8
	4 days	68	4.5
	5 days	16	1.1
	Missing	155	10.2
Hot meal at childcare center	Yes	315	20.6
	No	1189	77.9
	Missing	22	1.4

Between 19 and 67 (mean 41) food records were available per child. A food record comprises the consumption of a given quantity of a given food or beverage at a given occasion (e.g., breakfast). 14 children were breastfed (11 of whom were 12 months or younger).

3.2. Nutrient Intake

Table 2 displays the average daily intake of macronutrients (mean and standard deviation), both in absolute amount as in energy density. Boys had a higher mean energy intake than girls (5483 kJ versus 5271 kJ). All gender differences in intake of macronutrients were attributable to the higher energy intake by boys. However, the intake relative to energy was very similar for boys and girls (see supplementary materials Table S1). The absolute intakes of micronutrients (Table 2) were also somewhat higher for boys than for girls (see supplementary materials Table S1). According to their parents, 92% of the children had received a vitamin D supplement on at least one of the two study days.

Table 2. Mean daily nutrient intake by children attending childcare by age (mean of 2 days).

		Total Group (n = 1526) [1]		10–11 Months (n = 31)		1 Year (n = 411)		2 Years (n = 497)		3 Years (n = 410)	
Nutrient	**Unit**	**Mean**	**SD**	**Mean**	**SD**	**Mean**	**SD**	**Mean**	**SD**	**Mean**	**SD**
Energy	kJ	5383	958	4241	795	4954	822	5424	872	5841	923
Protein	g	45	9	32	8	43	9	45	8	48	10
	en%	14.1	2.2	12.6	2.2	14.6	2.4	13.9	2.0	13.9	2.1
Carbohydrates	g	174	34	136	27	159	30	177	32	189	33
	en%	54.4	5.1	54.2	5.9	54	5.3	54.8	5.0	54.5	4.8
Mono- and disaccharides	g	100	25	79	18	91	24	102	24	108	26
	en%	31.2	5.7	31.4	5.5	30.7	6.1	31.7	5.3	31.1	5.7
Polysaccharides	g	75	16	58	15	69	14	75	15	81	16
	en%	23.4	3.4	23.1	3.6	23.6	3.6	23.3	3.1	23.4	3.3
Fat	g	42	11	34	10	38	10	42	10	45	11
	en%	29.1	4.6	30.4	5.5	28.7	4.8	28.9	4.5	29.3	4.3
Saturated fatty acids	g	14.8	3.8	12.6	4.7	13.5	3.4	14.8	3.7	16.1	3.8
	en%	10.4	1.8	11.2	2.8	10.3	1.9	10.3	1.8	10.4	1.7
Monounsaturated fatty acids	g	14.4	4.5	11.7	4.3	12.9	4.2	14.4	4.5	15.8	4.4
	en%	10.0	2.3	10.4	3.0	9.8	2.4	9.9	2.3	10.2	2.2
Polyunsaturated fatty acids (PUFA)	g	8.6	3.2	6.7	2.3	8.0	3.1	8.6	3.0	9.4	3.4
	en%	6.0	1.8	5.9	1.5	6.1	1.9	5.9	1.7	6.0	1.7
n-3 PUFA	g	1.0	0.4	0.9	0.3	1.0	0.3	1.0	0.4	1.1	0.4
	en%	0.7	0.2	0.8	0.2	0.7	0.2	0.7	0.2	0.7	0.2
ALA (C18:3 (*n*-3) *cis*)	g	1.0	0.3	0.8	0.3	0.9	0.3	1.0	0.3	1.0	0.4
	en%	0.7	0.2	0.7	0.2	0.7	0.2	0.7	0.2	0.7	0.2
EPA (C20:5 (*n*-3) *cis*)	g	0.01	0.03	0.02	0.03	0.02	0.03	0.01	0.02	0.01	0.03
	en%	0	0	0	0	0	0	0	0	0	0
DHA (C22:6 (*n*-3) *cis*)	g	0.02	0.04	0.02	0.04	0.02	0.05	0.02	0.04	0.02	0.04
	en%	0	0	0	0	0	0	0	0	0	0
n-6 PUFA	g	7.3	2.8	5.4	2.0	6.8	2.7	7.3	2.6	8.0	3.0
	en%	5.1	1.6	4.8	1.4	5.1	1.7	5.0	1.5	5.1	1.5
Linoleic acid (C18:2 (*n*-6) *cis*)	g	7.3	2.8	5.4	2.0	6.7	2.7	7.2	2.6	7.9	3.0
	en%	5.0	1.6	4.8	1.4	5.1	1.7	5.0	1.5	5.1	1.5
Trans-unsaturated fatty acids	g	0.4	0.2	0.3	0.2	0.4	0.2	0.4	0.2	0.5	0.2
	en%	0.3	0.1	0.2	0.1	0.3	0.1	0.3	0.1	0.3	0.1
Cholesterol	mg	76.1	38.0	45.9	45.9	69.2	37.2	77.4	38.6	84.4	38.2

Table 2. *Cont.*

Nutrient	Unit	Total Group (*n* = 1526) [1] Mean	SD	10–11 Months (*n* = 31) Mean	SD	1 Year (*n* = 411) Mean	SD	2 Years (*n* = 497) Mean	SD	3 Years (*n* = 410) Mean	SD
Dietary fiber	g	12.6	2.7	12.4	2.6	12.4	2.7	12.5	2.6	13.1	2.7
	g/MJ	2.4	0.4	3.0	0.5	2.5	0.5	2.3	0.4	2.3	0.4
Water	g	1045	248	885	219	988	240	1047	231	1133	245
Sodium	mg	1273	359	790	266	1117	301	1317	340	1420	341
Potassium	mg	1923	405	1435	420	1864	391	1934	377	2010	402
Phosphorus	mg	943	199	715	190	907	189	941	186	997	206
Magnesium	mg	181	38	134	29	172	36	181	34	194	40
Iron	mg	6.3	2.0	8.4	2.5	6.5	2.4	6.0	1.7	6.1	1.7
Calcium	mg	735	186	684	200	734	177	720	177	745	202
Copper	mg	0.61	0.15	0.59	0.13	0.58	0.14	0.60	0.14	0.66	0.15
Selenium	µg	22	6	21	6	21	6	22	6	24	6
Zinc	mg	6.0	1.4	6.0	1.4	6.0	1.4	5.9	1.4	6.1	1.5
Iodine	µg	120	30	118	22	117	31	119	30	124	31
Vitamin A (RAE)	µg	846	568	753	448	746	483	834	568	902	626
Retinol	µg	731	560	648	434	636	479	712	558	787	618
Thiamin (Vitamin B_1)	mg	0.58	0.17	0.60	0.20	0.58	0.17	0.57	0.17	0.57	0.17
Riboflavin (Vitamin B_2)	mg	1.13	0.29	0.97	0.24	1.09	0.27	1.12	0.29	1.17	0.31
Niacin	mg	7.7	2.5	6.4	2.6	7.4	2.4	7.7	2.5	8.1	2.6
Vitamin B6	mg	0.80	0.27	0.69	0.28	0.79	0.25	0.81	0.28	0.82	0.28
Folate (DFE)	µg	156	47	177	49	162	47	154	50	154	46
Vitamin B_{12}	µg	2.95	1.06	1.95	0.79	2.73	0.90	2.94	1.00	3.18	1.19
Vitamin C	mg	93	35	105	29	94	35	92	35	92	35
Vitamin D	µg	3.7	2.8	8.4	3.7	4.7	3.5	3.2	2.1	2.8	1.8
Vitamin E	mg	6.8	2.8	8.0	2.9	6.8	3.0	6.6	2.7	7.0	2.7

[1] The total number of children does not equal the sum of those in the age groups, due to missing data on age. en%: energy percent, i.e., the energy that the nutrient contributes to the total energy intake of a person, expressed as percentage; ALA: alpha-linolenic acid; EPA: eicosapentaenoic acid; DHA: docosahexaenoic acid; RAE: retinol activity equivalents; DFE: dietary folate equivalents; SD: standard deviation

Comparing the transformed usual intake distribution with dietary reference values the following results were found. The intake of most of the assessed macro- and micronutrients was found to be adequate (see supplementary materials Table S2). Exceptions were encountered for:

- Energy: Mean daily intake, both for boys (5.5 MJ) and girls (5.3 MJ), was higher than the requirement established by the HCN (5 MJ for boys, 4.5 MJ for girls between 1 and 3 years old [16] and much higher than the intake considered adequate according to EFSA (3.3–4.9 MJ for boys, 3.0–4.6 MJ for girls [19]).
- Protein: Median usual intake (45 g, 14 energy percent) was approximately three times higher than the Adequate Intake of 5 energy percent [16] or the Population Reference Intake of 11–13 g [19]. Among the children below 1 year, 26% exceeded the TUIL of 15 energy percent for this age. If, among the children that used exclusively cow's milk, liquid cow's milk would be substituted by formula, median usual protein intake would decrease from 14.2 to 12.3 energy percent.
- Fat: Intake was relatively low (29 energy percent). The mean usual intake was within the recommended range (25–40 energy percent) according the HCN recommendation [16], although

11% of the population had an intake below 25 energy percent. The mean intake was lower than the more recent EFSA recommendation (35–40 energy percent for children under 4 years [19]). Less than 5% of the children achieved a usual fat intake of 35 energy percent. No children below the age of 1 year achieved a usual fat intake of 40 energy percent, as recommended by the HCN and EFSA.

- Dietary fiber: With a mean of 12.7 g or 2.3 g/MJ, the usual intake of the children of 1 year and older was below the intake considered as adequate by the HCN (2.8 g/MJ [17]) and not achieved by 92% of them. However, new reference intakes for young children established by EFSA are lower (10 g [19]). These were achieved by the large majority of the children.
- *n*-3 fatty acids from fish, i.e., eicosapentaenoic acid (EPA) and docosahexaenoic acid (DHA): the mean daily intake of DHA by children below 2 years and of EPA + DHA by children above 2 years was far below the intake considered adequate by the HCN or EFSA.
- Iron: The median usual iron intake of 6.0 mg was lower than the Adequate Intake of 8 mg/day [18] and also lower than the Population Reference Intake of 7 mg/day established by EFSA [22]. This implies that iron intake was possibly inadequate. Children receiving formula, most of them in combination with cow's milk, had a median usual intake of 6.8 mg iron, whereas exclusive cow's milk users had a median usual intake of 5.6 mg. If, in the latter group, liquid cow's milk products would be replaced by formula, median usual iron intake would increase to 8.5 mg.
- Sodium: The percentage of children with a usual sodium intake of more than 1200 mg, i.e., the upper limit established by the NNC for young children above 1 year, increased with age from 47% to 81%, whereas the usual intake of all children below 1 year exceeded the upper limit of 400 mg [23].
- Zinc: The median usual intake of 5.9 mg was adequate. However, 17% of the children exceeded the TUIL of 7 mg/day.
- Retinol: 30% of the children exceeded the TUIL of 800 mg retinol. The percentage increased from 27% in the youngest age group to 33% in the oldest age group. Liverwurst spread, popular among young children, appeared to be responsible for the excess intake.

3.3. Food Consumption

Almost all children (98%) had eaten a breakfast on both days, contributing to 20% of the daily energy intake. Only 12 out of 1526 (<1%) children did not have breakfast on any of the days.

Table 3 shows the mean daily consumption of food groups, classified according to type of food, across all age groups. Consumption of potatoes, vegetables, fruits, cereals, and cheese was similar across all age groups. In contrast, consumption of bread and, in accordance, fat spreads doubled over age, just as cakes and biscuits, and meat. Consumption of milk products increased slightly over age, with exception of the much lower consumption (176 g) by children under 1 year. However, this was compensated by the high consumption (411 mL) of follow-on formulae among the youngest age group, 87% of which used formula. Mean consumption of formulae (follow-on or young-child formulae) decreased from 111 mL among the 1-years old (41% users) to 15 mL among the 3-years old (7% users). Consumption of mixed dishes, including baby and young-child meals in jars, also substantially decreased over age. Mean fish consumption was rather low, and did not change with age. We calculated from the food records that the children ate fish once per 10 days on average.

Table 3. Mean daily consumption of food groups (g) by children attending childcare by age (mean of 2 days).

	Total Group (n = 1526) [1]		10–11 Months (n = 31)		1 Year (n = 411)		2 Years (n = 497)		3 Years (n = 410)	
Food Group	**Mean**	**SD**	**Mean**	**SD**	**Mean**	**SD**	**Mean**	**SD**	**Mean**	**SD**
Potatoes	29	27	25	25	31	28	28	27	28	26
Vegetables	58	39	48	45	60	41	58	39	61	38
Fruit	128	59	129	66	127	58	129	59	130	61
Legumes	1	7	1	4	2	9	1	6	1	6
Bread	100	35	57	29	86	33	103	33	114	33
Cereals (including rice and pasta)	29	29	21	26	30	30	28	28	30	28
Cakes and biscuits	13	12	6	8	11	10	14	12	16	13
Nuts, seeds, savory snacks	1	5	0	0	1	3	1	5	2	6
Milk and milk products	358	158	176	217	333	162	363	143	383	147
Follow-on and young children's formula	63	135	411	226	111	162	35	87	15	61
Cheese	14	11	14	10	15	11	14	11	15	12
Eggs	3	8	1	4	2	7	3	8	3	8
Fish	5	12	2	7	5	12	5	12	6	13
Meat, meat products, poultry	44	25	24	23	40	24	44	22	49	26
Soy and vegetarian products	8	49	0	2	8	54	8	47	10	55
Savory spreads	4	6	0	0	3	6	4	6	4	7
Mixed dishes	20	45	52	78	28	53	15	39	14	35
Soups	10	33	0	1	6	23	12	37	13	39
Sugar, confectionary, sweet spreads	18	13	6	7	13	10	20	12	23	14
Fat spreads, oils, savory sauces	24	11	11	8	20	10	24	11	27	12
Non-alcoholic beverages (excluding milk products)	427	222	182	145	367	204	446	209	508	220

[1] The total number of children does not equal the sum of those in the age groups, due to missing data on age; SD: standard deviation.

3.4. Consumption According to Food-Based Dietary Guidelines

Figure 1 displays the consumption of food groups by children from 1 year, classified according to the food-based dietary guidelines. Figure 1 shows for each defined food group the percentage of children with a consumption quantity (g or mL) below and above the recommended daily consumption. The majority of children did not comply with the recommendations for fruit and cooking fats. Around 40% of the children did not comply with the recommendations for vegetables, potatoes (including rice and pasta), cheese, meat (including poultry, fish and eggs) and beverages (including liquid milk products). Children who ate a hot meal at the childcare center ate more vegetables: Only 30% of them did not comply with the recommendation. A large majority of children complied with the recommendations for bread (including breakfast cereals), fat spreads and milk products.

The food groups were also subdivided into preferable or neutral foods and foods that should be eaten by exception only. Table 4 shows the mean consumption of each food group. More than half of the foods from the potatoes group were eaten as by-exception type. This was due to the consumption of white rice and refined pasta (instead of brown rice and wholemeal pasta). In contrast, bread and breakfast cereals were almost always eaten as wholemeal or "brown" type. Cheese was mostly eaten as full-fat type and therefore classified as by-exception type. Milk products were mostly (79%) consumed as preferable or neutral type, i.e., (semi-)skimmed, non-sweetened milk. Two thirds of the meat group was eaten as by-exception type, mostly because of the saturated fat content of the meat or the salt content of processed meats. Fats and oils, in contrast, were predominantly of the preferable (less-saturated fat) type. Sixty-two percent of the beverages were drunk as by-exception type, mostly because they contained sugars. This percentage is even higher as part of the water (in the preferable group) was used to mix it with fruit juice concentrate or syrup. Thirty-seven percent of the total foods (in g) consumed by the children were by-exception foods (35% at home and 40% at the childcare center). The higher consumption of by-exception foods at childcare centers was mainly attributable to by-exception beverages (see supplementary materials Figure S1).

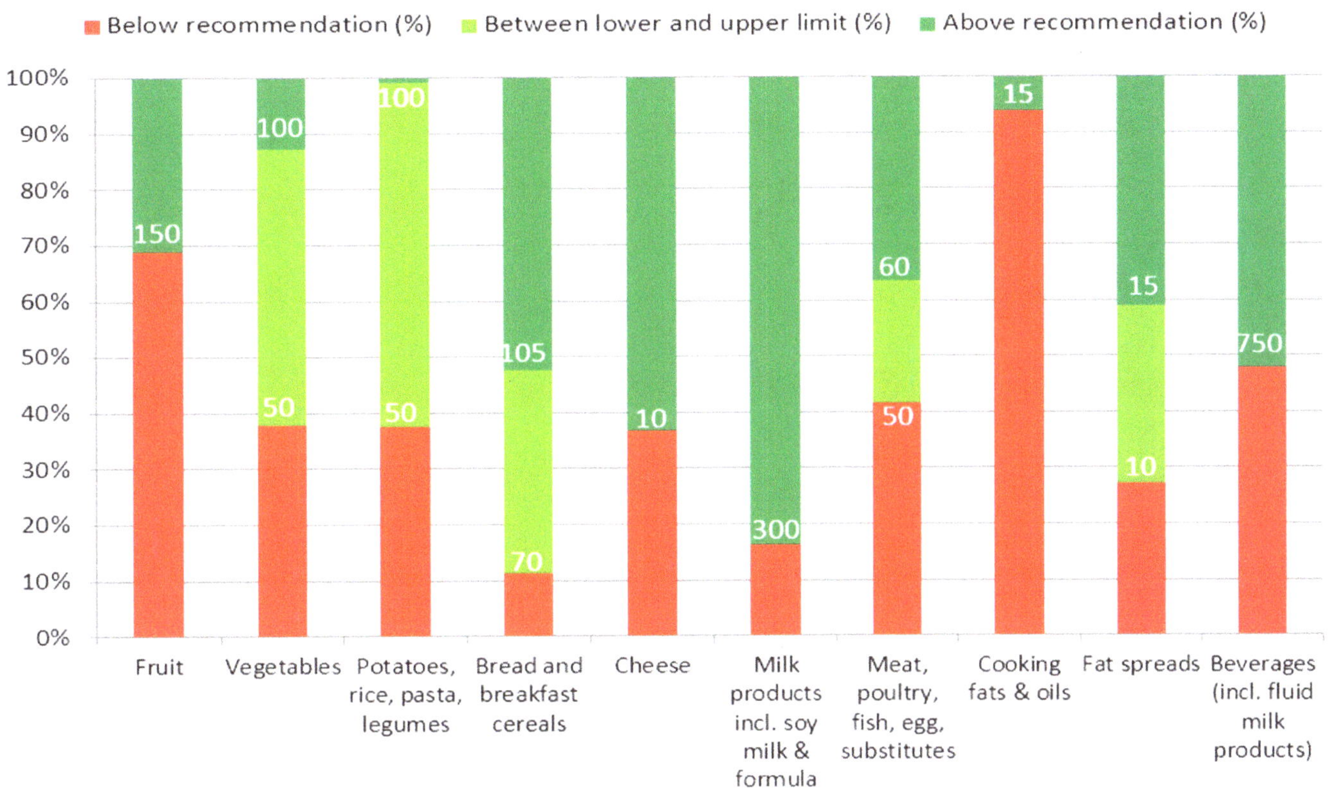

Figure 1. Percentage of children from 1 year old with a daily consumption (g) below, above or in within the range of the recommendation.

Table 4 also lists the contribution of the food groups to mean intake of selected nutrients. Bread, milk products and sweetened beverages were important contributors to energy intake. Milk products contributed most to protein intake, followed by bread and the meat group. Sweetened beverages were by far the largest contributors to intake of sugars, at a distance followed by milk products (contributes mainly lactose), fruit, and sugar and sweet spreads. Bread and potatoes were the main contributors to polysaccharides. Milk products, meats, and fats and oils contributed mostly to intake of fat and saturated fatty acids. However, almost half of the intake of polyunsaturated fatty acids originated from fats and oils. Dietary fiber came mainly from bread and breakfast cereals, followed by vegetables and fruit. Bread was also responsible for one third of the daily sodium intake (which excluded salt added at cooking and at the table), followed by processed meats, cheese and milk products. Fruit, followed at a distance by sweetened beverages (including fruit syrups and juices) and vegetables and milk, contributed most to vitamin C intake.

Table 4. Consumption of food groups [1] and their contribution to intake of selected nutrients among children 1–3 years old.

	Mean	Energy	Protein	MDS	PS	Fat	SFA	PUFA	Water	Dietary Fiber	Sodium	Vitamin C
Basic Foods	g/day	%	%	%	%	%	%	%	%	%	%	%
Fruit	123	6	2	13	3	1	1	2	10	16	0	42
Vegetables	58	1	2	1	1	1	0	1	5	10	1	11
Potatoes, rice, pasta, legumes	23	2	1	0	5	0	0	1	2	4	0	2
Potatoes, rice, pasta, legumes (exception)	30	3	3	0	10	2	1	2	2	3	0	1
Bread and breakfast cereals	98	19	22	3	54	4	3	7	3	42	34	2
Cheese	1	0	0	0	0	0	1	0	0	0	1	0
Cheese (exception)	13	3	5	0	0	8	13	1	1	0	10	0
Milk products including soy milk and formula	333	13	23	16	1	13	21	4	26	4	10	11
Milk products incl. soy milk (exception)	90	6	7	9	2	5	8	2	7	2	4	1
Meat, poultry, fish, egg, substitutes	18	2	9	0	0	2	2	2	1	0	4	0
Meat, poultry, fish, egg, substitutes (exception)	35	8	15	0	2	18	18	12	2	1	13	6
Fats, oils	18	8	0	0	0	26	15	47	1	0	2	0
Fats, oils (exception)	1	0	0	0	0	1	1	1	0	0	0	0
Beverages, excluding milk products	165	0	0	0	0	0	0		16	0	0	1
Beverages, excluding milk products (exception)	267	12	1	39	0	0	0	0	22	3	4	21
Mixed dishes	12	1	1	0	1	1	1	2	1	2	1	0
Mixed dishes (exception)	7	1	1	0	2	1	2	1	0	1	2	0
Non-Basic Foods												
Sugar, sweet spreads	18	5	1	12	1	4	4	2	0	3	0	0
Cakes and biscuits	13	4	2	4	7	3	4	2	0	3	3	0
Confectionary	3	1	0	1	0	1	1	0	0	0	0	0
Nuts, seeds, savory snacks	1	0	0	0	1	1	1	1	0	0	1	0
Sauces	5	1	0	0	0	2	1	4	0	0	2	0
Savory spreads	4	2	2	0	0	5	2	5	0	2	1	0
Soups	9	0	0	0	0	0	0	1	1	0	2	1
Miscellaneous [2]	14	3	2	1	8	1	1	1	1	4	4	0

[1] Division in food groups according to food choice guidelines by the Netherlands Nutrition Center [21]; [2] The sum of all not listed food groups that were consumed in small quantities; MDS: mono- and disaccharides; PS: polysaccharides; SFA: saturated fatty acids; PUFA: polyunsaturated fatty acids.

4. Discussion

This study showed that Dutch children aged 10 to 48 months, at the days they attended childcare, appeared to have an adequate nutrient intake according to national and European reference values with exception of intakes of total fat, n-3 fatty acids from fish and possibly iron which were all lower than the reference values. Intakes of energy and protein were substantially higher than recommended and part of the population exceeded the Tolerable Upper Intake Levels for sodium, zinc and retinol. Consumption of fruit and fats was substantially less than recommended according to food-based dietary guidelines. So were, to a lesser extent, components of the hot meal (vegetables, potatoes/rice/pasta, and meat/fish/poultry/eggs) and fluids. The children consumed milk products and bread mostly as recommended with respect to type (i.e., low fat and high fiber types, respectively), but milk consumption was on average higher than recommended. A notably high consumption of sugar-containing beverages contributed substantially to energy intake. Almost all children ate breakfast and received vitamin D supplements at the recorded days.

Results presented here are from a large dataset, which covers a very large variety of childcare centers, located across the country. Some limitations should be mentioned. Firstly, the authors were not involved in the design of the data collection methods, nor in the execution of the data collection. It was therefore difficult to evaluate the quality of the data. However, based on the documentation provided and the performed data checks, we assessed the data to be of sufficient quality to merit publication. Missing data on gender, age, and body weight and height reduced the usefulness of the data. However, comparing our results with those of the Dutch National Food Consumption Survey conducted among young children in 2005/2006 in the age categories of 2- and 3-years old overlapping between the studies, we observed that mean energy intake was very similar between the surveys (5632 kJ/day versus 5645 kJ/day, respectively). The Dutch National Food Consumption Survey concluded, based on comparison of energy intake and energy requirement, that underreporting was not an issue in their survey [24]. We conclude therefore that substantial underreporting is unlikely in our study either. Secondly, there are considerations with respect to the study population and design. During the period of data collection (2011–2014) approximately 40% of Dutch children under the age of 4 attended a childcare center on one or more days per week [6]. Although formal childcare in the Netherlands is partly subsidized depending on family income, parents (in particular mothers) of children attending a childcare center had on average a higher family income, were more educated and worked more hours per week than parents of other children of the same age [25]. The study population was therefore not representative of the total Dutch population of 10 to 48 months old. In addition, response rates were not formally monitored. Furthermore, food consumption was only recorded on days that the children attended the childcare center. Although we assumed—to compare the children's usual nutrient intake distribution with dietary reference values—that the recorded days were representative of a child's diet, this can be questioned, considering the structure of the day, the food provider, and possible peer pressure. Nevertheless, the data are valuable in their own right. They were mostly observed and recorded directly by the food providers, both at home and at the childcare center. The latter is unusual in food consumption surveys.

As concluded from other studies and countries, reviewed by EFSA [19], intake of n-3 fatty acids, in particular DHA and EPA, and iron and vitamin D is low among the Dutch young children. The low dietary intake of vitamin D was largely remedied through the high proportion of children (92%) that received a vitamin D supplement. Although some practitioners doubt whether such a high percentage of supplement users is real, communication about the recommendation has improved since 2012. Intake of n-3 fatty acids was much lower than recommended. Mean DHA intake by children younger than 2 years is only one fifth of the intake considered as adequate (100 mg/day). Children receiving formula, fortified with DHA, more or less double their DHA intake. If the children of 2 to 4 years old would eat 50 g lean fish and 50 g fatty fish such as salmon per week, as recommended by the NNC, they would easily achieve an adequate intake of DHA and EPA combined. Whether the low n-3 fatty acid intake has health consequences is uncertain. As for iron, there is evidence that iron deficit at young age may interfere with cognitive development [26,27]. However, while the usual iron intake of all children in this survey is above the Average Requirement of 3 mg/day for 1–3 years old established by the US Institute of Medicine [28], 25% of the children from 1 year do not achieve the Average Requirement of 5 mg/day recently proposed by EFSA [22]. Recent research in a well-defined, healthy population of 400 young children in The Netherlands has shown that iron deficiency and iron deficiency anemia was detected in 18.8% and 8.5% of the children, respectively, with a lower iron deficiency prevalence among children receiving formula and a higher prevalence among children receiving a large amount (more than 400 mL/day) of cow's milk after adjustment for age [29]. However, iron intake was not assessed in this study.

The high intake of energy and protein among young children is also a universal observation across Europe [19]. They both increase the risk for overweight [30,31]. In particular the 1-year-old are at risk: they use a lot of milk, mostly cow's milk and also formula, and have the highest protein intake. Although no reference value for sugars has been established by the HCN or by EFSA, increasing evidence shows that in particular sugar-sweetened beverages increase the risk of overweight [32]. We also found that usual intake exceeded the Tolerable Upper Intake Level for zinc (17%) and retinol (30%). As the Adequate Intake and TUIL for zinc are very close, such an excess is inevitable and is unlikely to be harmful. The TUIL for retinol intake among young children is based on the relatively low TUIL for pregnant women owing to its teratogenic effects and adjusted to children. Some excess intake is therefore not likely to be harmful for young children. Also, vitamin A intoxication has not been reported in young children in The Netherlands. Excess retinol intake can nevertheless be avoided if childcare centers and parents restrict the consumption of liverwurst (spread) by their young children, in accordance with the NNC guideline. Dietary sodium intake—70% of the children exceeded the TUIL set by the NNC—is difficult to reduce without endangering a balanced diet. Even though the Dutch bread sector made a major effort to reduce the salt content of bread, bread is a main contributor to young children's sodium intake. According to EFSA, however, sodium intake is not a matter of concern [19].

The results of this survey are in particular informative to nutrition policy and education, both for childcare organizations as for parents and youth health care providers. They demonstrate that the young children's food consumption pattern could be substantially improved by a few changes, such as a replacement of sugared beverages by water and some reduction of milk products. For example, milk-based desserts could be replaced by fruit. Childcare centers that serve a hot meal are able to increase the children's daily vegetable consumption. All in all, these changes would result in lower energy and protein intake and higher vegetable and fruit consumption, which may in turn lower the risk of overweight. Reduction of a high milk consumption should be able to enhance iron absorption from the diet, as calcium hampers iron absorption. Stimulating fish consumption, both at home and at day care, is a feasible way to increase intake of *n*-3 fatty acids. Only if, in specific situations, a recommended diet is difficult to achieve, replacement of cow's milk by formula may help to meet some of the dietary recommendations.

5. Conclusions

Dutch 10 to 48-month-old had, at least on the days they attended childcare, mostly an adequate nutrient intake. The intake of *n*-3 fatty acids and of iron however was low, which is in line with European findings. This seems a matter of concern in young children in this survey and most likely in all young children in the Netherlands, although more research is needed on their potential health effects. The high intakes of energy and protein in this population are also a matter of concern as they may increase the risk of becoming overweight.

Almost all children ate breakfast and received vitamin D supplements. They used mostly (semi-) skimmed types of milk products and non-refined bread and cereals, as recommended. However, their relatively high milk consumption and very high consumption of sugared beverages are undesirable and the latter should be replaced mostly by water. The relative low consumption of fruit, vegetables and fish, on the other hand, should be increased.

Acknowledgments: We thank the staff of the participating childcare centers and the parents of the children as well as the dieticians from Berdien van Wezel Dieticians for their roles in data collection. This study, including this publication, was funded by Nutricia Nederland BV.

Author Contributions: R.A.G. and C.M.R. designed the data analysis plan. C.M.R. carried out the data processing and analysis, R.A.G. drafted the manuscript. C.I.L. and K.F.M.J. contributed important intellectual content and expert advice, and critically reviewed the draft manuscript. All authors read and approved the final manuscript.

References

1. Hoyland, A.; Dye, L.; Lawton, C.L. A systematic review of the effect of breakfast on the cognitive performance of children and adolescents. *Nutr. Res. Rev.* **2009**, *22*, 220–243. [CrossRef] [PubMed]
2. Florence, M.D.; Asbridge, M.; Veugelers, P.J. Diet quality and academic performance. *J. Sch. Health* **2008**, *78*, 209–215. [CrossRef] [PubMed]
3. Singh, A.S.; Mulder, C.; Twisk, J.W.; van Mechelen, W.; Chinapaw, M.J. Tracking of childhood overweight into adulthood: A systematic review of the literature. *Obes. Rev.* **2008**, *9*, 474–488. [CrossRef] [PubMed]
4. Lanting, C.I.; de Vroome, E.M.; Elias, S.G.; van den Brandt, P.A.; van Leeuwen, F.E.; Kampman, E.; Kiemeney, L.A.; Peeters, P.H.; de Vries, E.; Bausch-Goldbohm, R.A. Contribution of lifestyle factors to cancer: Secondary analysis of Dutch data over 2010 and a projection for 2020. *Ned. Tijdschr. Geneeskd.* **2014**, *159*, A8085. [PubMed]
5. Singer, M.R.; Moore, L.L.; Garrahie, E.J.; Ellison, R.C. The tracking of nutrient intake in young children: The Framingham children's study. *Am. J. Public Health* **1995**, *85*, 1673–1677. [CrossRef] [PubMed]
6. Statistics Netherlands. Minder Kinderen naar Kinderdagverblijven (Less Children in Day Care), 2014. Available online: http://www.cbs.nl/nl-NL/menu/themas/dossiers/jongeren/publicaties/artikelen/archief/2014/2014-4024-wm.htm (accessed on 20 May 2015).
7. Gubbels, J.S.; Raaijmakers, L.G.M.; Gerards, S.M.P.L.; Kremers, S.P.J. Dietary intake by Dutch 1- to 3-year-old children at childcare and at home. *Nutrients* **2014**, *6*, 304–318. [CrossRef] [PubMed]
8. Gubbels, J.S.; Gerards, S.M.; Kremers, S.P. Use of food practices by childcare staff and the association with dietary intake of children at childcare. *Nutrients* **2015**, *7*, 2161–2175. [CrossRef] [PubMed]
9. WebArchitecten vof. FoodFigures. Available online: http://www.foodfigures.nl/ (accessed on 2 May 2015).
10. SAS. *Version 8.2*; SAS Institute Inc.: Cary, NC, USA, 1999–2001.
11. SAS. *Version 9.3*; SAS Institute Inc.: Cary, NC, USA, 1999–2001.
12. Kistemaker, C.; Bouman, M. *Voedselconsumptiepeiling Met SAS. de Ontwikkeling van een Geautomatiseerd Systeem voor de Verwerking van Voedingsenquetes. Deel 2: Beschrijving Functioneel en Systeem Ontwerp (Vertrouwelijk). Rapportnummer V98.799*; TNO Voeding: Zeist, The Netherlands, 1999.
13. NEVO-Online Versie 2013/4.0. Available online: http://nevo-online.rivm.nl/ (accessed on 20 May 2015).
14. Dekkers, A.L.M.; Verkaik-Kloosterman, J.; Rossum, C.T.M.; Ocke, M.C. SPADE, a new statistical program to estimate habitual dietary intake from multiple food sources and dietary supplements. *J. Nutr.* **2014**, *144*, 2083–2091. [CrossRef] [PubMed]
15. EFSA Panel on Dietetic Products, Nutrition and Allergies (NDA). Scientific opinion on principles for deriving and applying dietary reference values. *EFSA J.* **2010**, *8*, 1458.
16. Health Council of The Netherlands. *Dietary Reference Intakes: Energy, Proteins, Fats and Digestible Carbohydrates*; Health Council of The Netherlands: The Hague, The Netherlands, 2001.

17. Health Council of The Netherlands. *Guideline for Dietary Fibre Intake*; Health Council of The Netherlands: The Hague, The Netherlands, 2006.
18. Voedingscentrum (Netherlands Nutrition Centre). Aanbevelingen voor Vitamine, Mineralen en Spoorelementen: Factsheet (Recommendations for Vitamins, Minerals, and Trace Elements), 2014. Available online: http://www.voedingscentrum.nl/nl/pers/factsheets.aspx (accessed on 20 May 2015).
19. EFSA NDA Panel (EFSA Panel on Dietetic Products, Nutrition and Allergies). Scientific opinion on nutrient requirements and dietary intakes of infants and young children in the European Union. *EFSA J.* **2013**, *11*, 3408.
20. Gezond eten met de Schijf van Vijf. Available online: http://www.voedingscentrum.nl/nl/schijf-van-vijf/schijf.aspx (accessed on 20 May 2015).
21. Voedingscentrum (Netherlands Nutrition Centre). *Richtlijnen Voedselkeuze, 1 Maart 2011, Update 12 April 2011 (Guidelines for Food Choice, 12 April 2011)*; Voedingscentrum: Den Haag, The Netherlands, 2011.
22. EFSA NDA Panel (EFSA Panel on Dietetic Products, Nutrition and Allergies). Scientific opinion on dietary reference values for iron. *EFSA J.* **2015**, *13*, 4254.
23. Encyclopedie. Available online: http://www.voedingscentrum.nl/encyclopedie/zout.aspx (accessed on 20 May 2015).
24. Ocké, M.C.; van Rossum, C.T.M.; Fransen, H.P.; Buurma, E.M.; de Boer, E.J.; Brants, H.A.M.; Niekerk, E.M.; van der Laan, J.D.; Drijvers, J.J.M.M.; Ghameshlou, Z. *Dutch National Food Consumption Survey—Young Children 2005/2006*; RIVM: Bilthoven, The Netherlands, 2008.
25. Portegijs, W.; Cloïn, M.; Merens, A. *Krimp in de Kinderopvang*; Sociaal en Cultureel Planbureau: The Hague, The Netherlands, 2014.
26. Lozoff, B.; Jimenez, E.; Smith, J.B. Double burden of iron deficiency in infancy and low socioeconomic status: A longitudinal analysis of cognitive test scores to age 19 years. *Arch. Pediatr. Adolesc. Med.* **2006**, *160*, 1108–1113. [CrossRef] [PubMed]
27. Qubty, W.; Renaud, D.L. Cognitive impairment associated with low ferritin responsive to iron supplementation. *Pediatr. Neurol.* **2014**, *51*, 831–833. [CrossRef] [PubMed]
28. Trumbo, P.; Yates, A.A.; Schlicker, S.; Poos, M. Dietary reference intakes: Vitamin A, vitamin K, arsenic, boron, chromium, copper, iodine, iron, manganese, molybdenum, nickel, silicon, vanadium, and zinc. *J. Am. Diet. Assoc.* **2001**, *101*, 294–301. [CrossRef]
29. Uijterschout, L.; Vloemans, J.; Vos, R.; Teunisse, P.P.; Hudig, C.; Bubbers, S.; Verbruggen, S.; Veldhorst, M.; de Leeuw, T.; van Goudoever, J.B.; et al. Prevalence and risk factors of iron deficiency in healthy young children in the southwestern Netherlands. *J. Pediatr. Gastroenterol. Nutr.* **2014**, *58*, 193–198. [CrossRef] [PubMed]
30. Weber, M.; Grote, V.; Closa-Monasterolo, R.; Escribano, J.; Langehendries, J.; Sain, E.; Giovannini, M.; Verduci, E.; Gruzfeld, S.; Socha, P.; et al. Lower protein content in infant formula reduces BMI and obesity risk at school age: Follow-up of a randomized trial. *Am. J. Clin. Nutr.* **2014**, *99*, 1041–1051. [CrossRef] [PubMed]
31. Hebestreit, A.; Börnhorst, C.; Barba, G.; Siani, A.; Huybrechts, I.; Tognon, G.; Eiben, G.; Moreno, L.A.; Fernández Alvira, J.M.; Loit, H.M.; et al. Associations between energy intake, daily food intake and energy density of foods and BMI *z*-score in 2–9-year-old european children. *Eur. J. Nutr.* **2014**, *53*, 673–681. [CrossRef] [PubMed]
32. De Ruyter, J.C.; Olthof, M.R.; Seidell, J.C.; Katan, M.B. A trial of sugar-free or sugar-sweetened beverages and body weight in children. *N. Engl. J. Med.* **2012**, *367*, 1397–1406. [CrossRef] [PubMed]

17

A Comparison by Milk Feeding Method of the Nutrient Intake of a Cohort of Australian Toddlers

Jane Scott [1,*], Kristina Davey [2], Ellen Ahwong [2], Gemma Devenish [2], Diep Ha [3] and Loc Do [3]

1. Collaboration for Evidence, Research and Impact in Public Health (CERIPH), School of Public Health, Curtin University, Perth 6102, Australia
2. School of Public Health, Curtin University, Perth 6102, Australia; kristina.davey@postgrad.curtin.edu.au (K.D.); ellen.pearce@postgrad.curtin.edu.au (E.A.); gemma.Devenish@curtin.edu.au (G.D.)
3. Australian Research Centre for Population Oral Health, University of Adelaide, Adelaide 5000, Australia; diep.ha@adelaide.edu.au (D.H.); loc.do@adelaide.edu.au (L.D.)

* Correspondence: jane.scott@curtin.edu.au

Abstract: Breastfeeding is recommended beyond 12 months of age, but little is known about the contribution of breastmilk and infant formula to the nutritional intake of toddlers as they transition to a family diet in the second year of life. This study is a cross-sectional analysis of data collected from a birth cohort study in Adelaide, Australia. Dietary intake data were collected when children were approximately 1 year of age by an interviewer-administered multi-pass 24 h recall and a mother-completed 2 days food diary. Children were categorized according to their milk feeding method, i.e., breastmilk, infant formula, combination or other, and their nutrient intakes compared with recommended nutrient reference values. Complete data were available for 832 children, of which 714 had plausible energy intakes. Breastmilk and formula made a substantial contribution to the nutrient intake of those toddlers, contributing 28% and 34% of total energy, and 16% and 26% of protein intake, respectively when not drunk in combination. In general, Australian toddlers transitioning to the family diet consumed nutritionally adequate diets, although almost one quarter of all children and half of breastfed children with plausible intakes had iron intakes below the estimated average requirement, placing them at risk of iron deficiency.

Keywords: nutritional adequacy; diet; toddler; breastmilk; formula; iron

1. Introduction

Breastfeeding is recommended beyond 12 months of age [1–3], but relatively little is known about the contribution of breastmilk and infant formula to the nutritional intake of toddlers as they transition to a family diet in the second year of life. Similarly, little is known about the nutritional content and adequacy of the diets of Australian children under the age of 2 years. While the Australian National Infant Feeding Survey studied this age group, its focus was on breastfeeding and age of introduction of complementary foods and it did not investigate what and how much children in this age group ate [4]. On the other hand, the 2011–2012 Australian National Nutrition and Physical Activity Survey (NNPAS) [5] and the 2007 Australian National Children's Nutritional and Physical Activity Survey (NCNPAS) [6] only studied the diets of children aged 2 years and older. What data are available on the diets of Australian infants and toddlers aged less than 2 years come from a number of single-center or state-based studies of infants and toddlers of varying ages [7–12]. Relatively little is known about the diets of children as they enter their second year of life [9] and much of what we know about the diets of this age group comes from international studies [13–15].

The objectives of this paper were therefore to (1) estimate the usual intake of a cohort of Australian toddlers and to evaluate their diets relative to the Nutrient Reference Values (NRVs) for Australia and New Zealand [16]; (2) identify the contribution that breastmilk and formula make to the nutrient intake of toddlers; and (3) investigate the relationship between milk feeding method and nutrient adequacy.

2. Materials and Methods

2.1. Design

This study is a cross-sectional analysis of dietary data collected as part of the Study of Mothers' and Infants' Life Events Affecting Health (SMILE), a population-based longitudinal birth cohort study [17]. This study has recruited and is following a cohort of socioeconomically-diverse South Australian newborns from birth and into their third year of life. The primary health outcomes of this study are two related conditions: dental caries and obesity/overweight of young children.

2.2. Setting and Recruitment

In total, 2147 mothers and 2181 newborns, including 34 pairs of twins, were recruited from the three major maternity hospitals in Adelaide, Australia from July 2013 until August 2014. All new mothers who were sufficiently competent in English to be able to understand the description and instructions of the study were invited to participate. Those mothers who indicated their intention to move out of the greater Adelaide area within a year were excluded.

Mothers were recruited, usually within 48 h of giving birth, from the postnatal wards of the participating hospitals. Those agreeing to participate in the study were invited to complete a baseline questionnaire designed to collect mother and family-related information including socio-demographic details such as age, income, education, occupation and postcode. Further details of sample size and recruitment procedures have been reported elsewhere [17].

2.3. Ethical Considerations

The study was approved by the Southern Adelaide Clinical Human Research Ethics Committee (HREC/50.13, approval date: 28 February 2013) and the South Australian Women and Children Health Network (HREC/13/WCHN/69, approval date: 7 August 2013), and received clinical governance clearance from the three participating maternity hospitals. Signed informed consent was obtained from mothers who were advised that their participation was voluntary and that they could withdraw at any time without prejudice.

2.4. Collection and Handling of Dietary Data

Once their child had reached 12 months of age, mothers of the 1919 infants remaining in the study were mailed a food diary and a cover letter explaining that a member of the research team would telephone them to collect a 24 h dietary recall (24 HDR) of their child's intake and explain how to complete the food diary. The 24 HDR was conducted via a telephone interview by a trained dietitian using the five-step multi-pass method [18]. At the end of the 24 HDR interview mothers were allocated two days in the following week to record their child's food intake in the food diary. The days allocated ensured that, together with the 24 HDR, three nonconsecutive days (2 week days and one weekend day) of dietary intake over a 10-day period were recorded. The food diary booklet contained instructions for recording their child's intake and included a detailed example of a one-day food record, as well as photos of food portion sizes and examples of household measures (cups, bowls and spoons), to help mothers estimate amounts consumed when completing both the 24 HDR and the food diary.

The dietary data were entered into FoodWorks® version 8 (Xyris Software) and analyzed using the AUSNUT 2011–2013 food composition database [19]. Foods consumed by children but not included in the AUSNUT database were added utilizing nutrient information gathered from the nutrition information panels of product labels and manufacturer websites. The 24 HDR and the two-day food diary were entered together as a food record by a team of four nutritionists. For quality management purposes, standardization training was conducted and data were entered following a detailed data entry protocol. Cross-checking between the 24 HDR and food diary was conducted for data clarification purposes—for example, where a type of bread (e.g., wholegrain) had been collected as part of the 24 HDR but not recorded by the mother in the food diary.

Breastmilk intake was estimated using the method employed for this age group in the UK 2011 Diet and Nutrition Survey of Infants and Young Children (DNSIYC) [14]. Breastfeeds were recorded in minutes and the amount of milk consumed was calculated as 10 g/min to a maximum of 100 g per feed, as the contribution to nutrient intake after 10 min of breastfeeding is considered minimal in this age group [20]. If within 30 min of the start of the previous feed a second breastfeed was started, it was not considered a new feed, and the breastfeeding time was added to the previous feed to a maximum of 10 min [14]. If the child was breastfed for less than two minutes, this was not considered long enough to contribute to their nutrient intake and was not included [14].

Children were grouped initially into four categories of milk feeding method on the basis of whether or not they had consumed breastmilk and/or formula on one or more days. Formulas included infant formula, defined as suitable for children up to 12 months, and toddler formula. The 'breastmilk group' included toddlers who had received breastmilk but no formula. The 'formula group' included toddlers who had received infant or toddler formula but no breastmilk. The 'combination group' included toddlers who had received both breastmilk and infant or toddler formula. Children in these first three groups may also have consumed (usually in small amounts) animal milk or animal milk substitutes in addition to breastmilk and/or formula. Children in the 'other' group had consumed neither breastmilk nor infant or toddler formula.

2.5. Statistical Analysis

Once entered into FoodWorks® version 8 (Xyris Software, High Gate Hill, Qld, Australia), data were downloaded into an Access database (Microsoft Office, 2013) and imported into SPSS version 22 (IBM SPSS Statistics for Windows, Armonk, NY, USA) for statistical analysis. Descriptive statistics were run to identify outliers and improbable intakes of weight of food, energy and macronutrients, and data were checked and cleaned appropriately. As the child's current weight was unknown, a plausible energy intake was estimated for each child using a sex specific estimated energy requirement (EER) for a reference child of the participant's age [16]. The child's date of birth and the date when the 24 HDR was completed was used to calculate their age. The degree of under and over-reporting was assessed by calculating the ratio of reported energy intake to the EER for each child. Children were deemed to have an implausible intake if they had an average daily energy intake below 0.54 or above 1.46 for their age and sex specific reference EER [7].

Descriptive statistics, including mean values and standard deviations as well as 25th and 75th percentiles, were derived for children with plausible intakes for nutrient intakes averaged across the three days. The data were then transformed to determine the proportion of children with inadequate and excessive intakes compared with the NRVs for children aged 1–3 years [16]. Inadequate intakes were considered to be any value below the Estimated Average Requirement (EAR) and excessive intakes were considered to be any value above the Upper Limit of intake (UL), where relevant.

The mean intake of energy, macronutrients and those micronutrients for which more than 10% of the total sample had inadequate or excessive intakes were reported for each milk feeding group. A one-way ANOVA with a *post hoc* Bonferonni test was used to determine any significant between-group differences in mean intake of each nutrient. The percentage contribution of breastmilk and formula to total intake of energy and nutrients was determined for each group. Due to the small numbers of children with inadequate intakes in some groups, those children who received any formula whether in combination with breastmilk or not were collapsed into a single group for further analysis. The proportion of children with inadequate or excessive intakes in each of these three milk feeding group was then determined. Multivariate binary logistic regression, adjusting for maternal age, education and infant sex, was employed to determine the relationship of milk feeding group and inadequate or excessive intakes of nutrients. A p-value of < 0.05 was considered to be statistically significant for all analyses.

3. Results

Of the 1919 children who were mailed a food diary, 1165 had a completed 24 HDR interview (61% response rate) and 844 had returned food diaries (44% response rate). Usable, complete 3 day records were available for 832 children (43%). The participant flow chart is presented in Figure A1.

3.1. Participant Characteristics

Mothers who provided baseline data but did not provide complete dietary data at 12 months were younger ($p < 0.001$), less educated ($p < 0.001$), more socially disadvantaged ($p < 0.001$) and more likely to have been born outside of Australia ($p < 0.001$). However, due to the deliberate over-recruitment of disadvantaged women into the SMILE study [17], women who provided complete dietary data were generally representative of the socioeconomic profile reported by the Pregnancy Outcome Unit for South Australian for births in 2013 with regards to parity and country of birth, but our sample consisted of fewer younger (<25 years) and overweight or obese mothers [21] (Table S1).

The mean age of participant children was 13.1 $\pm$ 0.8 months and 54.7% were boys. In total, 118 children had implausible energy intakes (3 under-reporters and 115 over-reporters) and those 714 children with plausible energy intakes represent the analysis population in this study. The characteristics of mother-child dyads with and without plausible dietary data are presented in Table 1. There was no significant association between over-reporting and any of the maternal or child characteristics investigated, with the exception of milk feeding method.

Table 1. Characteristics of mother–child dyads with complete dietary data and of the subsets with plausible and implausible energy intake.

	Total		Plausible		Implausible		
	(n = 832)		(n = 714)		(n = 118)		
Maternal characteristics	n	%	n	%	n	%	p [a]
Maternal age at birth (years)							
<25	74	8.9	62	8.7	12	10.3	0.583
25–29	259	31.2	227	31.9	32	27.4	
≥30	496	59.8	423	59.4	73	62.4	
Maternal education completed							
School/vocational	358	43.4	310	43.7	48	41.0	0.585
Some university and above	468	56.7	399	56.3	69	59.0	
IRSAD score [b]							
Deciles 1–2	120	14.5	104	14.7	16	13.7	0.941
Deciles 3–4	175	21.2	147	20.7	28	23.9	
Deciles 5–6	172	20.8	147	20.7	25	21.4	
Deciles 7–8	161	19.5	140	19.7	21	17.9	
Deciles 9–10	198	24.0	171	24.1	27	23.1	
Mother's country of birth							
Australia and N. Zealand	613	74.1	519	73.1	94	80.3	0.061
Asia—other	57	6.9	35	4.8	5	1.7	
India	50	6.0	47	6.6	3	2.6	
China	36	4.4	34	3.2	2	6.8	
UK	31	3.7	23	7.3	8	4.3	
Other	40	4.8	35	4.7	5	4.3	
Maternal BMI [c] (kg/m^2)							
<25	476	60.6	413	60.8	63	58.9	0.217
25–29.99	170	21.6	151	22.2	19	17.8	
>30	140	17.8	115	16.9	25	23.4	

Table 1. *Cont.*

	Total		Plausible		Implausible		
	(n = 832)		**(n = 714)**		**(n = 118)**		
Parity							
Primiparous	388	48.2	336	48.7	52	45.2	0.489
Multiparous	417	51.8	354	51.3	63	54.8	
Child characteristics							
Child age (mean SD)	13.1	0.8	13.1	0.8	13.0	0.7	0.660 [d]
Infant sex							
Boy	455	54.7	395	55.3	60	50.8	0.366
Girl	377	45.3	319	44.7	58	49.2	
Milk feeding method							
Breastmilk	219	26.3	201	28.3	18	15.3	<0.001
Breastmilk and formula	68	8.2	59	8.3	9	7.6	
Infant formula	314	37.7	275	38.5	39	33.1	
Other	231	27.8	179	25.1	52	44.1	

[a] Chi Square p value; [b] Index of Relative Socio-Economic Advantage and Disadvantage (IRSAD) where decile 1 = most disadvantaged and decile 10 = most advantaged; [c] Body Mass Index; [d] Independent t-test.

3.2. Nutrient Intake of Children

3.2.1. Comparison of Nutrient Intakes with Nutrient Reference Values

Overall, children had adequate daily intakes of energy, protein and micronutrients, with a few notable exceptions (Table 2). Roughly one in ten children had intakes below the EAR for vitamin C (14.0%), thiamin (14.4%) and calcium (12.6%), while just over two out of ten (22.5%) had intakes below the EAR for iron (Figure 1). Conversely, 18.2% and 14.1% had intakes which exceeded the UL for sodium and zinc (Figure 2), respectively. Dietary fibre intake was generally low in this group.

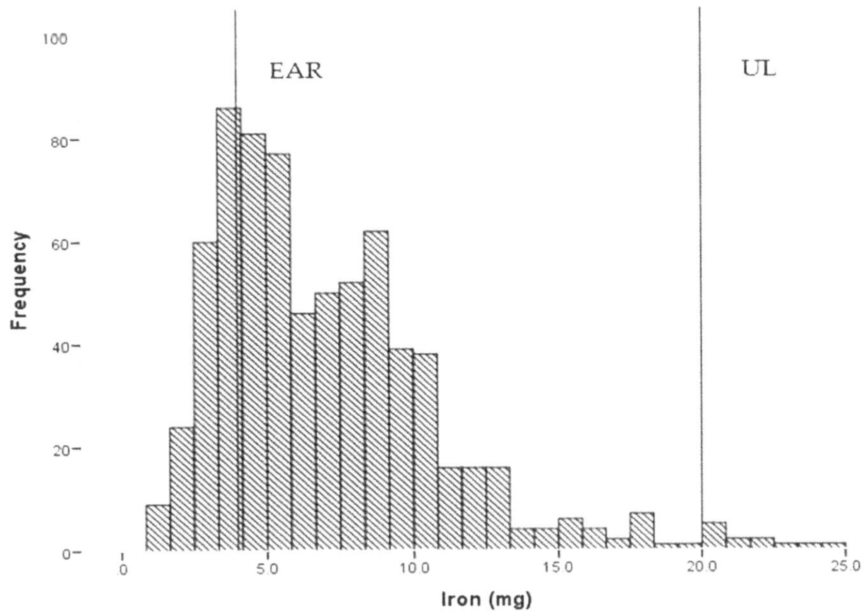

Figure 1. Frequency of intake of iron (n = 714) showing estimated average requirement (EAR = 4 mg) and upper limit of intake (UL = 20 mg).

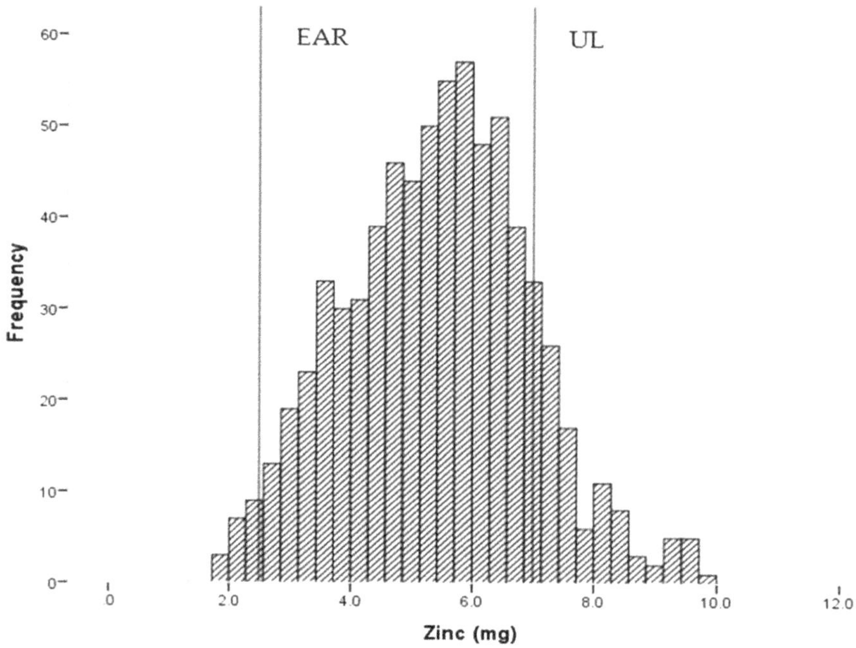

Figure 2. Frequency of intake of zinc ($n = 714$) showing estimated average requirement (EAR = 2.5 mg) and upper limit of intake (UL = 7 mg).

Table 2. Nutrient intakes of children [a] (mean age 13.1 months) and comparison with selected Nutrient Reference Values for children aged 1–3 years.

Average Intake/Day	Mean	SD	25	75	EAR	<EAR%	UL	>UL%
Total mass (kg)	1179	393	993	1322				
Energy (kJ)	3803	714	3297	4378				
Protein (g)	36	11	28	44	12.0	0.0		
Total carbohydrate (g)	107	23	89	123				
Sugar (g)	63	17	51	73				
Total fat (g)	36	9	29	42				
Saturated fat (g)	16.5	5.1	12.8	20.1				
Polyunsaturated fat (g)	4.2	1.6	3.1	5.0				
Monounsaturated fat (g)	12.3	3.4	10.0	14.3				
Dietary fibre (g)	9.6	4.0	6.7	11.8				
Water (g)	1013	386	809	1100				
Sodium (mg)	725	324	487	916			1000	18.2
Potassium (mg)	1467	433	1171	1745				
Calcium (mg)	650	235	481	812	360	12.6	2500	0.0
Phosphorous (mg)	736	229	573	888	380	6.3	3000	0.0
Magnesium (mg)	137	38	110	164	65	2.0		
Iron (mg)	7.1	4.0	4.2	9.0	4	22.5	20	1.5
Zinc (mg)	5.4	1.5	4.4	6.4	2.5	2.2	7	14.1
Vitamin A RE [b] (µg)	726	492	487	851	210	0.4	NA [c]	
Thiamin (mg)	0.8	0.5	0.5	1.0	0.4	14.4		
Riboflavin (mg)	1.4	0.6	1.0	1.8	0.4	2.1		
Niacin equivalents (mg)	16.6	5.5	12.8	19.8	5	0.0	NA [d]	
Folate (µg)	321	130	226	404	120	3.1	NA [d]	
Vitamin C (mg)	61	46	36	80	25	14.0		

NA—not applicable. [a] Children with plausible energy intakes; [b] Retinol equivalents; [c] Upper limit refers to vitamin A from retinol; [d] Upper limit refers to intake from supplements.

3.2.2. Comparison of Nutrient Intakes by Milk Feeding Method

The majority of all 832 children were still receiving breastmilk (n = 334, 36%) and/or formula (n = 374, 53%); only 26 children (4%) were consuming toddler formula. Of those with plausible energy intakes, 260 children (36%) were consuming breastmilk and 334 children (47%) were consuming formula. Children were categorized according to whether or not they consumed breastmilk and/or formula and the mean intakes of energy, macronutrients and those micronutrient for which more than 10% of children had inadequate or excessive intakes were compared (Table 3). There were a number of significant between-group differences for all nutrients but in general children who did not drink either breastmilk and/or formula had significantly higher intakes of energy, protein, sodium, calcium and a lower intake of vitamin C than the other groups. There was no significant difference in the mean protein and energy intakes of those children in the breastmilk group compared with those in the formula group, although formula made a greater contribution to the total protein (26% vs. 16%) and energy intake (34% vs. 28%) of children than did breastmilk. Those children who drank only breastmilk had significantly lower intakes of zinc than all other groups, while those children who drank only formula had significantly higher intakes of calcium than those children who consumed breastmilk either with or without formula, and significantly higher intakes of zinc and iron than all other groups. Formula contributed 31% and 50% of the total iron intake in those who drank formula with or without breastmilk, respectively.

3.3. *Relationship of Milk Feeding Method and Adequacy of Selected Nutrients*

Due to the small number of children with inadequate intakes in some groups, those children who received any formula, whether in combination with breastmilk or not, were collapsed into a single group. Those children who were in the breastmilk-only group were significantly more likely than the other milk feeding groups to have intakes of calcium, iron, and thiamin below the EAR (Table 4). Children who drank neither breastmilk nor formula were almost 10 times more likely (AOR 9.64, 95% CI 5.27–17.62) than the breastmilk-only group to have intakes of vitamin C below the EAR, but children who drank formula were less likely (AOR 0.23, 95% CI 0.09–0.59) to have inadequate vitamin C intakes. Almost half (48.8%) of the children in the breastmilk-only group had iron intakes below the EAR while children who consumed formula were less likely (AOR 0.04, 95% CI 0.02–0.07) to have inadequate iron intakes than those who drank breastmilk. Conversely, children in the breastmilk-only group were less likely than all other groups to have intakes of zinc above the UL and less likely than the group that drank neither breastmilk nor formula to have sodium intakes above the UL.

Table 3. Comparison of the mean nutrient intakes of children ‡ by milk feeding group.

	Milk Feeding Method														
	Breastmilk (n = 201)				**Combination—Breastmilk & Formula § (n = 59)**					**Formula § (n = 275)**				**Other (n = 179)**	
Average intake/day	Mean	SD	% CF	% BM	Mean	SD	% CF	% BM	% F	Mean	SD	% CF	% F	Mean	SD
Total mass (g)	1102 [a]	263	67	33	1214	1047	58	21	21	1186	264	62	38	1240 [a]	253
Energy (kJ)	3708 [a]	747	72	28	3557 [b]	783	62	20	18	3723 [c]	656	66	34	4111 [a,b,c]	646
Protein (g)	33 [a]	10	84	16	30 [b,c]	10	73	12	15	35 [b,d]	9	74	26	45 [a,c,d]	9
Total carbohydrate (g)	100 [a,b]	25	75	25	102	21	65	16	19	110 [a]	21	66	34	111 [b]	22
Total fat (g)	38 [a]	9	60	40	35	12	49	30	21	33 [a,b]	8	58	42	38 [b]	9
Na (mg)	700 [a,b]	393	89	11	546 [a,c,d]	183	79	8	13	687 [c,e]	279	78	22	872 [b,d,e]	284
Ca (mg)	467 [a,b]	175	72	28	522 [c,d]	191	50	17	33	703 [a,c,e]	177	50	50	815 [b,d,e]	229
Fe (mg)	5.0 [a,b]	3.3	97	3	7.8 [a,c,d]	4.3	68	1	31	9.3 [b,c,e]	3.1	50	50	5.9 [d,e]	4.2
Zinc (mg)	4.2 [a,b,c]	1.2	84	16	5.1 [a,d,e]	2	63	10	27	6.2 [b,d,f]	1.2	56	44	5.6 [c,e,f]	1.2
Thiamin (mg)	0.7 [a,b]	0.5	89	11	0.7 [c]	0.3	72	6	22	0.9 [a,c]	0.4	64	36	0.9 [b]	0.6
Vitamin C (mg)	52 [a,b,c]	21	62	38	69 [a,d]	30	44	20	36	83 [b,e]	58	40	60	36 [c,d,e]	30

‡ Children with plausible intakes; § Infant or toddler formula, CF = Complementary foods and beverages, BM = Breastmilk, F = Infant or toddler formula; Shared superscript letters indicate significant between group differences in the mean intake of that nutrient.

Table 4. Association between milk feeding method and intakes of selected ‡ micronutrients below the estimated average requirement (EAR) or above the upper level (UL) of intake.

	Total (n = 714)		Breastmilk (n = 201)		Formula (n = 334)		Other (n = 179)	
Calcium								
Number (%) below EAR	90	(12.6)	64	(31.8)	19	(5.7)	7	(3.9)
Adjusted # odds ratio (95% CI)			Ref		0.13	(0.07–0.22)	0.09	(0.04–0.19)
Iron								
Number (%) below EAR	161	(22.5)	98	(48.8)	11	(3.3)	52	(29.1)
Adjusted # odds ratio (95% CI)			Ref		0.04	(0.02–0.07)	0.42	(0.27–0.64)
Thiamin								
Number (%) below EAR	103	(14.4)	62	(30.8)	19	(5.7)	22	(12.3)
Adjusted # odds ratio (95% CI)			Ref		0.13	(0.07–0.23)	0.30	(0.17–0.51)
Vitamin C								
Number (%) below EAR	100	(14.0)	15	(7.5)	6	(1.8)	79	(44.1)
Adjusted # odds ratio (95% CI)			Ref		0.23	(0.09–0.59)	9.64	(5.27–17.62)
Zinc								
Number (%) above UL	101	(14.1)	4	(2.0)	75	(22.5)	22	(12.3)
Adjusted # odds ratio (95% CI)			Ref		13.5	(4.85–37.66)	6.35	(2.14–18.85)
Sodium								
Number (%) above UL	130	(18.2)	33	(16.4)	45	(13.5)	52	(29.1)
Adjusted # odds ratio (95% CI)			Ref		0.79	(0.49–1.29)	2.10	(1.28–3.44)

‡ Nutrients for which 10% or more of children had intakes below the EAR or above the UL; # Adjusted for maternal age, education and infant sex.

4. Discussion

In this study we have described the diets of a cohort of Australian toddlers aged approximately 1 year, an age by which they should have transitioned predominantly to family foods. More than one half and one third of children continued to consume formula or breastmilk, respectively. These 'milks' contributed up to roughly one third of their total energy intake and one quarter of their protein intake when consumed either alone or in combination. A relatively high prevalence of formula feeding (32%) has been reported in another Australian cohort of slightly older toddlers (12–16 months) [9] and 38% of children aged 12–18 months in the UK-based DNSIYC were receiving formula of some kind [14]. The higher prevalence of formula use in our study can be attributed to the younger age of this birth cohort, which had a mean age of 13.1 months at the time that dietary intake was assessed. The Australian Infant Feeding Guidelines (AIFG) encourage the continuation of breastfeeding beyond the first year of life, and while it is recommended that cow's milk not be given as a main drink to infants under the age of 12 months, this restriction is lifted once children enter their second year of life. Furthermore, the AIFG specifically state that "special complementary foods or milks for toddlers are not required for healthy children" [1] (p. 89).

It is unclear why contemporary Australian mothers continue to feed their children formula beyond 12 months of age. However, the advertising of toddler formulas has become increasingly prevalent [22] since Australia became a signatory to the International Code of Marketing of Breastmilk Substitutes (WHA 34.22 1981) which prohibits the advertising of infant formulas. With both products sharing common visual packaging elements such as colour, shape, typeface and logo, toddler milk advertisements appear to function as *de facto* infant formula advertisements with most women not being able distinguish between toddler and infant formulas and referring to both as 'formula' [23,24]. While most toddlers in this study were still consuming 'infant' versions of formula the advertising of toddler formula may have promulgated the perception amongst mothers that formulas of any kind are beneficial to the health of toddlers and are essential to meet the needs of developing toddlers that cannot be met by cow's milk and family foods.

In general, toddlers in this study consumed diets that either met or exceeded their nutritional requirements, with relatively small numbers failing to meet the EAR for any nutrient. A notable exception was our finding that roughly one in five toddlers consumed diets below the EAR of 4 mg/day for iron [16] which placed them at risk of iron deficiency. This is consistent with the findings of a recent Australian study of slightly older toddlers (mean age: 19.6 months) which reported a similar mean iron intake of 6.6 mg/day and that 18.6% of toddlers had inadequate iron intakes [8]. Comparison with international studies is difficult due to differences in the nutrient recommendations between countries and methodological differences in the way in which dietary data are collected. Nevertheless, just over one in 10 (13%) of UK children aged 12–18 months had iron intakes below the Lower Recommended Nutrient Intake (LRNI) of 3.7 mg/day [25]. When this slightly lower cut point was applied to our data, 17.8% of the SMILE cohort had intakes below the UK LRNI for iron. In comparison, less than 1% of toddlers aged 12 to 23 months in the US Feeding Infants and Toddlers Survey (FITS) reportedly consumed diets below the EAR for iron, which for the USA is set lower, at 3 mg/day for this age group [13]. Nevertheless, when the USA cut-off point was used, 8.3% of the SMILE cohort had an average daily iron intake below this level, which remains appreciably higher than that reported in the FITS.

Children in this study who consumed formula, either with or without breastmilk, were unlikely to have inadequate iron intakes. Conn et al. reported a significant difference in the average daily iron intake of breastfed and non-breastfed infants in a younger cohort of children aged 9 months (6.3 mg/day vs. 11.9 mg/day, $p < 0.001$) [7]. Infant formulas are required by law to be fortified with iron, and in our study toddlers consuming formula either in combination with breastmilk or alone received one third to one half of their iron from formula, respectively. On the other hand, while the iron in breastmilk is highly absorbable, the overall levels are low [26] and breastmilk contributed only 3% of the total iron intake in those who were breastfed and not consuming formula. The Euro-Growth study investigated the determinants of iron status in 12-month-old infants and reported that the most important factor positively associated with iron status was the duration of feeding of iron-fortified formula [27].

Foods that children transition to are often poor sources of iron or they may consume low amounts of those foods which are rich in iron [9]. For instance, Byrne et al. reported that the median intake of meat and alternatives amongst a group of Australian toddlers aged 12–16 months was 56 g/day and one quarter had intakes of 28 g/day or less, which is well below the recommended daily intake for this age group of a single 65 g serve of this food group [28]. A low intake of this food group, which is the primary source of iron in the diets of toddlers, is likely to be more of an issue for breastfed toddlers than those who continue to consume appreciable amounts of either infant or toddler formula. Almost one half of children who were breastfed and not consuming formula and one third of children who were not consuming either formula or breastmilk had iron intakes below the EAR, compared with less than 5% of children consuming formula.

While roughly one in ten of all children had calcium and thiamin intakes below the EAR, almost one third of children who were breastfed without receiving formula failed to meet the EAR for both these nutrients. Children from the other milk feeding groups were significantly less likely than those in the breastfed only group to fail to meet the EAR for calcium and thiamin. As with iron, formula contributed a larger proportion of the overall intake of both calcium (50%) and thiamin (36%) in the formula only group than did breastmilk (28% and 11%, respectively) in the breastmilk-only group. This finding is partly explained by the fact that the formula group consumed on average more formula (443 g) than the breastmilk group consumed breastmilk (352 g), and that formula is typically fortified with vitamins and minerals at levels which exceed the highly variable levels of these nutrients found in breastmilk.

The primary limitations of this study are that usual intake of nutrients was estimated by summing and averaging the three days of intake, though this method does not adjust for the day-to-day variability in intake within individuals, which can be achieved with the use of specialist software that was not available to the researchers [29]. Nevertheless, this method is likely to provide more reliable estimates of usual nutrient intake than estimates derived from a single 24 h recall. While less than half of the mothers returned complete dietary data on the intake of their child, the deliberate oversampling of participants from disadvantaged groups means that the sample of women and children in this study are generally representative of the population from which they were drawn.

5. Conclusions

This is one of the first studies to report the contribution of breastmilk and formula to the diets of Australian children as they transition to family foods at the beginning of their second year of life. While the majority of children had intakes which met or exceeded their nutrient requirements, those children who consumed breastmilk only as their milk feed were at greater risk of having intakes below the EAR for iron, calcium and thiamin. This finding should, however, be interpreted with caution and women should continue to be encouraged to breastfeed their children beyond 12 months of age. However, it is possible that breastfeeding mothers may have a misplaced faith in the nutritional superiority of breastmilk over formula and cow's milk as they transition to the family meal. All mothers, regardless of the milk they feed their child, must be educated and encouraged to feed their infant a varied and high-quality diet with adequate serves of the core food groups. In particular, health professionals should advise mothers of the importance of incorporating iron- and calcium-rich complementary foods into their child's diets, both of which are important nutrients required for adequate growth and development of toddlers.

Acknowledgments: The SMILE study was supported by a National Health and Medical Research Council Project Grant (APP: 1046219). These funds were not used to cover the costs of this open access publication. We would like to acknowledge Courtney Mizen and Tanya Coelho who assisted with entry of dietary records.

Author Contributions: L.D., J.S. and D.H. conceived and designed the SMILE cohort study; K.D. and E.A. entered and analyzed the data; G.D. wrote the data entry protocol and supervised the data entry; J.S. planned and supervised the analysis of the data and wrote the paper. All authors contributed to the interpretation of results and writing the manuscript, and read and approved the final version.

Abbreviations

The following abbreviations are used in this manuscript:

AIFG	Australian Infant Feeding Guidelines
CI	Confidence interval
EAR	Estimated average requirement
IRSAD	Index of Relative Socio-Economic Advantage and Disadvantage
NRV	Nutrient reference value
OR	Odds ratio
RE	Retinol equivalents
UL	Upper level of intake

Appendix A

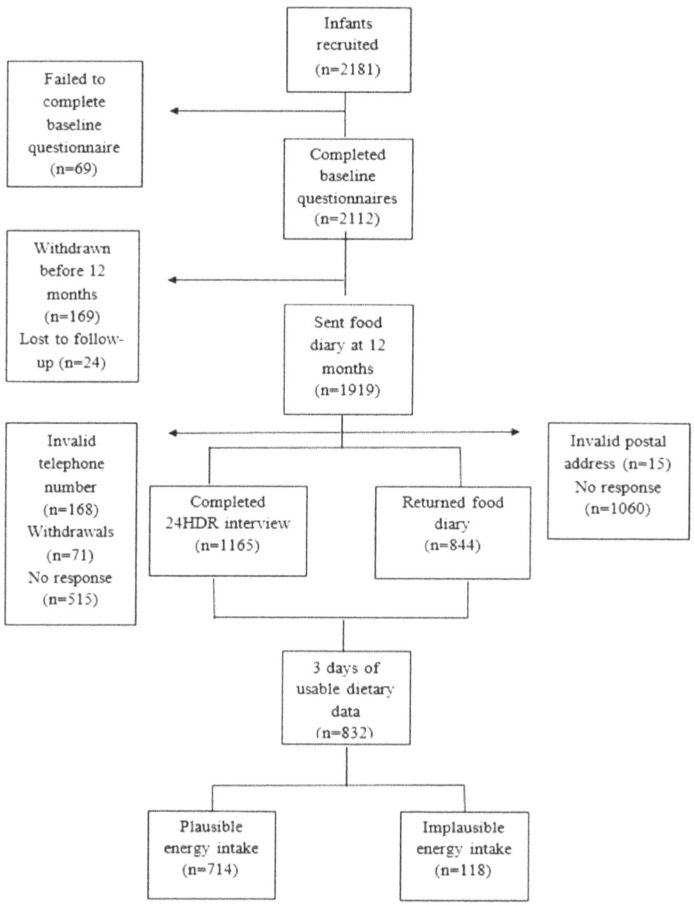

Figure A1. Participant Flow Chart.

1. National Health and Medical Research Council. *Infant Feeding Guidelines*; National Health and Medical Research Council: Canberra, Australia, 2012.
2. WHO/UNICEF. *Global Strategy for Infant and Young Child Feeding*; World Health Organization: Geneva, Switzerland, 2003.
3. Victora, C.G.; Bahl, R.; Barros, A.J.; França, G.V.; Horton, S.; Krasevec, J.; Murch, S.; Sankar, M.J.; Walker, N.; Rollins, N.C.; et al. Breastfeeding in the 21st century: Epidemiology, mechanisms, and lifelong effect. *Lancet* **2016**, *387*, 475–490. [CrossRef]
4. Australian Institute of Health and Welfare. *2010 Australian National Infant Feeding Survey: Indicator Results*; Cat. No. PHE 156; AIHW: Canberra, Australia, 2011.
5. Australian Bureau of Statistics and Food Standards Australia and New Zealand. *4364.0.55.008—Australian Health Survey: Usual Nutrient Intakes, 2011–2012*; Australian Bureau of Statistics: Canberra, Australia, 2015.
6. Commonwealth Scientific Industrial Research Organisation (CSIRO) Preventative Health National Research Flagship and the University of South Australia. *2007 Australian National Children's Nutrition and Physical Activity Survey: Main Findings*; Commonwealth of Australia: Canberra, Australia, 2008.
7. Conn, J.A.; Davies, M.J.; Walker, R.B.; Moore, V.M. Food and nutrient intakes of 9-month-old infants in Adelaide, Australia. *Public Health Nutr.* **2009**, *12*, 2448–2456. [CrossRef] [PubMed]
8. Atkins, L.A.; McNaughton, S.A.; Campbell, K.J.; Szymlek-Gay, E.A. Iron intakes of Australian infants and toddlers: Findings from the Melbourne Infant Feeding, Activity and Nutrition Trial (InFANT) Program. *Br. J. Nutr.* **2016**, *115*, 285–293. [CrossRef] [PubMed]
9. Byrne, R.; Magarey, A.; Daniels, L. Food and beverage intake in Australian children aged 12–16 months participating in the NOURISH and SAIDI studies. *Aust. N. Z. J. Public Health* **2014**, *38*, 326–331. [CrossRef] [PubMed]
10. Lioret, S.; Cameron, A.J.; McNaughton, S.A.; Crawford, D.; Spence, A.C.; Hesketh, K.; Campbell, K.J. Association between maternal education and diet of children at 9 months is partially explained by mothers' diet. *Matern. Child Nutr.* **2015**, *11*, 936–947. [CrossRef] [PubMed]
11. Kavian, F.; Scott, J.; Perry, R.; Byrne, R.; Magarey, A. Assessing dietary intake and growth of infants. *Matern. Paediatr. Nutr. J.* **2015**, *1*, 101.
12. Webb, K.L.; Lahti-Koski, M.; Rutishauser, I.; Hector, D.J.; Knezevic, N.; Gill, T.; Peat, J.K.; Leeder, S.R.; CAPS Team. Consumption of 'extra' foods (energy-dense, nutrient-poor) among children aged 16–24 months from western Sydney, Australia. *Public Health Nutr.* **2007**, *9*, 1035. [CrossRef]
13. Butte, N.F.; Fox, M.K.; Briefel, R.R.; Siega-Riz, A.M.; Dwyer, J.T.; Deming, D.M.; Reidy, K.C. Nutrient intakes of US infants, toddlers, and preschoolers meet or exceed dietary reference intakes. *J. Am. Diet. Assoc.* **2010**, *110*, S27–S37. [CrossRef] [PubMed]
14. Lennox, A.; Sommerville, J.; Ong, K.; Henderson, H.; Allen, R. Diet and Nutrition Survey of Infants and Young Children, 2011, 2013. Available online: http://webarchive.nationalarchives.gov.uk/20130402145952/http://transparency.dh.gov.uk/2013/03/13/dnsiyc-2011/ (accessed on 18 March 2016).
15. Smithers, L.G.; Brazionis, L.; Golley, R.K.; Mittinty, M.N.; Northstone, K.; Emmett, P.; McNaughton, S.A.; Campbell, K.J.; Lynch, J.W. Associations between dietary patterns at 6 and 15 months of age and sociodemographic factors. *Eur. J. Clin. Nutr.* **2012**, *66*, 658–666. [CrossRef] [PubMed]
16. National Health and Medical Research Council and Ministry of Health. *Nutrient Reference Values for Australia and New Zealand*; NHMRC: Canberra, Australia, 2005.
17. Do, L.; Scott, J.; Thomson, W.; Stamm, J.W.; Rugg-Gunn, A.J.; Levy, S.M.; Wong, C.; Devenish, G.; Ha, D.H.; Spencer, A.J. Common risk factor approach to address socioeconomic inequality in the oral health of preschool children—A prospective cohort study. *BMC Public Health* **2014**, *14*, 429. [CrossRef] [PubMed]
18. Australian Bureau of Statistics. 4363.0.55.001—Australian Health Survey: Users' Guide, 2011–2013. 24-h Dietary Recall 2014. Available online: http://www.abs.gov.au/ausstats/abs@.nsf/Lookup/0D6B1FE95EAB8FF3CA257CD2001CA113?opendocument (accessed on 18 March 2016).
19. Food Standards Australia and New Zealand. Ausnut 2011–2013. Australian Food, Supplement and Nutrient Database 2015. Available online: http://www.foodstandards.gov.au/science/monitoringnutrients/ausnut/pages/default.aspx (accessed on 18 November 2015).

20. Kent, J.C.; Mitoulas, L.; Cox, D.B.; Owens, R.A.; Hartmann, P.E. Breast volume and milk production during extended lactation in women. *Exp. Physiol.* **1999**, *84*, 435–447. [CrossRef] [PubMed]
21. Scheil, W.; Jolly, K.; Scott, J.; Catcheside, B.; Sage, L.; Kennare, R. *Pregnancy Outcome in South Australia 2013*; Pregnancy Outcome Unit SA Health, Ed.; Government of South Australia: Adelaide, Australia, 2015.
22. World Health Organization. *International Code of Marketing of Breast-Milk Substitutes*; WHO: Geneva, Switzerland, 1981.
23. Berry, N.J.; Jones, S.C.; Iverson, D. Toddler milk advertising in Australia: Infant formula advertising in disguise? *Australas. Market. J.* **2012**, *20*, 24–27. [CrossRef]
24. Cattaneo, A.; Pani, P.; Carletti, C.; Guidetti, M.; Mutti, V.; Guidetti, C.; Knowles, A. Advertisements of follow-on formula and their perception by pregnant women and mothers in Italy. *Arch. Dis. Child.* **2015**, *100*, 323–328. [CrossRef] [PubMed]
25. Department of Health. *Dietary Reference Values for Food Energy and Nutrients for the United Kingdom*; HMSO: London, UK, 1991.
26. Mcmillan, J.A.; Landaw, S.A.; Oski, F.A. Iron sufficiency in breast-fed infants and the availability of iron from human milk. *Pediatrics* **1976**, *58*, 686–691. [PubMed]
27. Male, C.; Persson, L.A.; Freeman, V.; Guerra, A.; van't Hof, M.A.; Haschke, F.; Euro-Growth Iron Study Group. Prevalence of iron deficiency in 12-mo-old infants from 11 European areas and influence of dietary factors on iron status (Euro-Growth study). *Acta Paediatr.* **2001**, *90*, 492–498. [CrossRef] [PubMed]
28. National Health and Medical Research Council. Eat for Health Educator Guide. National Health and Medical Research Council: Canberra, Australia, 2013. Available online: https://www.nhmrc.gov.au/_files_nhmrc/publications/attachments/n55b_educator_guide_140321.pdf (accessed on 26 June 2016).
29. Piernas, C.; Miles, D.R.; Deming, D.M.; Reidy, K.C.; Popkin, B.M. Estimating usual intakes mainly affects the micronutrient distribution among infants, toddlers and pre-schoolers from the 2012 Mexican National Health and Nutrition Survey. *Public Health Nutr.* **2016**, *19*, 1017–1026. [CrossRef] [PubMed]

Permissions

All chapters in this book were first published by MDPI; hereby published with permission under the Creative Commons Attribution License or equivalent. Every chapter published in this book has been scrutinized by our experts. Their significance has been extensively debated. The topics covered herein carry significant findings which will fuel the growth of the discipline. They may even be implemented as practical applications or may be referred to as a beginning point for another development.

The contributors of this book come from diverse backgrounds, making this book a truly international effort. This book will bring forth new frontiers with its revolutionizing research information and detailed analysis of the nascent developments around the world.

We would like to thank all the contributing authors for lending their expertise to make the book truly unique. They have played a crucial role in the development of this book. Without their invaluable contributions this book wouldn't have been possible. They have made vital efforts to compile up to date information on the varied aspects of this subject to make this book a valuable addition to the collection of many professionals and students.

This book was conceptualized with the vision of imparting up-to-date information and advanced data in this field. To ensure the same, a matchless editorial board was set up. Every individual on the board went through rigorous rounds of assessment to prove their worth. After which they invested a large part of their time researching and compiling the most relevant data for our readers.

The editorial board has been involved in producing this book since its inception. They have spent rigorous hours researching and exploring the diverse topics which have resulted in the successful publishing of this book. They have passed on their knowledge of decades through this book. To expedite this challenging task, the publisher supported the team at every step. A small team of assistant editors was also appointed to further simplify the editing procedure and attain best results for the readers.

Apart from the editorial board, the designing team has also invested a significant amount of their time in understanding the subject and creating the most relevant covers. They scrutinized every image to scout for the most suitable representation of the subject and create an appropriate cover for the book.

The publishing team has been an ardent support to the editorial, designing and production team. Their endless efforts to recruit the best for this project, has resulted in the accomplishment of this book. They are a veteran in the field of academics and their pool of knowledge is as vast as their experience in printing. Their expertise and guidance has proved useful at every step. Their uncompromising quality standards have made this book an exceptional effort. Their encouragement from time to time has been an inspiration for everyone.

The publisher and the editorial board hope that this book will prove to be a valuable piece of knowledge for researchers, students, practitioners and scholars across the globe.

List of Contributors

Elieke Demmer, Christopher J. Cifelli and Jenny A. Houchins
National Dairy Council, 10255 West Higgins Road, Suite 900, Rosemont, IL 60018-5616, USA

Victor L. Fulgoni III
Nutrition Impact, LLC, Battle Creek, MI 49014, USA

Maria Wik Markhus, Lisbeth Dahl, Jannike Øyen, Ingvild Eide Graff and Marian Kjellevold
Institute of Marine Research, 5817 Bergen, Norway

Vibeke Moe and Lars Smith
Department of Psychology, University of Oslo, 0316 Oslo, Norway

Marianne Hope Abel
Division of Infection Control and Environmental Health, Norwegian Institute of Public Health, 0456 Oslo, Norway
Department of Nutrition, TINE SA, 0902 Oslo, Norway

Anne Lise Brantsæter and Helle Margrete Meltzer
Division of Infection Control and Environmental Health, Norwegian Institute of Public Health, 0456 Oslo, Norway

Kjell Morten Stormark
Regional Centre for Child and Youth Mental Health and Child Welfare, Uni Research Health, Uni Research, 5020 Bergen, Norway

Iris Iglesia
Growth, Exercise, Nutrition and Development (GENUD) Research Group, University of Zaragoza, 50009 Zaragoza, Spain
Instituto Agroalimentario de Aragón (IA2), 50013, Zaragoza, Spain
Instituto de Investigación Sanitaria Aragón (IIS Aragón); 50009 Zaragoza, Spain
Red de Salud Materno-infantil y del Desarrollo (SAMID), Instituto de Salud Carlos III, Madrid, 50009 Zaragoza, Spain

Timm Intemann
Leibniz Institute for Prevention Research and Epidemiology—BIPS, 28359 Bremen, Germany
Institute of Statistics, Bremen University, 28359 Bremen, Germany

Pilar De Miguel-Etayo and Luis A Moreno
Growth, Exercise, Nutrition and Development (GENUD) Research Group, University of Zaragoza, 50009 Zaragoza, Spain
Instituto Agroalimentario de Aragón (IA2), 50013, Zaragoza, Spain
Instituto de Investigación Sanitaria Aragón (IIS Aragón); 50009 Zaragoza, Spain
Centro de Investigación Biomédica en Red de Fisiopatología de la Obesidad y Nutrición (CIBERObn), Instituto de Salud Carlos III, 28029 Madrid, Spain

Valeria Pala
Epidemiology and Prevention Unit, Department of Preventive & Predictive Medicine, Fondazione IRCCS Istituto Nazionale dei Tumori, 20133 Milan, Italy

Antje Hebestreit and Maike Wolters
Leibniz Institute for Prevention Research and Epidemiology—BIPS, 28359 Bremen, Germany

Paola Russo
Epidemology & Population Genetics, Institute of Food Sciences, National Research Council, 83100 Avellino, Italy

Toomas Veidebaum
Department of Chronic Diseases, National Institute for Health Development, 11619 Tallinn, Estonia

Stalo Papoutsou
Research and Education Institute of Child Health, 2018 Strovolos, Cyprus

Peter Nagy
Department of Pediatrics, University of Pécs, 7622 Pécs, Hungary

Gabriele Eiben
Department of Public Health and Community Medicine, University of Gothenburg, 405 30 Gothenburg, Sweden
Department of Biomedicine and Public Health, School of Health and Education, University of Skövde, 541 28 Skövde, Sweden

Patrizia Rise
Department of Pharmacological Sciences, University of Milan, 20122 Milan, Italy

Stefaan De Henauw
Department of Public Health, Ghent University, 9000 Ghent, Belgium

Daniel Munblit
Department of Paediatrics, Imperial College London, London W2 1NY, UK
International Inflammation (in-FLAME) Network of the World Universities Network, Sydney 2006, NSW, Australia
Faculty of Pediatrics, I. M. Sechenov First Moscow State Medical University, Moscow 119991, Russia

Marina Treneva and Alexander Pampura
International Inflammation (in-FLAME) Network of the World Universities Network, Sydney 2006, NSW, Australia
Allergy Department, Veltischev Clinical Pediatric Research Institute of Pirogov Russian National Research Medical University, Moscow 125412, Russia

Diego G. Peroni
International Inflammation (in-FLAME) Network of the World Universities Network, Sydney 2006, NSW, Australia
Department of Clinical and Experimental Medicine, Section of Paediatrics, University of Pisa, 56126 Pisa, Italy

Silvia Colicino
National Heart and Lung Institute, Imperial College London, London SW3 6NP, UK

Li Yan Chow, Priya Abrol and Shreya Sheth
Department of Paediatrics, Imperial College London, London W2 1NY, UK

Shobana Dissanayeke
Royal Holloway University of London School of Biological Sciences, Biomedical Sciences, London TW20 0EX, UK

Attilio L. Boner
Department of Life and Reproduction Sciences, Section of Paediatrics, University of Verona, 37124 Verona, Italy

Donna T. Geddes
International Inflammation (in-FLAME) Network of the World Universities Network, Sydney 2006, NSW, Australia
School of Chemistry and Biochemistry, The University of Western Australia, Perth 6009,WA, Australia

Robert J. Boyle and John O. Warner
Department of Paediatrics, Imperial College London, London W2 1NY, UK
International Inflammation (in-FLAME) Network of the World Universities Network, Sydney 2006, NSW, Australia

Zoya Gridneva, Anna R. Hepworth, Jacqueline C. Kent, Hazel Gardner, Wan J. Tie, Ching T. Lai and Peter E. Hartmann
School of Chemistry and Biochemistry, The University of Western Australia, Crawley, Perth, Western Australia 6009, Australia

Sambavi Kugananthan
School of Chemistry and Biochemistry, The University of Western Australia, Crawley, Perth, Western Australia 6009, Australia
School of Anatomy, Physiology and Human Biology, The University of Western Australia, Crawley, Perth, Western Australia 6009, Australia

Leigh C. Ward
School of Chemistry and Molecular Biosciences, The University of Queensland, St. Lucia, Brisbane, Queensland 4072, Australia

Geok Lin Khor, Sue Yee Tan and Kok Leong Tan
Department of Nutrition and Dietetics, International Medical University, Kuala Lumpur 57000, Malaysia

Pauline S. Chan and Maria Sofia V. Amarra
International Life Sciences Institute South East Asia Region, Singapore 238959, Singapore

Suchada Japakasetr
Department of Nutrition, Faculty of Public Health, Mahidol University, Bangkok 10400, Thailand

Chutima Sirikulchayanonta
College of Medicine, Rangsit University, Bangkok 10400, Thailand

Umaporn Suthutvoravut
Department of Pediatrics, Faculty of Medicine, Ramathibodi Hospital, Mahidol University, Bangkok 10400, Thailand

Busba Chindavijak
Department of Pharmacy, Faculty of Pharmacy, Mahidol University, Bangkok 10400, Thailand

Masaharu Kagawa
Institute of Nutrition Sciences, Kagawa Nutrition University, Saitama Prefecture 350-0288, Japan

Somjai Nokdee
Nursing Department, Buddhasothorn Hospital, Chachoengsao 24000, Thailand

Sambavi Kugananthan
School of Anatomy, Physiology and Human Biology, The University of Western Australia, Perth 6009, Australia
School of Chemistry and Biochemistry, The University of Western Australia, Perth 6009, Australia

Ching Tat Lai, Zoya Gridneva, Peter J. Mark and Foteini Kakulas
School of Chemistry and Biochemistry, The University of Western Australia, Perth 6009, Australia

Geraldine Huini Lim, Jia Ying Toh and Izzuddin M. Aris
Singapore Institute for Clinical Sciences (SICS), Agency for Science, Technology and Research (A*STAR), Singapore 117609, Singapore

Ai-Ru Chia
Department of Obstetrics & Gynaecology, Yong Loo Lin School of Medicine, National University of Singapore, Singapore 119228

Wee Meng Han
Department of Nutrition and Dietetics, KK Women's and Children's Hospital, Singapore 229899, Singapore

Seang Mei Saw
Saw Swee Hock School of Public Health, National University of Singapore, Singapore 117549, Singapore

Keith M. Godfrey
Medical Research Council Lifecourse Epidemiology Unit and National Institute for Health Research Southampton Biomedical Research Centre, University of Southampton and University Hospital Southampton National Health Service Foundation Trust, Southampton SO16 6YD, UK

Peter D. Gluckman
Singapore Institute for Clinical Sciences (SICS), Agency for Science, Technology and Research (A*STAR), Singapore 117609, Singapore
Liggins Institute, University of Auckland, Auckland 1023, New Zealand

Yap-Seng Chong
Singapore Institute for Clinical Sciences (SICS), Agency for Science, Technology and Research (A*STAR), Singapore 117609, Singapore
Department of Obstetrics & Gynaecology, Yong Loo Lin School of Medicine, National University of Singapore, Singapore 119228

Fabian Yap
Department of Paediatrics, KK Women's and Children's Hospital, Singapore 229899, Singapore
Department of Paediatrics, Duke-National University of Singapore Graduate Medical School, Singapore 169857, Singapore
Lee Kong Chian School of Medicine, Nanyang Technological University, Singapore 308232, Singapore

Yung Seng Lee
Singapore Institute for Clinical Sciences (SICS), Agency for Science, Technology and Research (A*STAR), Singapore 117609, Singapore
Departments of Paediatrics, Yong Loo Lin School of Medicine, National University of Singapore, Singapore 119228, Singapore
Division of Paediatric Endocrinology and Diabetes, Khoo Teck Puat-National University Children's Medical Institute, National University Hospital, National University Health System, Singapore 119074, Singapore

Michael S. Kramer
Department of Obstetrics & Gynaecology, Yong Loo Lin School of Medicine, National University of Singapore, Singapore 119228
Departments of Pediatrics and of Epidemiology, Biostatistics and Occupational Health, McGill University Faculty of Medicine, Montreal, QC H3A 1A2, Canada

Mary Foong-Fong Chong
Singapore Institute for Clinical Sciences (SICS), Agency for Science, Technology and Research (A*STAR), Singapore 117609, Singapore
Saw Swee Hock School of Public Health, National University of Singapore, Singapore 117549, Singapore
Clinical Nutrition Research Centre, Singapore Institute for Clinical Sciences, Agency for Science, Technology and Research, Singapore 117609, Singapore

Reyna Sámano, Rosa M. Hernández, Cristina Ramírez and María E. Flores Quijano
Departamento de Nutrición y Bioprogramación, Instituto Nacional de Perinatología, Secretaría de Salud Montes Urales 800, Miguel Hidalgo, Lomas Virreyes, Ciudad de México CP. 11000, Mexico

Hugo Martínez-Rojano
Departamento de Posgrado e Investigación, Escuela Superior de Medicina del Instituto Politécnico Nacional, Plan de San Luis y Díaz Mirón s/n, Colonia Casco de Santo Tomas, Delegación Miguel Hidalgo, Ciudad de México CP. 11340, Mexico
Coordinación de Medicina Laboral, Instituto de Diagnóstico y Referencia Epidemiológicos (InDRE) "Dr. Manuel Martínez Báez", Secretaría de Salud Francisco de P. Miranda 177, Lomas de Plateros, Ciudad de México CP. 01480, Mexico

José M. Espíndola-Polis
Departamento de Nutrición Humana, Universidad del Altiplano, Mirasol 1, Tlacomulco, Tlaxcala de Xicohténcatl CP. 90102, Mexico

Daniela Veruete
Universidad del Valle de México, campus Chapultepec Av. Constituyentes No. 151, Miguel Hidalgo, San Miguel Chapultepec I Secc, Ciudad de México CP. 11850, Mexico

Claudia Carletti, Paola Pani, Lorenzo Monasta, Alessandra Knowles and Adriano Cattaneo
Clinical Epidemiology and Public Health Research Unit, Institute for Maternal and Child Health IRCCS "Burlo Garofolo", Via dell'Istria 65/1, Trieste 34137, Italy

Ulrik K. Sundekilde and Hanne C. Bertram
Department of Food Science, Aarhus University, Årslev 5792, Denmark

Eimear Downey, James A. O'Mahony and Alan L. Kelly
School of Food and Nutritional Sciences, University College Cork, Cork T12 YN60, Ireland

Carol-Anne O'Shea and C. Anthony Ryan
Department of Paediatrics and Child Health, University College Cork, Cork T12 YN60, Ireland

Sergio Verd
Department of Primary Care, Balearic Health Authority, Health Sciences Research Institute IUNICS, 10 Alexandre Rosselló Ave, 07002 Palma de Mallorca, Spain
Department of Primary Care, Balearic Health Authority, 07003 Palma de Mallorca, Spain

Diego de Sotto
Endocrinology Unit, Department of Paediatrics, Hospital Son Espases, Valldemossa Road, 79, 07010 Palma de Mallorca, Spain

Consuelo Fernández
Department of Primary Care, Balearic Health Authority, 07003 Palma de Mallorca, Spain

Antonio Gutiérrez
Molecular Biology Unit, Division of Hematology, Son Espases University Hospital, Valldemossa Road, 79, 07010 Palma de Mallorca, Spain

Palma de Mallorca Institute of Health Research (IdISPa), Valldemossa Road, 79, 07010 Palma de Mallorca, Spain

Navnit Kaur Grewal, Cathrine Solheim Kolve, Ingrid Kverndalen and Liv Elin Torheim
Department of Nursing and Health Promotion, Faculty of Health Sciences, Oslo and Akershus University College of Applied Sciences, 4 St. Olavs Plass, 0130 Oslo, Norway

Lene Frost Andersen
Department of Nutrition, Institute of Basic Medical Sciences, University of Oslo, 0317 Oslo, Norway

R. Alexandra Goldbohm and Caren I. Lanting
Netherlands Organisation for Applied Scientific Research TNO, Schipholweg 77–89, Leiden 2316 ZL, The Netherlands

Carina M. Rubingh
Netherlands Organisation for Applied Scientific Research TNO, Utrechtseweg 48, Zeist 3700 AJ, The Netherlands

Koen F. M. Joosten
Erasmus University Medical Centre, Erasmus MC-Sophia Children's Hospital, Dr. Molewaterplein 60, Rotterdam 3015 GJ, The Netherlands

Jane Scott
Collaboration for Evidence, Research and Impact in Public Health (CERIPH), School of Public Health, Curtin University, Perth 6102, Australia

Kristina Davey, Ellen Ahwong and Gemma Devenish
School of Public Health, Curtin University, Perth 6102, Australia

Diep Ha and Loc Do
Australian Research Centre for Population Oral Health, University of Adelaide, Adelaide 5000, Australia

Index